Handbook
of Neurological
Therapy

HANDBOOK OF NEUROLOGICAL THERAPY

Edited by

Carlo Colosimo

*Department of Neurology and Psychiatry, Sapienza
University of Rome, Rome, Italy*

Antonio Gil-Nagel

*Hospital Ruber Internacional, Neurology Department,
Epilepsy Program, Madrid, Spain*

Nils Erik Gilhus

Department of Clinical Medicine, University of Bergen, Norway

Alan Rapoport

*The David Geffen School of Medicine at the University of California,
Los Angeles, CA, USA*

Olajide Williams

*Department of Neurology, Columbia University Medical Center,
Neurological Institute of New York, New York, NY, USA*

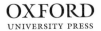
OXFORD
UNIVERSITY PRESS

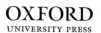

Oxford University Press is a department of the University of Oxford.
It furthers the University's objective of excellence in research,
scholarship, and education by publishing worldwide.

Oxford   New York
Auckland   Cape Town   Dar es Salaam   Hong Kong   Karachi
Kuala Lumpur   Madrid   Melbourne   Mexico City   Nairobi
New Delhi   Shanghai   Taipei   Toronto

With offices in
Argentina   Austria   Brazil   Chile   Czech Republic   France   Greece
Guatemala   Hungary   Italy   Japan   Poland   Portugal   Singapore
South Korea   Switzerland   Thailand   Turkey   Ukraine   Vietnam

Published in the United States of America by
Oxford University Press
198 Madison Avenue, New York, NY 10016

© Oxford University Press 2015

Library of Congress Cataloging-in-Publication Data
Handbook of neurological therapy / edited by Carlo Colosimo, Nils Erik Gilhus,
Antonio Gil-Nagel, Alan Rapoport, Olajide Williams.
      p. ; cm.
Includes bibliographical references.
ISBN 978–0–19–986292–4 (alk. paper)
I. Colosimo, Carlo, editor of compilation.   II. Gil-Nagel, Antonio, editor of compilation.
III. Gilhus, Nils Erik, editor of compilation.   IV. Rapoport, Alan M., 1942– editor
of compilation.   V. Williams, Olajide editor of compilation.
[DNLM: 1. Nervous System Diseases—therapy. WL 140]
RC349.8
616.8′046—dc23
2014001299

9 8 7 6 5 4 3 2 1
Printed in the United States of America
on acid-free paper

Contents

Section Nine: Movement Disorders and Dementia

Section Ten: Central Nervous System Tumors

Preface

When most of us chose neurology as their specialty (in the 1960s through the 1980s), this was interpreted as a sign of courage by the other newly qualified physicians. Neurology was seen as a fascinating and intellectual exercise in terms of diagnostic approach but also a *Cinderella* story in terms of therapeutic possibilities. Luckily, the situation has dramatically changed since then, with a plethora of effective pharmacological and nonpharmacological treatments for several of the most common neurological diseases. Striking examples of these new therapies are the newer dopaminergic medications and deep brain stimulation for Parkinson's disease, thrombolytics for acute ischemic stroke, interferons and other imunotherapies for multiple sclerosis, the new-generation antiepileptic drugs, and the triptans for migraine.

We always thought a volume like this would be timely and necessary. But we were also aware that one editor could not do the book alone, because the complexity of data has become too much for any neurologist to master. Thus, an internal collection of editors, from both sides of the Atlantic Ocean, with very different expertise on the treatment of neurological disorders, have come together to undertake this much-needed manual. Neurology has continued to evolve into so many different subspecialties, such that no adult neurologist can reasonably possess in-depth expertise in all areas, particularly in dealing with complex cases. Hence, we have asked for further help from more than forty international authors, who have been chosen for being opinion leaders in their respective fields. We are very grateful to all of them, for the enthusiasm and hard work they have instilled in writing their sections. This approach has also helped in shaping a book that is a truly international guide on how to treat neurological disorders.

The book is directed mainly to neurology specialists and residents, but we also believe that other physicians, such as neurosurgeons, psychiatrists, internists, pediatricians, and physical medicine specialists, will find it useful. The book has a practical approach; it was not meant to be kept on a bookshelf but rather to have it at hand when seeing patients in the ward, the outpatient clinic, or the emergency department. Our goal in preparing this book was to focus on the treatment of the main neurological conditions and to discuss the neurological therapy of adults. As a consequence, some rare neurological disorders (e.g., most of the early-onset inherited neurometabolic disorders) have not been discussed. For those conditions, we recommend any of the recent textbooks on neuropediatrics.

Each chapter has a consistent format: after an initial brief introduction on the main clinical features of each disease, the focus on therapy is then presented. The book offers detailed coverage of every available treatment option for each neurological disorder and includes categorized sections on medical management, surgical therapy, and neurorehabilitation. The use of tables and figures (including practical flowcharts) has been strongly implemented. We have decided to allocate more space to common conditions, especially on those in which there is more to discuss about symptomatic therapy (e.g., acute ischemic stroke, epilepsy, Parkinson's disease, and myasthenia and related disorders). An evidence-based approach has been used as a first step, but when we found no clear-cut evidence or the data were inconclusive (as occurs frequently in evidence-based medicine), an expert opinion has been given. This is a practical handbook that should always give concise and updated answers to busy practicing clinicians, so no chapter will conclude that more work has to be done before deciding that a treatment is effective! Key references have been added as suggested readings at the end of each chapter, without being directly cited in the text. These are general references, mainly consisting of recent European or North American guidelines or reviews from known opinion leaders.

We really hope to have met the initial aim of this volume; describing the advances in clinical neurology and the neurosciences and their impact on the understanding of neurological disorders, while providing practical output on patient care.

Carlo Colosimo
Nils Erik Gilhus
Antonio Gil-Nagel
Alan Rapoport
Olajide Williams

Contributors

Sachin Agarwal
Department of Neurology, Columbia University Medical Center,
Neurological Institute of New York
New York, NY

Mónica Álvarez
Neurological Department, University Hospital Fundación Alcorcón,
Madrid, Spain

Roberto Attanasio
Endocrinology, Galeazzi Institute IRCCS,
Milan, Italy

Veronica Biassoni
Pediatrics Unit, Fondazione IRCCS Istituto Nazionale dei Tumori,
Milan, Italy

Laurence Bindoff
Department of Neurology, Haukeland University Hospital,
Bergen, Norway

Barbara Borroni
Neurology Unit, Department of Medical and Experimental Sciences,
University of Brescia,
Brescia, Italy

Cecilia Casali
Neuro-oncology Unit, Fondazione IRCCS Istituto Neurologico C. Besta,
Milan, Italy

Comana Cioroiu
Department of Neurology, Columbia University Medical Center,
Neurological Institute of New York
New York, NY

Carlo Colosimo
Department of Neurology and Psychiatry, Sapienza University of Rome,
Rome, Italy

E. Sander Connolly, Jr
Department of Neurological Surgery, Columbia University Medical Center,
Neurological Institute of New York
New York, NY

Pietro Cortelli
IRCCS Istituto delle Scienze Neurologiche di Bologna, *Alma Mater Studiorum*,
University of Bologna,
Bologna, Italy

Renato Cozzi
Endocrinology, Niguarda Hospital,
Milan, Italy

Maria Cristina Martinez-Torrens
Department of Neurology and Psychiatry, Sapienza University of Rome,
Rome, Italy

Neha Dangayach
Department of Neurology, Columbia University Medical Center,
Neurological Institute of New York
New York, NY

Francesco Di Meco
Department of Neurosurgery, Fondazione IRCCS Istituto Neurologico C. Besta,
Milan, Italy

Nils Erik Gilhus
Department of Clinical Medicine, University of Bergen,
Bergen, Norway

Anna Fiumani
Neurology Unit, Alessandro Manzoni Hospital,
Lecco, Italy

Paola Gaviani
Neuro-oncology Department, Fondazione IRCCS Istituto Neurologico C. Besta,
Milan, Italy

Antonio Gil-Nagel
Hospital Ruber Internacional, Neurology Department, Epilepsy Program
Madrid, Spain

Marco A. Gonzalez Castellon
Department of Neurology, Columbia University Medical Center,
Neurological Institute of New York
New York, NY

Christopher P. Kellner
Department of Neurological Surgery, Columbia University Medical Center,
Neurological Institute of New York
New York, NY

Inna Keselman
The David Geffen School of Medicine at UCLA
Los Angeles, CA

Teresa Montojo
Neurological Department, University Hospital Fundación Alcorcón,
Madrid, Spain

Kjell-Morten Myhr
Norwegian Multiple Sclerosis Competence Centre,
Department of Neurology, Haukeland University Hospital,
Bergen, Norway

Luca Marsili
Department of Neurology and Psychiatry, Sapienza University of Rome,
Rome, Italy

Maura Massimino
Pediatrics Unit, Fondazione IRCCS Istituto Nazionale dei Tumori,
Milan, Italy

Alessandro Padovani
Neurology Unit, Department of Medical and Experimental Sciences,
University of Brescia,
Brescia, Italy

Juan A. Pareja
Sleep Disorders Center, Neurological Department, University Hospital Quirón,
Madrid, and Neurological Department, University Hospital Fundación Alcorcón,
Madrid, Spain

Alan Rapoport
The David Geffen School of Medicine at UCLA
Los Angeles, CA

Andrea Saladino
Department of Neurosurgery, Fondazione IRCCS Istituto Neurologico C. Besta,
Milan, Italy

Andrea Salmaggi
Neurology Unit, Alessandro Manzoni Hospital,
Lecco, Italy

Luisa Sambati
IRCCS Istituto delle Scienze Neurologiche di Bologna, *Alma Mater Studiorum*,
University of Bologna,
Bologna, Italy

Elisabetta Schiavello
Pediatrics Unit, Fondazione IRCCS Istituto Nazionale dei Tumori,
Milan, Italy

Brendan Scully
Department of Neurological Surgery,
College of Physicians and Surgeons of Columbia University
New York, NY

Antonio Silvani
Neuro-oncology Department, Fondazione IRCCS Istituto Neurologico C. Besta,
Milan, Italy

Elyse J. Singer
Department of Neurology, UCLA,
Los Angeles, CA

Aaron Sylvan Lord
Department of Neurology, Columbia University Medical Center,
Neurological Institute of New York
New York, NY

Rafael Toledano
Hospital Ruber Internacional, Neurology Department, Epilepsy Program
Madrid, Spain

Ole-Bjørn Tysnes
Department of Neurology, Haukeland University Hospital,
Bergen, Norway

Christina Ulane
Neurological Institute, Columbia University Medical Center,
New York, NY

Miguel Valdes-Sueiras
Department of Neurology, UCLA,
Los Angeles, CA

Christian A. Vedeler
Department of Neurology, Haukeland University Hospital,
Bergen, Norway

Joshua Z. Willey
Department of Neurology, Columbia University Medical Center,
Neurological Institute of New York
New York, NY

Olajide Williams
Department of Neurology, Columbia University Medical Center,
Neurological Institute of New York
New York, NY

SECTION ONE

HEADACHE

AND FACIAL PAIN

1 Primary Headaches

Inna Keselman and Alan Rapoport

INTRODUCTION

There are three main primary headache types (as well as several miscellaneous headaches) according to the Second Edition of *The International Classification of Headache Disorders* (ICHD-2):

1. Migraine
2. Tension-type headache (TTH)
3. Cluster headache (CH) and other trigeminal autonomic cephalalgias (TACs)

We first provide pointers, herein, on how to differentiate a primary headache from a secondary one and then we discuss each type of primary headache in terms of diagnosis and treatment.

DIAGNOSIS

The first step to successful treatment is an accurate diagnosis. Differentiating between a primary and a secondary headache is the key, as headache could be a presenting symptom of a systemic and sometimes life-threatening disease. A detailed history is the most important element in making the diagnosis of a headache problem, while physical examination (general and neurological) is often unrevealing but still required. An abnormal examination strongly suggests a secondary cause. Further testing is primarily needed to rule out secondary causes of headache, not to diagnose the primary headache disorder.

HISTORY

The history in a headache patient should be extensive and should encompass all the elements of pain (i.e., location, duration, severity, periodicity, triggers, response to past treatments), associated symptoms (photophobia/phonophobia, nausea, vomiting, reaction to exertion), and past history of headache (if more than one headache type, ask about each individually). It should also contain an extensive review of systems (i.e., fever, weight loss, rash, etc.), other past medical and surgical history (i.e., presence of known autoimmune or oncological conditions, history of brain surgery), habits and exposure to toxic substances, social and psychiatric history, and family history of headaches and other disorders. It helps to ask a patient to describe his or her typical headache and any disability resulting from it. Certain information from the history

Table 1.1 Primary Headaches Subtypes by ICHD-2 Criteria (Simplified)

Headache Type	Subtypes
1. Migraine	a. Without aura
	b. With aura
	Typical aura with migraine headache
	Typical aura without headache
2. Tension-type headache	a. Infrequent episodic
	b. Frequent episodic
	c. Chronic
3. Cluster and other trigeminal autonomic cephalalgias (TACs)	a. Cluster
	Episodic
	Chronic
	b. Paroxysmal hemicranias
	Episodic
	Chronic
	c. Short-lasting unilateral neuralgiform headache attacks with conjunctival injection and tearing: SUNCT or SUNA
4. Other primary headaches	Thunderclap headache
	Headache associated with sexual activity
	New daily persistent headache (NDPH)
	Hemicrania continua (HC) (Moving to the TAC section)
	Primary stabbing headache
	Primary cough headache
	Primary exercise headache
	Hypnic headache
	Nummular headache

can be a clue to the cause (menstruation-related headaches, headache caused by exertion or sleep apnea, etc.).

You can think of taking a headache history in two steps:

1. Make a primary headache diagnosis according to diagnostic criteria.
2. Rule out a secondary etiology.

Step 1. The first step is to figure out what type of primary headache the patient has by taking a complete history. Table 1.1 lists the primary headaches as given in ICHD-2.

Because most patients who come to a physician in an outpatient setting complaining about their headaches have migraine, one way to start the diagnostic tree is to differentiate headaches into "a migraine" or "a non-migraine headache." You can ask a patient to describe her or his typical headache and follow with a few specific questions covering all the diagnostic criteria. Table 1.2 lists key historical points.

It is important to note that headaches can be also subdivided into episodic and chronic. For migraine and tension-type headache, the term *chronic* means 15 or more days per month, for at least 3 months—so it really refers to frequency rather than chronicity. For cluster headache, *chronic* means it continues for 1 year without a remission for at least a month, and therefore means chronicity. Because primary chronic

Table 1.2 Key Points While Taking History

Component	Example
Headache description	
Location	Frontal, temporal, periorbital; does it change?
Radiation	To neck, to the other side
Type	Burning, stabbing, steady, throbbing, pressure-like
Timing	Time of the day/night, season
Precipitating event	History of trauma, viral illness, moving into a new house
How often	How many times per week or month
Associated symptoms	Nausea/vomiting, photophobia/phonophobia, blurry vision, weakness/numbness, etc.
Triggers	Menses, chocolate, wine, altitude, weather, stress
What makes it better	Sleeping, lack of sleep, walking around
What makes it worse	Exercise, bending down, standing up, coughing
Is there headache-free time	
Family history	Of migraine, other headaches, or other systemic disorders (autoimmune, cardiovascular)
Social history	Abuse, exposure
Past medical/surgical history	History of trauma, surgeries, dental work, systemic diseases
Allergies	May provoke headaches
Medications	Any medications known to cause/exacerbate headaches

headaches can be thought of as extensions/transformations of episodic ones into more frequent ones occurring 15 days or more per month, we will concentrate our discussion on episodic headaches and comment on chronic ones. The treatment of chronic headaches is somewhat similar to the treatment of episodic ones with some special adjustments, as you will read later.

Once the diagnosis is made, the treatment choices are discussed with the patient and vary from behavioral techniques to acute care treatment to daily prevention, most often being a combination of all treatment choices. Many treatments can be used for more than one headache type (i.e., calcium channel blockers work best in cluster prevention but could work in migraine), but some are very specific (i.e., indomethacin is used to treat the episodic and paroxysmal hemicranias [PHs] and other very specific indomethacin-responsive headaches).

Step 2. Look for red flags, or historical facts that would argue for a secondary cause. If ruled out, your patient will most likely have the primary headache diagnosis you have made. One of the most important questions to ask is: Is this a *new or changing headache*, or has this been going on for a while? Even if the patient has had headache all of their life, if this one is new or has changed, then that is a red flag that this could have a secondary cause.

When taking a history, look for red flags or features that would argue for a secondary cause, including:

- Abrupt onset reaching maximum intensity within 1 minute ("thunderclap headache")
- "The first or worst headache of my life"

- The presence of neurological symptoms/focal signs (confusion, weakness/numbness, balance problems, pupillary or eye movement abnormalities)
- A change in pattern (especially increasing frequency/severity or change in location)
- Systemic symptoms (fever)/risk factors (inflammatory/infectious conditions, HIV infection, malignancy)
- Atypical headaches (not meeting ICHD-2 criteria, waking up from sleep with headache, worsening with valsalva maneuver)
- Older age of onset (over age 40, suggesting a vascular or tumor etiology)

Dr. David Dodick of Mayo Clinic in Scottsdale developed a handy mnemonic for practitioners to use for ruling out organic pathology:

SSNOOP

Systemic symptoms (i.e., fever, weight loss)

Secondary risk factors—known underlying disease (i.e., cancer, HIV, high blood pressure)

Neurological signs/symptoms (i.e., confusion, weakness, focal findings)

Onset sudden—especially if it is severe, rapidly progressive

Onset after age 40—can be giant cell arteritis, cancer, vascular

Pattern change—existing headache with new quality/severity/location

Taken together with any abnormalities on the physical examination, the presence of these red flags should prompt an expedited workup that should include, at a minimum, blood work and brain and vessel imaging.

Table 1.3 lists useful diagnostic tools.

Table 1.3 Useful Diagnostic Tools in the Primary Care Setting: Labs and Imaging*

Diagnostic Study	Reason
CBC	Basic lab
Comprehensive metabolic panel (CMP)	Basic lab
Thyroid function tests	Headaches secondary to abnormal thyroid function
Erythrocyte sedimentation rate (ESR)	Inflammatory marker, elevated in vasculitis
C-reactive protein (CRP)	Inflammatory marker, elevated in vasculitis
Lyme antibody	Headache secondary Lyme infection
HIV test	Headache secondary HIV infection
Toxicology screen	Headache secondary to intoxication
Magnetic resonance imaging (MRI) vs. computer tomography (CT)† MR angiography (MRA) vs. CT angiography (CTA) MR venography (MRV) vs. CT venography (CTV)	Looking for space occupying lesion, arterial dissection, cerebral venous thrombosis, aneurysm, etc.
Lumbar puncture	Looking for opening pressure, chemistry, cellular content, antibodies, atypical cells
Electroencephalogram (EEG)	Looking for abnormalities such as focal abnormalities and seizures

* Table was adopted from the *Cleveland Clinic Manual of Headache Therapy* (CCMHT).

† MRI brain is considered to be a superior modality to CT brain.

Secondary headaches are a consequence of a condition/disease process and should improve with the treatment of an underlying disorder (please see above as well as Chapter 2 for more extensive discussion of secondary headaches). **If a secondary headache is suspected, a patient should be referred to a specialist for further evaluation.**

PRIMARY HEADACHES: MIGRAINE, TENSION-TYPE, AND TRIGEMINAL AUTONOMIC CEPHALALGIAS

Migraine

A Typical Patient

Anna is a 34-year-old, single, female teacher who is healthy and has a history of occasional motion sickness as a teenager. She presents to your office complaining of headache. She has been having infrequent headaches for the past 10 years, but over the past few months her headaches have become more frequent and she is worried she may have a brain tumor. She describes her headaches as "pressure-like" and severe (8–9/10), occurring mostly on the left side of her head. They last all day and into the next. A couple of her headaches have been preceded by visual changes, which she describes as seeing bright, curved, flickering lines on the left side of her vision, moving slowly to the left and lasting about 25 minutes. Her headaches are associated with nausea and sensitivity to both light and sound. She now experiences five to seven headaches a month, each lasting longer than a day. Some headaches are so bad she has to take time off work. Going to a dark quiet room and falling asleep usually will help the headache. Anna notes that she tends to have more headaches, which are more severe, after drinking red wine and just prior to her menstrual periods. She is not taking any medications except for an occasional ibuprofen tablet, which provides little help.

Her mother and older sister both have migraine, and her physical and neurological examinations are normal.

Diagnosis

Migraine is extremely common, affecting 12% of the population: 18% of women and 6% of men. Women have more migraine due to fluctuating estrogen and progesterone levels and genetic factors. It is important to point out that a migraine is a complex neurological disorder affecting the brain, blood vessels, and neurotransmitter release and it is not just a headache. The pathophysiology of migraine involves changes in cortical excitability and vascular tone, sensitization of peripheral nociceptors in the meninges, as well as alternations in transmitters including glutamate, serotonin, and calcitonin gene–related peptide, and remains an area of extensive research.

There are two main subdivisions of migraines: *migraine with aura* (in about 30% of migraineurs) and *migraine without aura* (more common), and its semiology tends to vary within, as well as between, individuals.

A typical migraine headache begins gradually and builds to a moderate or severe intensity over 30 minutes to several hours. It may be located on one side of the head, in or behind an eye or in the forehead or temples. Migraine can affect any part of the face or head and can be bilateral. The pain is often throbbing or pounding but it can be steady and associated with disability, nausea more than vomiting, and sensitivity to light and sound. It can be worsened with movement or exertion. Patients may have various triggers that can set off their pain (e.g., menses, delayed eating, lack of sleep, weather, alcohol, etc.), and they usually prefer to lie quietly in a dark, quiet room with no stimulation. They may have increased sensitivity to touch on the scalp or face on the side of the pain, or the skin all over the body, called allodynia, during which even a touch can be painful. Allodynia is a window into the brain as it usually occurs only when the brainstem has become involved (central sensitization). That tends to occur 90 to 120 minutes into the attack if it has not been well treated. The entire migraine attack lasts from 4 to 72 hours on average but is typically 12 to 24 hours in duration; if untreated or unsuccessfully treated, it can last for 3 days. It can occur a few times per year or several times per month, but it must have occurred five times previously before a diagnosis is made. Migraine usually begins between ages 8 and 25 and sometimes earlier in boys, but it can start at any age. After puberty, it is three times more common in women. A headache beginning over the age of 40 is a red flag for a secondary cause of headache.

Patients with migraine should have a normal neurological examination and workup, including brain imaging if indicated (magnetic resonance imaging [MRI] is the scan of choice). Abnormalities suggest other diagnoses, especially secondary causes of headache. Abnormalities are often incidental and not the cause of headache. It should be noted that a scan is not necessary to diagnose migraine, but it helps in ruling out secondary etiologies.

The ICHD-2 diagnostic criteria for migraine with and without aura follow:

Migraine without aura

At least five headache attacks lifetime with the following criteria:
- Duration 4 to 72 hours (untreated or unsuccessfully treated)
- Characteristics include two or more for the following:
  - Unilateral location (side often varies between attacks)
  - Pulsating or throbbing quality
  - Moderate to severe intensity
  - Worsened by routine physical activity
- Plus one of the following:
  - Nausea and/or vomiting
  - Photophobia *and* phonophobia
- Other causes have been eliminated

Migraine with aura

At least two attacks of migraine preceded by aura lifetime:
- Typical aura (visual, sensory, or speech disturbance—see below)
- Headaches similar to above

There are also atypical auras, as mentioned next.

Aura

The ICHD-2 separates migraine auras into two categories: *typical* and *atypical*

Typical aura—reversible, neurological event (with positive more than negative characteristics), which lasts 5 to 60 minutes and precedes a headache by less than 1 hour. The average aura lasts 20 minutes, and patients can start to have headache during or shortly after the aura.

Reversible neurological events are (based on ICHD-2 criteria):

- Reversible *visual symptoms* including positive features such as flickering lights, spots, zigzags, photopsias or flashes of light, lines, with or without negative features such as blind spots

OR

- Reversible *sensory symptoms* including positive features such as paresthesias or dysesthesias with or without negative features such as numbness, usually involving one arm and face on the same side

OR

- Reversible *speech disturbance*

Atypical (unusual) aura—as seen in hemiplegic and basilar-type migraine (ICHD-3 beta [the third revision of the classification now published as a beta version for field testing] changed the name of basilar type migraine to migraine with brainstem aura).

Migraine with brainstem aura requires two symptoms localizable to the brainstem and posterior circulation, such as dysarthria, vertigo, tinnitus, impaired hearing, diplopia, visual changes in all fields in both eyes, ataxia, bilateral paresthesias, and decreased level of consciousness. Two such events lifetime are required for diagnosis.

Hemiplegic migraine requires two attacks lifetime with an aura of weakness on one side of the body plus one other typical aura.

These migraine subtypes are diagnoses of exclusions and patients need to be thoroughly worked up to rule out secondary causes before making the diagnosis.

Remember—these symptoms have to be REVERSIBLE to be even considered as a migraine aura. At presentation of such symptoms, even a known migraineur should receive a workup for a stroke/transient ischemic attack/seizure, arteriovenous malformation, etc.

It is important to note that headache that follows an aura does not have to meet ICHD-2 criteria for migraine. Often a headache following an aura can be quite mild. Aura does not have to precede every headache, nor does it have to be the same every time. It can occur in isolation, i.e., even without a headache following, which tends to happen more often in patients over 50 years of age.

Interesting Facts About Migraine

- Frequent migraine triggers are menses, alcohol, weather shifts, stress, and altitude (every patient has their own set of migraine triggers).
- Neck pain is commonly present at start of an attack as referred pain or well into the attack due to allodynia.
- Attacks vary a lot in the same patient.
- Response to triptans/ergots should not be used as a diagnostic tool (see treatment section later).
- Migraine often has a negative impact on daily life, family, job, and school.
- The majority of migraineurs have a positive family history of migraine.
- Family history and patient history are often positive for motion sickness.
- Based on recent studies, 93% of patients who complain of "sinus headaches" in primary care offices actually have migraine and respond to triptans.

In the new ICHD-3 beta classification, Chronic migraine (CM) was moved to a separate category under migraine and taken out of the complications of migraine section. Chronic

Migraine is migraine that increases in frequency to 15 or more days per month of any type of headache, as long as there are 8 days that qualify for migraine, or would have qualified if the patient had not been treated with an ergot or triptan. These patients are difficult to treat, and the only treatment approved by the Food and Drug Administration (FDA) for CM is onabotulinumtoxinA injected into 31 sites at a dose of 155 units.

The four complications of migraine are status migrainosis (an attack that lasts longer than 3 days), persistent aura without infarction, migrainous infarction, and migraine aura-triggered seizures. We will not discuss these migraine complications further; for additional information, please see the Suggested Reading list for helpful sites and references.

Treatment

General Principles After the diagnosis of migraine is established, treatment should be initiated as soon as possible. Each patient requires an individualized approach, which should take into consideration attack frequency, duration, disability, and results of past treatments. A treatment plan should ideally consist of education, behavioral management (e.g., identifying and avoiding triggers, keeping a calendar of headaches, and going for biofeedback training, cognitive restructuring and stress management), and consideration of pharmacological therapy (prescription and nonprescription). A good strategy would target pain relief as well as associated symptoms (nausea, photophobia and phonophobia, etc) and should target disability as well as comorbid and co-occurring conditions.

Behavioral Medicine Approach and Non-pharmacological Therapies Migraineurs do best with a very regulated and consistent lifestyle. Any change from the ordinary may trigger an attack. Thus, one should always discuss the importance of a regular schedule with a migraineur. This should include consistent times for sleep, meals, and exercise routines, as well as identifying and avoiding triggers that are individual and specific to that patient. One should always think about stress as a powerful trigger, and stress management techniques can be discussed with every migraine sufferer. Biofeedback training can be very helpful, especially for children. Stress management, behavioral modification, and cognitive restructuring can all be useful. Keeping a headache calendar is a good way to identify triggers and monitor individual progress. It helps both the practitioner and the patient.

Some patients benefit from non-pharmacological adjunctive therapy consisting of specific vitamins, minerals, herbs, and additives (such as vitamin B2, magnesium, coenzyme Q-10, *petasites hybridus* [butterbur], feverfew, and melatonin), as well as Ayurvedic medicine techniques, classic Chinese medicine, and integrative medicine.

Pharmacological Treatment If behavior modifications and adjunctive therapies fail to control a patient's headaches, the next step is to consider pharmacological treatment. These can be divided into the following categories:

Acute care (abortive, symptomatic) therapy—taken when the patient has a headache and wants to stop it, improve it, or shorten it and get back to functioning.
Preventive (prophylactic) therapy—taken every day, to decrease frequency, intensity, and severity of attacks and maybe even stop them.

Acute Care Treatment of Migraine These are used to stop an attack once it starts. The key to acute treatment is to do it as early in the attack because once it is full blown and involves the brainstem with central sensitization, it becomes a lot more difficult to control. Thus, patients should be instructed to take an acute care medication at the first sign of an attack, which usually means when the pain is mild and just starting.

There are several classes of medications used to stop an attack. These range from simple medications a migraineur can buy over the counter (OTC) to prescription medications to emergency intravenous medications administered in the hospital, as follows:

Nonspecific migraine medications
- OTC simple analgesics (aspirin and acetaminophen)
- OTC nonsteroidal anti-inflammatory drugs (NSAIDs)
- OTC combination analgesics (i.e., aspirin, acetaminophen, and caffeine)
- Prescription NSAIDs (diclofenac potassium for solution [Cambia] the only NSAID approved for migraine) and others
- Butalbital-containing medication (i.e., aspirin/APAP, butalbital and caffeine [Fiorinal, Fioricet, Esgic])—note these have been approved only for tension-type headache, not for migraine
- Opiates and Tramadol
- Antiemetics
- Steroids

Migraine-specific medication
- Ergots (ergotamine tartrate and dihydroergotamine [DHE])
- Serotonin (5-HT)$_{1B/1D}$ receptor agonists (the 7 triptans)
- Diclofenac potassium for solution [Cambia] approved by the FDA for migraine with and without aura

Opioids and butalbital medications should be avoided, both because they are not migraine-specific medications and due to the high risk of dependency and chance of developing medication overuse headache (previously termed "rebound headaches"). Triptans are usually the drugs of choice. However, due to their vasoconstrictive properties, they should be avoided in people with coronary artery disease, uncontrolled hypertension, history of stroke or any vessel disease (cerebrovascular, peripheral, or ischemic bowel disease), basilar and hemiplegic migraine, pregnancy, and other conditions.

For optimal triptan response, look for a *"One and done"* strategy for triptan use by

- Ordering the optimal dose of a triptan (often the highest approved dose)
- Ordering the optimal formulation (often injectable or nasal)
- Suggesting early intervention, during mild pain, less than 30 minutes into attack
- Considering addition of an NSAID to the triptan to increase efficacy and decrease recurrence

Triptan have side effects that can be frightening for patients and thus should be discussed before their initiation. They also have known interactions with other classes of medications and should be avoided or given with care if the patient is already taking these. Table 1.4 lists currently available triptans and includes facts on differences in their pharmacokinetics.

Triptans' Side Effects Tightening of the throat, chest, jaw, neck, and limbs; paresthesias; hot/cold sensations; and dizziness are almost always non-cardiac as suggested by tests. Side effects may be slightly different between different triptans, and patients will respond to them and tolerate them differentially. It is helpful to warn patients about a transient worsening of pain and occasional chest or neck discomfort.

Special Considerations When Using Triptans Triptans interact with many other medications, so care should be taken when triptans are initiated. They are known to interact with:

- Ergots
- Selective serotonin reuptake inhibitors (SSRIs) and serotonin-norepinephrine reuptake inhibitors (SNRIs)
- Monoamine oxidase inhibitors (MAOIs)
- Cimetidine, quinolones, and fluvoxamine—due to *CYP1A2* interactions

Patients should not be given two triptans on the same day or an ergot and triptan on the same day.

Table 1.5 lists important points on what to watch for when prescribing triptans.

Preventive Treatment of Migraine The goal of preventive medications is to decrease the number, duration, and intensity of attacks. Initiating prevention should be considered if attacks are frequent (more than four a month), if they are infrequent but long lasting with poor response to acute care medication resulting in severe disability, if there is a risk of developing medication overuse headache (such as with frequent use of acute care medications) and if the patient desires to have fewer attacks. Although controversial, we prefer to use no medication at all during pregnancy or in the consideration of future pregnancy.

Table 1.4 Triptans Available in the United States

Triptans	Route, Dose (mg)	t_{max} (h)	$t_{\frac{1}{2}}$ (h)
Amerge (naratriptan)	Tablet 1, 2.5	2–3	5–6.3
Axert (almotriptan)	Tablet 12.5	1.4–3.8	3.2–3.7
Frova (frovatriptan)	Tablet 2.5	2–4	26
Imitrex (sumatriptan)*	Tablet 25, 50,100	2.5	2.5
	SC 4,6	0.2	2.5
	NS 20	1	2.5
Maxalt (rizatriptan)*	Tablet 5, 10	1.2	2
	ODT 5,10	1.6–2.5	2
Relpax (eletriptan)	Tablet 20, 40	1–2	3.6–5.5
Zomig (zolmitriptan)	Tablet 2.5, 5	1.5	2.5–3
	ODT 2.5, 5	3.3	2.5–3
	NS 5	2	2.5–3
Treximet (sumatriptan 85 mg and naproxen 500 mg)—see sumatriptan above			

Adapted from the *Cleveland Clinic Manual of Headache Therapy* (CCMHT) and Johnston and Rapoport, 2010.
SC, subcutaneous; NS, nasal spray; ODT, orally disintegrating tablet.
* Generic equivalent is available in the U.S.

Table 1.5 Treatment Tips on What to Watch Out for When Using Triptans

Do not use more than one type of triptans in a 24-hour period.

Do not use sumatriptan, rizatriptan. or zolmitriptan with a monoamine oxidase inhibitor (MAOI) or within 2 weeks of discontinuation of an MAOI.

Use half of zolmitriptan dose if a patient is on oral contraceptives, cimetidine, quinolones, fluvoxamine—due to *CYP1A2* interactions

Use half of naratriptan if patient is on oral contraceptives or is a smoker.

Eletriptan should be avoided if possible or used at a half dose when combined with macrolide antibiotics (clarithromycin, erythromycin), ketoconazole, verapamil. and other *CYP3A4* inhibitors.

Rizatriptan should be used at half dose (5 mg) when combined with propranolol.

Do not use with serotonin (5-HT$_2$) receptor antagonists (within 24 hours of each other) if the drug is an ergot such as methysergide (no longer available in most countries).

Because some patients will respond to supplements such as magnesium or riboflavin, we may try these first, prior to initiating a prescription medication. Sometimes we use them with prescription medication. Table 1.6 lists available supplements and their doses. We also like to try behavioral medicine techniques, sometimes prior to preventive medications and sometimes simultaneously.

There are multiple classes of preventive medications, all acting on one or more neurotransmitter pathways thought to play an important role in migraine pathophysiology. There are only five medications that are FDA approved to use for migraine prevention in the United States, but there are many more classes that are currently being used by headache specialists off label with good results. The five medications are propranolol, timolol, valproic acid (VPA), topiramate, and methysergide (no longer available in the United States and most other countries). OnabotulinumtoxinA is approved only for chronic migraine (CM is defined as migraine with at least 15 headache days per month, 8 of which must be migraine days.)

Classes of preventive medications

1. Antidepressants
   Tricyclic antidepressants (TCAs)
   SNRIs
   SSRIs*
   MAOIs
2. Antiepileptic drugs (AEDs)
3. Antihypertensive drugs

Table 1.6 Vitamins, Minerals, Herbs, and Supplements With Doses

Magnesium glycinate 375 mg in divided doses

Riboflavin (vitamin B2)—200 mg twice a day

Coenzyme-Q10—300 mg/day

Butterbur (*Petasites hydridus*)—75 mg twice a day of brand Petadolex

Melatonin 0.5 to 12 mg before sleep

* SSRI can worsen migraine so they should only be maintained if they help significant psychiatric problems in migraineurs and have not caused a worsening of headache. They should not be started to prevent migraine. Table 1.7 lists preventive migraine medications.

β-Blockers
Calcium channel blockers
Angiotensin-converting enzyme (ACE) inhibitors
Angiotensin receptor blockers (ARBs)
4. Serotonin (5-HT$_2$) antagonists
5. NSAIDs for a short time
6. Miscellaneous

NSAIDs should not be used daily for long-term migraine prevention except in special circumstances (some headaches are indomethacin responsive and patients must be kept on the drug for months). Patients should be placed on a proton pump inhibitor to protect their gastrointestinal tract. They can be considered for short-term prevention, after an exposure to a trigger or during menstruation.

Pointers on How to Choose and Use Preventive Medications

Use individualized approach and consider side effect profile—and sometime you can go for a "therapeutic 2-fer" (two for the price of one):
If the patient has hypertension—use a β-blocker, a calcium channel blocker, an ACE inhibitor, or an ARB
If anxiety—use a β-blocker
If depression and sleep disturbance—use a TCA
If pain disorder—use gabapentin
If weight loss is desired—use topiramate, zonisamide, or duloxetine

General Principles of Preventive Therapy

- Start with a low dose and increase slowly.
- Allow 2- to 3-month trial on a medication at an adequate dose before assessing efficacy.
- After 6 to 12 months, consider slowly tapering a medication to see if the patient still needs it.

How Should We Treat Anna?

Now back to our patient Anna. Based on what we discussed earlier in this chapter, Anna meets the diagnostic criteria for migraine with aura. Because her neurological examination results were normal and her headaches did not significantly change over the past 10 years, brain MRI is not indicated at this time (it should be explained to the patient that one can never be sure about brain abnormalities without a scan but the headache is caused by migraine). However, we would send her to the lab for a metabolic panel, inflammatory markers, thyroid function tests, CBC, ESR, Lyme titer, and pregnancy test. Then, we will talk to her about her diagnosis and how to decrease the frequency and severity of her attacks. Because her migraines are triggered by red wine, we will suggest that she avoid it. We will also ask her to fill out a headache calendar and bring it in to each office visit, which will help with identifying other triggers as well as help us to follow the response to treatment. Before discussing medications, we will talk with her about the importance of regular sleep, meals, and exercise routines, as well as talk about stress relief techniques.

Table 1.7 Preventive Migraine Medications

Medication	Group†	Starting Dose and Titration	Pluses and Minuses, Other Medications, Comments
Antidepressants			
Tricyclics			
Amitriptyline	1	General: 10 mg PO at bedtime and up to 50 mg (higher if response and no significant side effects)	Good for patients with other chronic pain, insomnia, low cost Side effects: dry mouth, constipation, sedation, wt gain, orthostatic hypotension, urinary retention, confusion in elderly, syndrome of inappropriate antidiuretic hormone secretion (SIADH), tachycardia and arrhythmias, mania *Migraine doses are less than doses needed to treat depression Other tricyclic antidepressants (TCAs): imipramine, doxepin, desipramine, protriptyline (stimulating, no weight gain)
Nortriptyline (less sedating)	3	General: 10 mg PO at bedtime and up to 50 mg (higher if response and no significant side effects)	
Serotonin–Norepinephrine Reuptake Inhibitors (SNRIs)			
Venlafaxine	3	37.5–225 mg/day may be divided into 2 doses	Good for patients with comorbid anxiety and depression as well as other chronic pain syndromes including fibromyalgia. Tend to be stimulating. Clinically SNRIs—appear to be more effective Side effects: increase blood pressure, weight gain, sexual dysfunction, withdrawal, SIADH, gastrointestinal effects, sweating, sedation or insomnia, lower seizure threshold, serotonin syndrome, mania, dry mouth, nervousness, tremor Other SNRIs: desvenlafaxine, milnacipran (approved for fibromyalgia)

(continued)

Table 1.7 (Continued)

Medication	Group†	Starting Dose and Titration	Pluses and Minuses, Other Medications, Comments
Duloxetine (weight neutral)		20–120 mg/day	

Selective Serotonin Reuptake Inhibitor (SSRI)

Fluoxetine	2	10–80 mg/day	Other SSRIs: paroxetine, fluvoxamine

Monoamine Oxidase Inhibitor

Phenelzine		15 mg/day to start Last resort due to potential serious side effects	Hypotension, weight gain, sexual dysfunction, urinary retention, hypertensive crisis (when combined with SSRI)

Antiepileptic Drugs

Topiramate	3	Start at 25 mg at night and up every week by 25 to total of 100 mg/day. If no adverse effects and not effective, slowly push up to 200 mg/day	Renal excretion Weight loss, paresthesia (resolves), cognitive dysfunction at 100 mg Rare: calcium phosphate renal stones, hyperchloremic acidosis, oligohydrosis, narrow angle glaucoma
Valproic acid	1	250 mg twice a day up to 1500 mg/day (use extended-release form and give at night)	Not for women of child-bearing age (tetratogenic and increased risk in polycystic ovarian syndrome)
Gabapentin	2	Start at 100 mg 3 times a day and up as needed/tolerated (typical doses are 900–2400 mg)	Drowsiness, dizziness, and weight gain
Zonisamide		25 mg at night and may go up to 300 mg	Other antiepileptic drugs: lamotrigine (rash, Steven Johnson syndrome), levetiracetam, pregabalin, lacosamide

Antihypertensives

β-Blockers

Timolol	1	10 mg twice a day, may go up to 15 mg twice s day	Others: atenolol, metoprolol, nadolol
Propranolol	1	20 mg twice a day, may go up to 80 mg twice a day or higher	

(continued)

Medication	Group†	Starting Dose and Titration	Pluses and Minuses, Other Medications, Comments
Calcium Channel Blocker			
Verapamil	2	80 3 times a day and can double	Others: diltiazem, amlodipine
Angiotensin-Converting Enzyme Inhibitor			
Lisinopril		Start with 10 mg/day for 1 week, then 20 mg/day	
Angiotesin Receptor Blocker			
Candesartan		16 mg/day	
Serotonin (5-Ht₂) Receptor Antagonists			
Methysergide		4–8 mg/day in divided doses	*Do not use within 24 hours of a triptan. Not available in most countries.
Cyproheptadine		4 mg 3 times daily; not to exceed 0.5 mg/kg/day	
Other			
Memantine-glutamate receptor blocker		Start at 5 mg PO daily and go up to 5 mg or 10 mg twice daily as needed	Usually well tolerated
Quetiapine—atypical antipsychotics		Usually start at 12.5 mg at night and increase as tolerated/needed	Consider in a patient who has trouble sleeping
Acetazolamide—carbonic anhydrase inhibitor		250 mg/day and increase as needed tolerated	Consider in a patient with vertiginous symptoms

*Group (based on evidence as separated by US Headache Consortium).

As for medications, given that she has five to seven attacks per month, she would need acute care medication as well as daily preventive treatment.

For acute care, we could start with a triptan tablet—sumatriptan because it is generic and inexpensive or one of the other triptan tablets.. If she does not respond we can switch to zolmitriptan, rizatriptan, eletrptan or others. We might also give her diclofenac potassium for solution (Cambia), which works faster than a tablet of the same medication, to take early in the migraine attack or after the triptan if it is not effective or even to take with the triptan.

For adjunctive treatment, we would start with magnesium glycinate 375 mg and riboflavin 200 mg twice a day, which we will try for 1 month before considering a prescription medication (which in Anna's case will most likely be topiramate 25 mg increasing slowly to 100 mg to be taken at night). Also, because we know that Anna tends to have her migraines around her period, we will start naproxen sodium 500 mg three times a day with food starting 2 days before her projected menstrual headache and until the end of her susceptibility. She could also try pulsed estrogen or a milder longer-acting triptan (frovatriptan) as mini-prophylaxis around her period.

Special Issues for Women

Migraine and Changing Estrogen and Progesterone Levels Migraine affects 18% of the female population, partially related to fluctuating estrogen and maybe progesterone levels. Thus, it is not surprising that migraine frequency and severity change when women are undergoing hormonal changes as happens during menarche and throughout reproductive age (during the cycle and mid-period), pregnancy, lactation, and menopause. Migraine patterns also change with any pathological or other physiological condition that influences hormonal levels including starting/stopping contraceptive use.

Our favorite treatment of attacks during menses is to give a fast-acting triptan shortly after the attack begins. We often prefer a nasal spray (such as zolmitriptan) or injection of sumatriptan (such as the needle free one Sumavel DosePro). Only if these fail do we need special techniques.

Thus, when questioning a woman with headaches, it is important to find out if she is undergoing any of the changes listed earlier as that will help with diagnosis and management. In fact, some women will only have migraine attacks around their periods (these are called Pure Menstrual Migraine). These patients have attacks that occur exclusively on days −2 to +3 of menstruation in at least two of three menstrual cycles. If migraine attacks occur with menses and at other times in the month as well, this is called Menstrually Related Migraine. Treatment goals for these are same as for other forms of migraine. Short-term preventive measures can be used around the period with either NSAIDs or triptans, especially those with longer half-lives such as frovatriptan. These are started 2 days prior to the onset of menstrual headache and continued for 5 to 7 days depending on the patient. Lower doses of tripans are tried first. Oral magnesium, taken preventively, can be especially helpful in women with these forms of migraine.

Continuous Hormonal Contraception There is a lot of discussion about the use of continuous estrogen delivery for menstrual migraine. There are three types of oral contraception (OCPs): fixed dose, triphasic, and progesterone only. Thus far, there have been no randomized controlled studies showing benefit of using a specific type. However, generally speaking, OCPs with constantly changing hormonal levels, such as triphasics, are more likely to worsen migraines and low-dose single estrogens should be used whenever possible. If a woman gets an attack invariably a day or two after stopping her estrogen-containing pill each month, it makes sense to switch to a 3-month birth control pill with continuous estrogen. That way, she will only have 4 attacks per year rather than 12.

Menopause/Perimenopause The incidence of headaches in women tends to increase around perimenopause due to irregular hormonal fluctuations. However, neither menopause nor hormone replacement therapy has clear effects on migraine as studies show variable outcomes. In most cases, it is best to wait out the increase or consider preventive and acute care medication for migraine.

Pregnancy It is important to discuss treatment plans for women who are pregnant or lactating or are considering pregnancy, due to poorly studied teratogenic effects of regular migraine medications. During pregnancy, possibly due to high steady levels of estrogen, migraineurs tend to experience few headaches in their second two trimesters. They might actually be worse early in the pregnancy before it is known that they are pregnant; thus, is it always best to be certain that a woman of child-bearing potential is not pregnant before instituting treatment. *It is our philosophy to urge women to use no acute care or preventive medication during pregnancy.* If the patient is attempting to get pregnant, she can take acute care medications from day 1 in her cycle after the start of menses until day 10. We do recommend that pregnant women take vitamin B2 and magnesium daily and have biofeedback training. If they insist on medication, we would consider the following current recommendations for acute medications *during pregnancy*:

- Stop triptans (although they are often prescribed in Europe during pregnancy).
- The use of NSAIDs is recommended only in the first and second trimesters.
- Acetaminophen can be used.
- Low-dose opioids—said to be acceptable (beware of rebound) but we do not recommend or use them.
- Antiemetics that are class B such as ondansetron ODT are acceptable.
- Steroids can be used in a short course.
- Hydration and rest are always good.

Table 1.8 summarizes migraine medications and associated pregnancy risk categories. In general, check pregnancy category prior to prescribing anything to a pregnant patient and consider checking with her obstetrician/gynecologist. Moreover, discuss any new medication with a migraineur of child-bearing age due to a risk for unplanned pregnancy; 50% of all pregnancies are unplanned.

Lactation In general, the same medications used in pregnancy are acceptable to use while breastfeeding except diphenhydramine. Sumatriptan is safe.

TENSION-TYPE HEADACHE

A Typical Patient

Boris is a 63-year-old software engineer who comes to you for a regular checkup without complaints. When performing his review of systems, you find out that he has been having daily headaches for the past 6 months. These headaches are not severe and he can perform his daily tasks without difficulty. The headaches start in the afternoon; are constant, nonthrobbing, and mostly bilateral and occipital; and radiate down his neck. He sometimes experiences mild photophobia but denies any phonophobia, nausea, or vomiting. The intensity is 3/10 and rarely goes over 5/10. Working out at home seems to help. He states that he has had a lot of deadlines at work over the past several months and has been stressed out more than usual, spending many hours on the computer producing some neck and shoulder dyscomfort. He denies headaches in the past and is otherwise healthy.

His general and neurological examinations are both normal, except for some tenderness in his upper cervical neck muscles and his trapezei.

Diagnosis

Tension-type headache (TTH) is the most common headache in the general population, and most people have experienced these on occasion. It can be infrequent (less than 1 day per month), frequent (1 to 14 days per month), or chronic (15 to 30 days

Table 1.8 Medications/Pregnancy Risk Categories

Acute	**B***
	Acetaminophen, caffeine, IV magnesium sulfate, ibuprofen, metoclopramide, ondansetron
	Naproxen—*first and second trimesters*
	IV solumedrol—*second and third trimesters*
	C*
	Codeine, quetiapine, indomethacin, triptans
	Aspirin (ASA)—*first trimester*
	Prednisone/methylprednisolone—*first trimester*
	D*
	Butalbital, butorphanol, ibuprofen, naproxen, IV VPA
	ASA—*second and third trimesters*
	X*
	Ergots
Preventive	**B***
medications	Cyproheptadine
	C*
	Propranolol, atenolol, gabapentin, lamotrigine, zonisamide, bupropion, fluoxetine, sertraline, doxepin, protriptyline, venlafaxine, desvenlafaxine, duloxetine, milnacipran, tizanidine
	D*
	Amitriptyline, nortriptyline, paroxetine, VPA, lithium, topiramate

*Categories: **B**: chance of fetal harm is remote but possible (controlled human studies show no risk, or animal studies showed adverse effects, but adequate studies in pregnant women failed to show risk); **C**: cannot rule out risk (no adequate human or animal trials); **D**: positive evidence of fetal risk; **X**: contraindicated.

Adapted/table from the *Cleveland Clinic Manual of Headache Therapy* (CCMHT).

per month). A typical TTH is of mild to moderate intensity, squeezing or pressing (nonthrobbing) pain, usually on both sides of the head. It can be in or over or behind the eyes, on the top of the head, in the back, or like a band around the head. It is rarely on one side. There is usually no nausea, vomiting, sensitivity to light or sound, or worsening of the headache with movement or exertion. Some patients have sensitivity to either light or sound. In the chronic form, which can be daily or frequent but at least 15 days per month, mild nausea is sometimes present.

One can think of TTH as being *NOT* a migraine (i.e., it is not severe, not unilateral, not throbbing, not worse with activity, not associated with nausea, and generally not associated with photophobia/phonophobia). TTH tends NOT to have a negative impact on one's life, so patients tend not to complain about it to their physician. Instead, they either relax or exercise, or they take OTC simple analgesics or combination analgesics with caffeine or NSAIDs. Stress may exacerbate this type of headache, just like migraine. If patients use pain medication or NSAIDs up to 2 to 3 days per week, they should be fine. But if they have chronic TTH and use these medications almost daily, they will probably develop medication overuse headache eventually. Interestingly, most people with chronic TTH also have occasional migraine, so pure TTH is hard to find. Episodic TTH is very common but not usually a problem for most patients.

ICHD-2 lists the following to diagnostic criteria for TTH (10 or more episodes of the following):

- Intensity: mild to moderate
- Duration: 30 minutes to 7 days
- Two or more characteristics must be present:
  Not unilateral
  Not throbbing
  Not severe
  Not aggravated by physical activity
- Both of these must be present:
  No nausea
  Acceptable to have either photophobia or phonophobia but not both
- Not due to a secondary cause

Treatment

General Principles These headaches, especially if infrequent, are easy to treat with simple OTC analgesics, stress avoidance, and exercise. When they occur frequently (more than 2 days per week) or cause disability or are associated with medication overuse headache, they can be treated with behavioral therapy and TCAs such as nortriptyline in low doses. We would start biofeedback training before daily preventive medication, or at the same time.

Acute Care Therapy Acute care therapy consists of a combination of non-pharmacological therapies plus simple analgesics if needed. Non-pharmacological therapies include relaxation techniques, biofeedback training, massage, exercise, acupuncture, and yoga.

Simple analgesics
- Aspirin 325 to 1000 mg
- Acetaminophen 325 to 1000 mg
- NSAIDs
  - Ibuprofen 200 mg, 400 mg
  - Naproxen 275 to 550 mg
  - Ketoprofen 12.5 to 75 mg

Analgesics are even more effective in combination with caffeine (64 to 200 mg). Hence, it is common to try pills containing 250 mg aspirin, 250 mg acetaminophen, and 65 mg of caffeine (Excedrin or Excedrin Migraine, which are the same formulation).

Triptans tend to work for TTH days in patients who also have migraine, but they do not work for pure TTH and are not recommended.

Preventive Therapy Amitriptyline or nortriptyline are the drugs of choice but do not always work. Start either medication at 10 mg at about 8 PM and go up by 10 mg every 1 to 2 weeks as tolerated until relief or 50 mg is reached. Some patients may need more but adverse events become more problematic over 50 mg. The drug is given at night, and patients must be warned that they could be drowsy in the morning or have dry mouth and an increased appetite and gain weight. Consider starting preventive medications when frequency and severity increase and simple analgesics do not have an effect, or the patient is in danger of developing medication overuse headache.

How Should We Treat Boris?

Boris most likely has TTH partially brought on by stress at work. His headaches do not bother him enough to cause him to seek medication, but he admits to taking medications, when he is asked. Because these headaches are new, secondary causes need to be ruled out with brain imaging and laboratory studies, including basic metabolic panel, white count, inflammatory markers (ESR, CRP), Lyme titer, and thyroid function tests.

With regard to treatment, we will talk to Boris about regular sleep and exercise as well as stress-relieving techniques and advise him to take an NSAID of his choice with or without a caffeinated drink as needed. Behavioral medicine consultation with starting biofeedback training is one of our favorite treatments. At this point, we would not advise him to take a TCA, unless he strongly wishes to do so. However, if his NSAID use escalates, we will have to revisit the issue of a preventive medication.

CLUSTER HEADACHE AND OTHER TRIGEMINAL AUTONOMIC CEPHALALGIAS

A Typical Patient

Cliff is a 47-ear-old healthy man, married, accountant with two boys, who complains of occasional heartburn and presents to your office complaining about bouts of severe head pain. The pain started 1 week ago and has been occurring every night since, waking him up at exactly 1 AM. It is so severe that it wakes him up suddenly from a deep sleep and causes him to jump out of bed and pace around the house. It is located behind and above his right eye. When the pain begins, his right eye begins to tear and turns red and his right nostril stuffs up. Sometimes he notes that his right eyelid is drooping, which happens only when the pain is present. The pain rapidly escalates from mild (3–4/10) to incapacitating (10/10) in 5–10 minutes and then persists for a bit over 1 hour and slowly disappears. When the pain is at its height, he rocks back and forth and rubs his eye. It returns at the same time nightly. He sometimes has a second attack after getting home from work. He realized that after having an alcoholic drink a couple of nights ago, his pain was a lot more severe and came on just afterward. He never had this type of pain before, nor does he complain of having any other headaches in the past. He denies any weakness in his face or anywhere else in his body; he also denies any numbness or tingling in his face and visual problems. He tried to take Tylenol, ibuprofen, and Afrin (nasal decongestant) with no relief.

His physical and neurological examinations are both normal, except for ptosis and miosis on the side of the pain, only during the pain.

Diagnosis

The TACs are a specific group of primary headaches characterized by unilaterality, associated cranial autonomic features, and specific duration of pain (5 seconds to 3 hours depending on the type), which tends to be brief and very severe.

Although little is understood about the pathophysiology of TACs, the posterior hypothalamus is thought to be involved in the pathogenesis of these disorders.

ICHD-2 lists the main types of TACs:

i.   Cluster (CH) (listed in ICHD-2 under Section 3.1)
ii. The Paroxysmal Hemicranias (PH) (listed in ICHD-2 under Section 3.2)
iii. Short-lasting Unilateral Neuralgiform headache attacks with Conjunctival injection and Tearing/Short-lasting Unilateral Neuralgiform headache attacks with cranial Autonomic symptoms (SUNCT/SUNA) (listed in ICHD-2 under Section 3.3*)

These headaches all cause severe pain in and over one eye and have similar autonomic findings but are differentiated by duration, frequency, associated symptoms, and response to medication.

Duration/Frequency
1. CH: longest duration, 15 to 180 minutes/one to eight times per day, usually three or fewer attacks, occurring at least once every other day during a cluster period of 4 to 8 weeks.
2. PH: intermediate, 2 to 30 minutes/5 to 15 times per day for at least half of the days.
3. SUNCT/SUNA: shortest, 5 seconds—4 minutes/3 to 200 times per day for at least half of the days. ICHD-3 beta has changed the duration to 1 to 600 seconds in a single stab or a series.

All three are rare disorders, with CHs being most common and occurring in less than 0.1% of population. It occurs in 3–4 times more men than women, and PH is slightly more common in women. We will discuss how to diagnose and treat CHs and comment on PH and SUNCT/SUNA.

Cluster

CH is rare, occurring in less than 0.1% of the population (compared with migraine, which occurs in 12% of the population). It is one of the few headaches that is more prevalent in men than in women, at a ratio of about 3 to 4:1. The typical patient with CH has the episodic form of cluster and is a tall, thin, 20- to 50-year-old man with deep facial lines who has episodes of headache about once or twice per year, called cluster periods. These periods last about 4 to 8 weeks, and during this time, patients have headache on most days, often one to three times per day. Sometimes the headache occurs in the middle of the night, waking them up from sleep in about 90 minutes, coexistent with the first rapid eye movement (REM) cycle. Pain is short, sharp, and severe (triple S, Tepper and Tepper, 2011) and comes on suddenly, reaching maximum intensity within minutes. It is located around one eye, the temple, or the upper jaw and can involve upper teeth, the back of the head, or the neck. It does not usually change sides during cluster periods or from one to the next, but it can. Attacks are

---

* SUNA is not listed in ICHD-2 but experts consider SUNCT to be a subset of SUNA in which patients can have other autonomic symptoms instead of just red and tearing eye. In ICHD-3 beta, 3.3 is Short-lasting unilateral neuralgiform headache attacks with autonomic features, and it is further subdivided into: Episodic and chronic SUNCT as well as episodic and chronic SUNA.

usually associated with ipsilateral autonomic symptoms: red and tearing eye, stuffed and running nostril, sweating and redness of the forehead, small pupil, and drooping of the eyelid. Patients tend to be irritable and agitated during an attack and tend to pace around the room. During a cluster period, an attack can be precipitated by alcohol or sleep. Most patients have remission periods, which are headache-free periods, even in the presence of triggers, that last 6 months to 1 year or more. It is termed *chronic cluster* if there is not a remission period of 1 month or longer in the year.

Cluster attacks in a cluster period tend to occur at the same time every day or night (circadian pattern). Cluster periods tend to restart at the same week or month each year, often in some relationship to clock changes in the spring and fall (circannual pattern). This suggests involvement of the biological clock in the hypothalamus as suggested by Lee Kudrow of Los Angeles many years ago and proven with a positron emission tomography study done by Arne May working with Peter Goadsby at the Queen Square Institute of Neurology in London.

Obstructive sleep apnea, tobacco, and alcohol use are associated with CHs, but cluster patients should have a normal neurological examination (unless done during an attack, when the earlier-mentioned eyelid and pupillary changes can be noted). Workup, including brain imaging (MRI is the scan of choice), should also be normal. Abnormalities in the examination or on imaging would suggest other diagnoses, especially secondary causes of headache that include arterial dissection, sinusitis, glaucoma, and intracranial lesions (pituitary/parasellar).

ICHD-2 diagnostic criteria for the diagnosis of CH follows.

Cluster Headache More than five attacks of the following:

- 15 to 180 minutes (untreated) of unilateral orbital/supraorbital/temporal pain
- Plus one or more of the following autonomic symptoms ipsilateral to pain:

  Conjunctival injection/lacrimation
  Nasal congestion/rhinorrhea
  Eyelid edema
  Facial/forehead sweating or flushing
  Miosis or ptosis
  Sense of restlessness/agitation (usually more specific for CH and does not usually apply to other TACs)

  NOTE: Current criteria require either one autonomic symptom or only sense of restlessness In ICHD-3 beta a new criterion was added: sense of fullness in the ear.

- Attacks can occur from every other day and up to eight per day (they average one to three per day).
- Exclude secondary causes.

Treatment
General Principles

CHs, just like other TACs, are short and severe; thus, treatment is designed for fast relief. Some patients need preventive treatment, which is often started with bridge/transition therapy, depending on the length of a typical cluster period. Because of the severity of CH and other TACs, its treatment should be fast and effective, so a tablet is not be the best solution. Thus other routes of drug delivery are being used to abort these headaches.

Acute Care Treatment Options

100% oxygen inhalation at 7 to 10 L/min (12 L/min proved to be effective versus room air and up to 15 L/min if refractory) (based on Peter Goadsby's publication out of UCSF)

Sumatriptan 6 mg subcutaneously (SQ) or 20 mg via nasal spray (NS) at headache onset

Dihydroergotamine (DHE) 0.5 to 1.0 mg SC, IM, IV

Zolmitriptan 5 mg or 10 mg NS (nasal spray approved in the European Union for CH but not in the United States)

Ergotamine tartrate 2 mg sublingual (SL), by mouth (PO), or by rectum (PR)

Lidocaine 4% to 6% nasal drops at headache onset and 14 minutes later

Methylphenidate 5 mg as needed for headache (not available in most countries)

Transitional/Bridge Therapy

The goal of this therapy is to institute treatment that starts to work before prevention kicks in. Because of seasonal periodicity of CHs in some patients, this kind of therapy can potentially make the cluster more tolerable or even prevent it from occurring. The decision to try a transitional therapy should be left to a specialist, thus in this chapter we will only list available therapies, which are:

- Occipital nerve block/including lidocaine and steroid injection
- Systemic steroids: oral prednisone starting at 60 mg and tapering over 1 to 2 weeks
- Daily preventive DHE injections at bedtime

Preventive/Maintenance Therapy

This therapy is used during the cluster period to shorten attack duration and frequency.

Verapamil (240 mg to 720 mg/day) is the drug of choice with Class I evidence available. Check the electrocardiogram first because verapamil can cause heart block.

Others medications include:

Lithium carbonate (150 mg to 300 mg 3 times a day)

Melatonin (10 mg), when added to verapamil

Divalproex sodium ER form 500 to 1500 mg/day

Topiramate 100 to 200 mg a night (titrate up by 15 to 25 mg every 3 days)

Gabapentin 1800 to 3000 mg/day (start with 300 to 900 mg/day)

Indomethacin 75 to 300 mg/day

Methysergide (2 mg 3 times a day, up to 12 mg daily) *Not available in the United States*

Methylergonovine (Methergine) 0.2 mg three times a day to start; maybe doubled.

Paroxysmal Hemicranias

There are two types of PHs, chronic and episodic. Chronic PH has no remissions and goes on for months or years. Episodic PH stops at some point and totally disappears, often to return again. PH is a type of TAC that is defined by its *absolute responsiveness to indomethacin*. The pains are shorter than CH and usually last 2 to 30 minutes but tend to occur more frequently, more than 5 per day and often up to 12 (versus 1 to 3 in the case of CH). Pain location is similar to that in CH but usually less agitation is present. Unlike CH, PH is more common in women. And unlike CH, these attacks occur at random.

ICHD-2 diagnostic criteria for PH follow.

Paroxysmal hemicranias
- More than 20 attacks with the following characteristics
- Duration 2 to 30 minutes of severe unilateral orbital/supraorbital/temporal
- Plus one or more of the following autonomic symptoms ipsilateral to the pain:
  Conjunctival injection/lacrimation
  Nasal congestion/rhinorrhea
  Eyelid edema
  Facial/forehead swelling or flusing
  Miosis or ptosis
  Sense of fullness in the ear (new in ICHD 3 beta)
- Frequency more than 5 per day (periods with lower frequency may occur) and can be up to 15.
- *Absolute responsiveness to indomethacin*
- Secondary causes are excluded.

Treatment PH is defined as absolutely responsive to indomethacin. Thus, if PH is suspected, indomethacin should be started.

Start at 25 mg 3 times a day for 48 hours to 1week
Increase by 25 mg 3 times a day every 72 hours to 2 weeks
Maximum 100 mg 3 times a day

Indomethacin is an NSAID; thus, one has to be aware of its gastrointestinal side effects and a proton pump inhibitor should be considered. We always start a proton pump inhibitor if an NSAID will be given daily for a month or longer. If a patient is indomethacin intolerant or is unresponsive, one can consider celecoxib, other NSAIDs or aspirin, topiramate, or gabapentin (starting at the lowest dose and increasing as necessary).

Short-Lasting Unilateral Neuralgiform Headache Attacks With Conjunctival Injection and Tearing/Short-Lasing Unilateral Neuralgiform Headache Attacks With Cranial Autonomic Symptoms (SUNCT/SUNA)

These headaches are the shortest (5 to 240 seconds in duration; now 1 to 600 seconds according to ICHD-3 beta) and the rarest type of TAC. The quality of pain is similar to both CH and PH but occurs 3 to 200 times a day. However, unlike the other TACs, these may have cutaneous triggers.

SUNCT is associated with a red and/or tearing eye on the side of the pain. SUNA is any combination of autonomic symptoms. Because SUNCT/SUNA is extremely rare, secondary causes, especially intracranial pathology (pituitary tumors, brainstem stroke, arteriovenous malformation, vertebral arterial dissections, demyelination), must be ruled out in every patient who presents with these symptoms. The workup should include brain imaging (preferably MRI) as well as peripheral bloodwork (further discussed under secondary headaches).

ICHD-2 diagnostic criteria for SUNCT/SUNA follow.

SUNCT/SUNA

- More than 20 attacks of the following
- Attacks lasting 5 seconds to 4 minutes of (now 1 to 600 seconds) moderate or severe unilateral orbital/supraorbital/temporal stabbing or pulsating pain
- Pain is accompanied by ipsilateral conjunctival injection/lacrimation (different autonomic findings for SUNA, and the same as in PH).
- Frequency 3 to 200 per day, either isolated or in volleys of several one after the other
- Secondary causes are excluded.

Treatment Unlike CH and PH, SUNCT/SUNA do not respond to many medications preventively. AEDs, IV lidocaine, and greater occipital nerve (GON) block can be tried:

- Lamotrigine, 100 to 400 mg/day (first reported by Giovanni D'Andrea of Vicenza, Italy)
- Topiramate 50 to 400 mg/day
- Gabapentin 600 to 3000 mg/day
- IV lidocaine 1.3 to 3.3 mg/kg/hr
- GON block

How Should We Treat Cliff?

Based on what we discussed earlier in this chapter, Cliff most likely has CHs but we will order MRI of the head to rule out pituitary tumors and other intracranial pathology. Without waiting for the MRI results, we will start him on acute, bridge, and preventive therapies.

Acute Care Therapy A 100% oxygen inhalation at 7 L/min at headache onset and increase to 12 to 15 L/min if not responsive. The oxygen should be give through a non-rebreathing mask over the nose and mouth. The patient should sit on the edge of the bed, bend at the waist, and breathe normally for 10 to 15 minutes. In the United States, we have the patient rent a D cylinder of oxygen to be kept in the bed room as cluster attacks tend to occur after work or at night.

If oxygen alone does not abort the headache, we will also prescribe 6 mg sumatriptan injections SQ often as the needle-free Sumavel Dose Pro or zolmitriptan NS 5 mg taken at headache onset.

Bridge Therapy (Transitional) Prednisone 60 to 80 mg/day tapering over 7 to 14 days. We used to prescribe it for 3 weeks, but some patients can develop aseptic necrosis of bone quickly so the duration was shortened and we prefer no more than 7 days. The risk is still present and should be discussed with the patient.

Preventive Therapy Our goal is to shorten the duration of ongoing cluster attacks:

Verapamil, starting at 80 mg 3 times a day, is increased to 480 mg/day if needed. We always start with the short-acting medication and increase it slowly, checking electrocardiograms to rule out secondary heart block. Some patients need a dose as high as 720 mg if they can tolerate the side effects of constipation and pedal edema. Cliff will continue receiving verapamil for 1 to 2 weeks after cessation of his cluster attacks. We will then slowly taper the verapamil. Otherwise, if cluster continues, we might consider adding melatonin 10 mg to take at night to the verapamil or change to another preventive such as topiramate, gabapentin, or lithium.

We will give him our pager numbers so he can reach us emergently if acute medications are not working for him, so that we can try something else. Otherwise, we will tell him to call us the day his cluster period begins again, and he will have prednisone, verapamil, and sumatriptan injections at home ready to start.

When patients with daily Chronic Cluster are intractable and do not respond to treatment, various types of surgery can be tried. So far, the best type is occipital nerve stimulation and deep brain stimulation of the posterior hypothalamus.

Other Primary Headaches

ICHD-2 includes a forth category of primary headache disorders that encompasses the remaining primary headaches. We will briefly discuss a few of these and list the rest.

Primary thunderclap headache—defined as extremely rapid onset to extreme peak pain, reaching maximum intensity in less than 1 minute, often in a second. Most patients, after experiencing such a headache, will present to an emergency department, where they should be worked up to rule out secondary causes including but not limited to intracranial hemorrhage, sentinel bleed, arterial dissection, cerebral venous thrombosis, stroke, reversible cerebral vasoconstriction syndrome, and pituitary apoplexy. For a detailed description of the workup, please see Chapter 2 on secondary headaches.

Primary headache associated with sexual activity (preorgasmic and orgasmic types no longer recognized in ICHD-3 beta)—these headaches occur mostly in younger patients just prior to or during orgasm and can be short lived or can last for hours. They tend to present as a thunderclap or "worst headache in patient's life" and, as such, should be worked up as any new headache. Given the sudden severe characteristic of this headache, special care should be taken to rule out a subarachnoid hemorrhage. Otherwise, please see discussion on secondary headaches in Chapter 2 for detailed description of the workup.

New daily persistent headache—these headaches are daily and may resemble any chronic type headache with one exception, abrupt onset over a 3-day period, with patients able to recall almost an exact moment when a headache started. Half the patients remember a specific trigger (i.e., viral illness) and half have family history of frequent headaches. The headache type is variable but usually some TTH days and some migraine days. It is of unknown etiology, and there is no known effective treatment.

Hemicrania continua (HC)—This is a constant, mild to moderate, steady pain on one half of the head. At times there are periods of worsening or exacerbation that can last minutes to hours. During these times, patients develop autonomic findings on the same side of the head as the pain. ICHD-2 does not classify HC under TACs because it differs in that it is constant; however, other qualities of HC mimic PH. ICHD-3 beta moved HC to the TAC section.

Other in this category include primary stabbing headache, primary cough headache, primary exercise headache, hypnic headache, and a new entry in ICHD-3 beta, nummular headache.

For further information about primary headaches, please see the Suggested Reading list.

ACKNOWLEDGMENTS

The authors give special thanks to Roland McFarland for helpful comments on this chapter.

SUGGESTED READING

Bigal ME, Rapoport AM. Obesity and chronic daily headache. Curr Pain Headache Rep 2012; 16(1): 101–109.

Chang M, Rapoport AM. Acute treatment of migraine headache. Techn Regional Anesth Pain Manage 2009;13:9–15.

Cutrer FM, Bajwa ZH, Sabahat A. Pathophysiology, clinical manifestations, and diagnosis of migraine in adults, Garza, I Central craniofacial pain. Up to Date 2012.

Johnston MM, Rapoport AM. Triptans for the management of migraine. Drugs 2010;70:1505–1518.

Loder E. Triptan therapy in migraine. N Engl J Med 2010;363:63–70.

Michail V, Rapoport AM. Role of antiepileptic drugs as preventive agents for migraine. CNS Drugs 2010;24:21–33.

Olesen J, Tfelt-Hansen P, Welch KMA, Goadsby PJ, Ramadan NM. *The headaches*, 3rd ed. Philadelphia, PA: Lippincott Williams and Wilkins; 2006.

Purdy A, Rapoport A, Tepper S, Sheftell F, editors. *Advanced therapy of headache*, 2nd ed. Toronto, Canada: BC Decker; 2005.

Rapoport AM. Acute treatment of migraine: established and emerging therapies. Headache 2012;52:60–64.

Silberstein SD, Lipton RB, Dodick DW. *Wolff's headache*. New York, NY: Oxford University Press; 2007.

Sun-Edelstein C, Bigal ME, Rapoport AM. Chronic migraine and medication overuse headache: clarifying the current International Headache Society classification criteria. Cephalalgia 2008;29:445–452.

Tepper SJ, Tepper DE. *The Cleveland Clinic manual of headache therapy*, 3rd ed. New York, NY: Springer Science and Business Media; 2011.

The International Classification of Headache Disorders (ICHD) II. Cephalalgia 2004;24 (Suppl 1):1–160.

The International Classification of Headache Disorders (ICHD) 3rd edition (beta version). Cephalalgia 2013;33:1–808.

2 Secondary Headaches

Inna Keselman and Alan Rapoport

INTRODUCTION

There are numerous types of secondary headaches listed and described in the Second Edition of *The International Classification of Headache Disorders* (ICHD-2), including but not limited to, those headaches related to infection, changes in cerebrospinal fluid pressure, systemic causes, trauma, intracranial or vascular pathology, and medications. We will review only the ones that we consider to be most relevant:

1. Headache secondary to giant cell arteritis (listed in ICHD-2 under Section 6.4)
2. Headache secondary to idiopathic intracranial hypertension (previously known as pseudotumor cerebri) (listed in ICHD-2 under Section 7.1)
3. Headache secondary to low cerebrospinal fluid (CSF) pressure (listed in ICHD-2 under Section 7.2)
4. Medication overuse headache (listed in ICHD-2 under Section 8.2)

An important point to note: Headache is often a presenting symptom of a secondary headache disorder; red flags may be present, which should suggest prompt evaluation and treatment. Headache may be due to such serious neurological disorders such as intracranial neoplasm, stroke, cerebral venous thrombosis, brain aneurysm, or carotid artery dissection. Thus, any patient presenting to your office with red flags in the history (see SNOOP mnemonic below) should warrant an expedited workup and prompt referral for a neurological evaluation. A sudden headache, especially if it is severe and quickly escalates in frequency or severity, or a new or changing headache should be quickly and fully evaluated. Even patients with stable primary headache disorders can develop a secondary headache. A detailed history and neurological examination is a must in every patient, and additional workup should be initiated in those with a concerning history or abnormal examination.

As mentioned in Chapter 1, the **SSNOOP** mnemonic for troubling historical facts (adopted from Dr. David Dodick) is as follows:

Systemic symptoms (i.e., fever, weight loss)
Secondary risk factors—know underlying disease (i.e., cancer, HIV infection, high blood pressure)
Neurological signs/symptoms (i.e., confusion, weakness, eye movement problems)
Onset sudden—especially if it is severe, rapidly progressive
Onset after age 40—can be giant cell arteritis, cancer, vascular
Pattern change—excising headache with new quality/severity

Next, the tests listed in Table 1.2 should be considered.

In this chapter, we will briefly discuss a few types of commonly encountered secondary headaches. **Any headache that is associated with worrisome signs and symptoms, especially if it is sudden and severe or quickly escalating in frequency, as well as abnormal neurological examination or imaging, should be promptly evaluated or referred to a specialist for further workup.**

HEADACHE SECONDARY TO GIANT CELL ARTERITIS (TEMPORAL ARTERITIS)

Giant cell arteritis is a vasculitis of large and medium-sized arteries that affects people over age 50, women more commonly than men. Its former name was temporal arteritis, due to inflammation of the temporal artery, which is a branch of an external carotid artery in the scalp.

Giant cell arteritis presents with headache, scalp tenderness, and jaw claudication and may lead to visual loss if not promptly treated. These patients will have markers of systemic inflammation: elevated erythrocyte sedimentation rate (ESR; >50 mm/hr), and increased C-reactive protein (CRP). These headaches can present with or without myalgias, which are symptoms of polymyalgia rheumatica, a related condition of proximal weakness and pain. Diagnosis is made clinically and by abnormal blood tests, but temporal artery biopsy is still the gold standard. When giant cell arteritis is suspected, treatment with high-dose corticosteroids should be started immediately and a rheumatology consult should aid with the diagnosis (for temporal artery biopsy) and treatment. If you are consulting on the patient, starting steroids, arranging for the biopsy, and calling a primary physician is appropriate.

The ICHD-2 diagnostic criteria for giant cell arteritis are as follows:

Giant Cell Arteritis
A. Any new persisting headache filling criteria C and D
B. At least one of the following:
- Swollen tender scalp artery with elevated ESR and/or CRP
- Temporal artery biopsy demonstrating giant cell arteritis
C. Headache develops in close temporal relation to other symptoms and signs of giant cell arteritis
D. Headache resolves or greatly improves within 3 days of high-dose steroid treatment

Note: In any patient over age 50, a new headache should make you think of this condition.

HEADACHE SECONDARY TO IDIOPATHIC INTRACRANIAL HYPERTENSION, PREVIOUSLY KNOWN AS PSEUDOTUMOR CEREBRI

Normal CSF pressure is 70 to 200 mm H_2O. When it is elevated, headache can be the major symptom. If elevated intracranial pressure is suspected, secondary causes must be ruled out with blood work and imaging as described earlier. If no secondary causes can be found, this pressure elevation is most likely idiopathic and may be due to poor reabsorption of CSF into the venous system.

The ICHD diagnostic criteria for idiopathic intracranial hypertension (IIH) as follows:

Idiopathic Intracranial Hypertension

A. Progressive headache with at least one of the following:
- Daily occurrence
- Diffuse and/or constant (nonpulsating) pain
- Aggravated by coughing or straining

And fulfilling criteria C and D

B. Intracranial hypertension fulfilling the following criteria
1. Alert patient with normal neurological examination but acceptable to have:
   - Papilledema
   - Enlarged blind spot
   - Visual field defect (progressive if untreated)
   - Sixth cranial nerve palsy, unilateral or bilateral
2. Increased CSF pressure (>200 mm H_2O in the non-obese and >250 mm H_2O in the obese) measured via lumbar puncture in the recumbent position or by epidural or intraventricular pressure monitoring
3. Normal CSF chemistry and cellularity
4. Intracranial disease is ruled out.
5. No metabolic, toxic, or hormonal cause is found.

C. Headache develops in close temporal relation to increased intracranial pressure.

D. Headache improves after withdrawal of CSF to reduce pressure to 120 to 170 mm H_2O and resolves within 72 hours of persistent normalization of intracranial pressure.

A typical patient with IIH is a young obese female with diffuse headache of moderate severity worsened by valsalva. Patients may complain of visual symptoms, including blurred vision, transient visual obscurations, and/or diplopia, as well as hearing a sound in their ears (pulsatile tinnitus). If untreated, this can lead to permanent vision loss.

Evaluation requires extensive history and neurological examination that could be normal or show papilledema, enlarged blind spot, visual field defect, and/or sixth cranial nerve palsy.

Any patient in whom IIH is suspected requires brain magnetic resonance imaging (MRI; which is usually normal or can show an empty sella or slit-like lateral ventricles), MRV with contrast, and a neuro-ophthalmological examination to evaluate visual fields. IIH diagnosis requires lumber puncture documenting increased intracranial pressure greater than 200 mm H_2O in the non-obese and greater than 250 mm H_2O in the obese. CSF studies in IIH are normal (low protein is acceptable). The following are conditions with increased intracranial pressure:

- Central venous thrombosis
- Mass lesion
- Meningitis
- Hypothyroidism/hyperthyroidism
- Vitamin A intoxication/deficiency
- Renal disease
- Iron deficiency

The following are risk factors for developing IIH:
Female gender
Obesity

Medication
- Steroids
- Oral contraceptives
- Growth hormone
- Tetracycline
- Lithium

These headaches respond to drainage of CSF, but this response is short lasting; thus daily preventive medication is usually prescribed. Acetazolamide, a carbonic anhydrase inhibitor, is the drug of choice and is started at 250 mg 3 times a day and increased up to 1500 mg to 2 grams a day or more as needed/tolerated. Obese patients should be told to lose a significant amount of weight.

Other medications used include:

- Topiramate, which is a weak carbonic anhydrase inhibitor, at 100 to 200 mg/day
- Furosemide, which is a diuretic and can be used alone or in addition to acetazolamide, at 40 to 120 mg/day

Patient should also be referred to an ophthalmologist for frequent visual field testing.

If these treatments fail, more invasive options may be considered; optic nerve sheath fenestration, and ventriculoperitoneal or lumboperitoneal shunts. Patients should be referred to a neurologist prior to considering any of these.

HEADACHE SECONDARY TO LOW CSF PRESSURE

These types of headaches can result from previous lumbar puncture, CSF fistula, or trauma or may be idiopathic. It is the idiopathic ones that often go undiagnosed. They are usually bilateral, throbbing, occipital or frontal and strikingly positional early on. The classical presentation is for the headache to get worse with sitting or standing and improve on lying down. The position aspect may disappear with time making a diagnosis much harder. Post–lumbar puncture headaches are the most common reason for a low CSF pressure headache as it develops in one-third of patients undergoing lumbar puncture. It usually starts in 2 to 5 days after the procedure and should spontaneously resolve in 1 week. However, it may develop into a chronic condition when headache persists even while lying flat.

Post–lumbar puncture headaches can be associated with tinnitus, hearing impairment, phonophobia, photophobia, nausea/vomiting, dizziness/vertigo, stiffness, and pain and parethesias in the neck. They can also have significant associated neurological findings including cranial nerve dysfunction (i.e., horizontal diplopia), gait imbalance, and facial numbness.

MRI with contrast in this case may show diffuse pachymeningeal enhancement (without leptomeningeal involvement) and brain sag with flattening of the pons, small prepontine cistern and descent of the cerebellar tonsils into through the foramen magnum. These MRI findings are subtle and should be reviewed with a neuroradiologist. But finding the leak is often difficult, and computed tomography (CT) myelography is the most reliable diagnostic study. Most hidden leaks are in the cervical area.

Treatment includes bedrest, oral or intravenous hydration, and caffeine. Epidural blood patch with at least 20 cc of autologous blood is performed in those patients who continue to have headaches despite conservative treatment. It is successful more than 95% of the time. Spontaneous CSF leaks are difficult to manage, especially when the source of a leak cannot be found.

ICHD-2 diagnostic criteria for low CSF pressure headache are as follows:

Low CSF Pressure Headache

A. Diffuse and/or dull headache that worsens within 15 minutes after sitting/standing and has one or more of the following characteristics:
   - Neck stiffness
   - Tinnitus
   - Hypacusia (diminished hearing)
   - Photophobia
   - Nausea

B. At least one of the following:
   - Evidence of low CSF pressure on MRI
   - Evidence of CSF leakage on conventional myelography, CT myelography or cisternography
   - CSF opening pressure <60 mm H_2O water in sitting position
C. No history of dural puncture or other causes of CSF fistula
D. Headache resolves within 72 hours after epidural blood patch

MEDICATION-OVERUSE HEADACHE (PREVIOUSLY KNOWN AS REBOUND HEADACHE)

Medication-overuse headaches, which were first described in 1979 by Dr. Lee Kudrow from Los Angeles, are daily or near-daily headaches that occur as a consequence of episodic headaches (most often migraine) that are associated with overuse of acute medications (i.e., barbiturates, opioids, nonsteroidal anti-inflammatory drugs [NSAIDs], acetaminophen, triptans, ergots, etc.). The headache does not usually have specific characteristics and are phenotypically similar to both migraine and tension-type headache. *Overuse* is defined in terms of duration and frequency of use, and risk of developing medication-overuse headache depends on the specific medications overused.

The risk is high when the follow medications are used:

Opioids more than 8 days per month
Barbiturates more than 5 days per month
Triptans/NSAIDs more than 10 days per month

The ICHD-2 revised criteria of medication-overuse headache are as follows:

Medication Overuse Headache

A. Headache on 15 or more days per months
B. Regular overuse for 3 or more months of one of these acute medications:

   - Ergotamine, triptan, opioid, butalbital-containing medication or combination analgesic medication on 10 days or more per month

OR

- Simple analgesics (i.e., aspirin, acetaminophen, NSAIDs) or any combination of ergotamine, triptan, and opioids on 15 days per month (this last group of combinations has been changed in ICHD-3 beta to 10 or more days per month).

C. Headache has developed or markedly worsened during medication overuse.

Note that a patient can be taking too many medications, but if the headaches do not worsen or a new headache begins, then it is not considered medication overuse headache at that time, even though the patient is using too many medications and may develop the syndrome.

Treatment includes educating your patient on the consequences of overuse and tapering off an offending medication. This is done slowly and can be aided by adding a preventive medication like a tricyclic antidepressant, β-blocker, antiseizure medication, or onabotulinumtoxinA, if chronic migraine is present (see prior sections for discussion and Table 1.7 for the list of preventive medications). Behavioral therapy services can be helpful, and some patients may need sleeping medication. If the patient has difficulty during the tapering due to escalating headache, a short course of steroids can be considered. Most patients can be treated on an outpatient basis. For some patients who are overusing high-dose opioids, benzodiazepines, or butalbital or have significant medical or psychiatric problems, it may be appropriate to consider an inpatient setting.

OTHER SECONDARY HEADACHES

ICHD-2 lists many *other types of secondary headaches,* which include headaches due to head or neck trauma, headache related to a metabolic condition or neoplasm, reversible cerebral vasoconstriction syndrome, and primary central nervous system angiitis. As mentioned, we cannot cover them all. For further information on resourses about headaches described here or other secondary headaches, please see the reference list.

Before we discuss the next category of headaches, we will review general principles of pain.

ACKNOWLEDGMENTS

The authors give special thanks to Roland McFarland for helpful comments on this chapter.

SUGGESTED READING

Schievink WI. Spontaneous spinal cerebrospinal fluid leaks and intracranial hypotension. JAMA 2006;295:2286–2296.

Olesen J, Tfelt-Hansen P, Welch KMA, Goadsby PJ, Ramadan NM. The headaches, 3rd ed. Philadelphia, PA: Lippincott Williams and Wilkins; 2006.

Purdy A, Rapoport A, Tepper S, Sheftell F, editors. Advanced therapy of headache, 2nd ed. Toronto, Canada: BC Decker; 2005.

Silberstein SD, Lipton RB, Dodick DW. Wolff's headache. New York, NY: Oxford University Press; 2007.

Smith HS. Definition and pathogenesis of chronic pain. Up to Date, 2012. http://www.upto-date.com/contents/definition-and-pathogenesis-of-chronic-pain?source=search_resu lt&search=Definition+and+pathogenesis+of+chronic+pain&selectedTitle=1%7E150

Sun-Edelstein C, Bigal ME, Rapoport AM. Chronic migraine and medication overuse headache: clarifying the current International Headache Society classification criteria. Cephalalgia 2008;29:445–452.

Tepper SJ, Tepper DE. The Cleveland Clinic manual of headache therapy, 3rd ed. New York, NY: Springer Science and Business Media; 2011.

The International Classification of Headache Disorders (ICHD) II. Cephalalgia 2004; 24(Suppl 1):1–160.

The International Classification of Headache Disorders (ICHD) 3rd edition (beta version). Cephalalgia 2013;33:1–808.

3 Facial Pain

Inna Keselman and Alan Rapoport

INTRODUCTION

Pain is one of the most common complaints encountered by physicians. If persistent, pain is often debilitating, causing functional impairment, disability, and psychological distress not only to the patient but also the surrounding family and friends. In the United States, pain is the most common cause of long-term disability, with more than 75 million of 312 million Americans suffering from chronic pain. Great efforts are being spent on pain research every year, yet our understanding of its mechanisms remains limited. Here we will briefly discuss a few key points on pain pathogenesis and how it may be related to headaches and craniofacial pain.

Acute pain—vital, protective mechanism that ensures our survival in an environment full of potential dangers. It can be divided into *adaptive* and *maladaptive*, with adaptive pain serving a protective role (protects from injury), while maladaptive or chronic pain is a pathological malfunctioning of the nervous system.

Chronic pain—pain that lasts beyond the ordinary duration of time that an insult or injury to the body needs to heal

There are two broad categories of pain:

Nociceptive—due to noxious/damaging stimulus (i.e., postoperative pain or injury)

Neuropathic—can be thought of as *non*-nociceptive, meaning there is no damaging stimulus required to trigger this type of pain; instead neuropathic pain originates from a dysfunction of the nervous system itself, either a central nervous system (CNS) process or a peripheral nerve lesion.

Differentiating between nociceptive and neuropathic pain is important and clinically significant in that these two types of pain respond differently to medications, with neuropathic pain being less responsive to opioids and more likely to respond to other drugs like anticonvulsants and antidepressants.

Neuropathic pain can be stimulus evoked or stimulus independent and is further subdivided into the following:

- *Sympathetically mediated,* arising from a peripheral nerve lesion and associated with autonomic changes (i.e., complex regional pain syndrome)
- *Peripheral*, from damage to a peripheral nerve without autonomic symptoms (i.e., postherpetic neuralgia)
- *Central*, from abnormal CNS activity (i.e., phantom limb pain)

Neuralgia is a form of neuropathic pain that is defined by the following characteristics:

- Brief, paroxysmal (seconds to minutes)
- Without objective neurological deficit in the distribution of an affected nerve
- Attacks may be provoked by non-painful stimuli
- Refractory period follows an attack (this refractory period gets shorter as the disease progresses)

Mechanisms of neuropathic pain are complex and still not well understood. Nerve injury can lead to changes in peripheral and central nervous systems, which result in persistent pain even after injury heals (peripheral and central sensitization). These changes are consequences of multiple processes including inflammation and changes in neuronal excitability. Understanding these processes is key to developing more targeted approaches to treat pain.

It is also important to mention that some structures are sensitive to pain, while others are not. The following is the list of intracranial and extracranial structures currently believed to be *pain sensitive* (adopted from Dr. David Dodick):

> *Intracranial:* Dura; venous sinuses; proximal intracranial arteries; cranial nerves V, VII, IX, and X; and upper cervical nerves
> *Extracranial:* Carotid, vertebral, and basilar arteries; blood vessels within scalp and skin; skin; mucosa; muscles; fascia; synovia within the temporomandibular joint (TMJ); teeth; and periosteum

HEADACHE

The pathogenesis of headache is thought to be generated by a combination of peripheral and central processes and involves different brain structures (i.e., hypothalamus, thalamus, cortex, sphenopalatine ganglion, pons, and the trigeminal nucleus caudalis), blood vessels (intracranial and extracranial arteries and veins), glial cells (i.e., astrocytes and microglia), and different types of neurons. Cortical spreading depression is an electrical phenomenon that may precede migraine in some or all cases. Most headaches are thought to involve the trigeminal nerve and its terminals in the meninges, especially the first division, and/or upper cervical nerves.

CRANIAL NEURALGIAS AND TMJ DISORDERS

Cranial Neuralgias

Cranial neuralgias are a group of disorders that involve pain in the head and neck that is mediated by sensory pain fibers of cranial nerves (CNs) V, VII, IX, and X as well as upper cervical roots connecting with CN V through the trigeminocervical complex. Damage or pathological stimulation of these nerves (i.e., irritation, compression, exposure to cold/hot) will result in pain. This group of disorders is classified in ICHD-2 separately from primary or secondary headaches due to the fact that a problem source cannot be found in many patients. Thus, the term "secondary" is used for patients in whom a source, such as vascular compression or a neuroma, is found, while the term "classical," rather than primary, is used for those patients who present with a typical history but without an identifiable source. ICHD-2 lists multiple neuralgias; here, we will only discuss two most common ones: trigeminal and occipital.

Classical Trigeminal Neuralgia

Description Trigeminal neuralgia (TN) consists of brief (lasting from a fraction of a second up to 2 minutes or longer), electric shock–like pains that are unilateral, severe, repetitive pains in the distribution of sensory divisions of the trigeminal nerve (V2 and V3 are more common, affecting the cheek or jaw). Pain is often triggered by touching, chewing, and talking as well as occurring spontaneously. TN tends to affect older individuals.

Any patient presenting with these complaints should be evaluated for secondary causes, which include an underlying lesion, aneurysms, or multiple sclerosis, especially if TN is bilateral and sarcoid. These patients should have blood work to include complete blood cell count, erythrocyte sedimentation rate, and C-reactive protein, as well as brain magnetic resonance imaging (MRI) with contrast and MR angiography of the brain vessels, especially near the three branches of the trigeminal nerve to rule out vascular compression (for a detailed description of a workup to evaluate secondary causes, please see Chapter 2 on secondary headache disorders).

The ICHD-2 diagnostic criteria for TN are as follows:

Trigeminal Neuralgia
A. Paroxysmal attacks of pain lasting from a fraction of a second to 2 minutes, affecting one or more divisions of the trigeminal nerve and fulfilling criteria B and C
B. Pain has a least one of the following characteristics:
- Intense, sharp, superficial, or stabbing
- Precipitated from trigger areas or by trigger factors
C. Attacks are stereotyped in the individual patient.
D. There is no clinically evident neurological deficit.
E. Not attributed to another disorder

Treatment
1. Carbamazepine—start at 100 mg twice a day and build up to about 600 mg to 1200 mg/day as tolerated. The target maintenance dose is 1200 mg/day, but lower doses may be effective without adverse events. Hyponatremia is a potential side effect of carbamazepine.
2. Oxcarbazepine, a structural derivative of carbamazepine, has a better side effect profile— start at 300 mg twice a day and increase as tolerated in 300-mg increments every 3 days to a total of 1200 to 1800 mg/day.
3. Gabapentin—start at 300 mg/day and escalate as needed/tolerated; can go up to at least 900 mg 3 times a day. Beware of sedating and weight gain side effects of gabapentin.

Patients usually respond well to these medications. If necessary, second-line treatment with lamotrigine, baclofen, or onabotulinumtoxinA can be tried. The older drug diphenylhydantoin was often effective at 400 mg/day. If medications fail, surgical procedures are possible and include vascular decompression, during which a branch of the fifth cranial nerve is separated from a nearby vascular loop by a soft substance (the Janetta procedure), and percutaneous thermal denervation of one or more divisions of CN V on the same side as the pain.

If the workup produces a source of TN, a patient can be started on these medications and referred to a neurologist/neurosurgeon for further evaluation.

Occipital Neuralgia

Description Occipital neuralgia (ON) can be considered a variation on the theme of TN with pain occurring in the distribution the greater, lesser, and/or third occipital nerves in the back of the head. The nerve is usually very tender to the touch and pressure on the nerve can produce pain radiating to the ipsilateral eye. Examination should show tenderness to palpation in the ipsilateral suboccipital area. Again, patients presenting with any head or neck pain should be worked up as described earlier and, if needed, referred to a neurologist/neurosurgeon.

The ICHD-2 diagnostic criteria for ON are as follows:

Occipital Neuralgia
A. Paroxysmal stabbing pain, with or without persistent aching between paroxysms, in the distribution(s) of the greater, lesser, and/or third occipital nerves
B. Tenderness over the affected nerve
C. Pain is eased temporarily by local anesthetic block of the nerve.

Treatment Occipital nerve block with local anesthetic is usually tried first, before systemic (oral) therapies. If that fails, the same oral medications used for TN can be tried for ON. There is no clear consensus as to whether the block should be done with local anesthetic alone or combined with a steroid. The result are sometimes good either way.

If nerve block and PO medications fail, one can try steroids or cervical onabotulinumtoxinA injections as well as physiotherapy concentrating on the cervical area.

Headache and Facial Pain Due to TMJ Disorders

These disorders are common and result either from damage to the TMJ (i.e., disk displacement, joint hypermobility, arthritis), or to muscular abnormalities which lead` to headaches and facial pain.

Headaches are usually frontotemporal with pain localized to preauricular region, mandible, and TMJ region. Patients report jaw locking and popping as well as bruxism during sleep and may complain of otalgia, tinnitus, or dizziness. An examination may show limited jaw opening and tenderness of the muscles of mastication. In our experience, most patients referred to specialists in orofacial pain were told they had different problems from those their dentists had diagnosed. The majority of headache patients exhibiting these symptoms do not have significant pathology in the TMJ but instead have muscular problems of the face and jaw, and should be diagnosed with myofascial pain. Orofacial pain specialists know how to treat these symptoms and rarely resort to any type of surgery.

The ICHD-2 diagnostic criteria for TMJ disorders are as follows:

Temporomandibular Joint Disorders
A. Recurrent pain in one or more regions of the head and/or face fulfilling criteria C and D

B. Radiography, MRI, and/or bone scintigraphy demonstrates TMJ disorder
C. Evidence that pain can be attributed to the TMJ disorder, based on at least one of the following:
   • Precipitated by jaw movement and/or chewing of hard food
   • Reduced range of or irregular jaw opening
   • Noise from one or both TMJs during jaw movement
   • Tenderness of the joint capsule(s) of one or both TMJs
D. Headache resolves within 3 months and does not recur after successful treatment of TMJ disorder

Treatment

TMJ-related headache and pain are usually self-limited, and treatment is reserved for moderate to severe symptoms. The treatment usually involves rest, avoidance of loading, control of contributing factors, mobility exercises, mild analgesics or NSAIDs (such as ibuprofen or naproxen sodium), muscle relaxants, occlusal splints, stretching and spraying muscles, and physical therapy. Most dentists like to treat TMJ problems but, in our experience, difficult patients with possible TMJ disorders should be seen by orofacial pain specialists.

ACKNOWLEDGMENTS

The authors give special thanks to Roland McFarland for helpful comments on this chapter.

SUGGESTED READING

Olesen J, Tfelt-Hansen P, Welch KMA, Goadsby PJ, Ramadan NM. The headaches, 3rd ed. Philadelphia, PA: Lippincott Williams and Wilkins; 2006.

Purdy A, Rapoport A, Tepper S, Sheftell F, editors. Advanced therapy of headache, 2nd ed. Toronto, Canada: BC Decker; 2005.

Silberstein SD, Lipton RB, Dodick DW. Wolff's headache. New York, NY: Oxford University Press; 2007.

Smith HS. Definition and pathogenesis of chronic pain. Up to Date, 2012. http://www.upto-date.com/contents/definition-and-pathogenesis-of-chronic-pain?source=search_resu lt&search=Definition+and+pathogenesis+of+chronic+pain&selectedTitle=1%7E150

Tepper SJ, Tepper DE. The Cleveland Clinic manual of headache therapy, 3rd ed. New York, NY: Springer Science and Business Media; 2011.

The International Classification of Headache Disorders (ICHD) II. Cephalalgia 2004; 24(Suppl 1):1–160.

The International Classification of Headache Disorders (ICHD) 3rd edition (beta version). Cephalalgia 2013;33:629-808.

4 Childhood and Adolescent Headaches

Inna Keselman and Alan Rapoport

INTRODUCTION

Childhood headache has a major impact on the child and the family and is one of the most common complaints for which children are referred to a neurologist. Just like for adults, making a correct diagnosis for children is essential to good treatment. Although most children do not have secondary causes of headache, it is vital to rule them out if present (see Chapter 1 for details on obtaining history and workup).

Primary headaches in children are also divided into the same categories as in adults and possess the same features, although diagnosis may be more difficult depending on the patient's age. Two main primary pediatric headaches are migraine and tension-type headache (TTH). A recent analysis of children and adolescents by Abu-Arefeh et al. (2010) showed the overall prevalence of migraine to be 7.7% in that population, with females being more likely than males to develop migraine. Others have found a slight prevalence in boys from ages 8 to 12. Trigeminal autonomic cephalalgias (TCAs) are extremely uncommon in the pediatric population. Other pediatric headaches are similar to their adult counterparts and include chronic daily headache, new daily persistent headache, and post-traumatic and exertional headaches.

CHILDHOOD PERIODIC SYNDROMES

There are three childhood periodic syndromes coded in the migraine section, and they are all commonly precursors of migraine. The Third Edition of *The International Classification of Headache Disorders* (ICHD-3 beta) has changed the terminology to Episodic syndromes that may be associated with migraine:

1. Cyclical vomiting (listed in ICHD-2 under Section 1.3.1)
2. Abdominal migraine (listed in ICHD-2 under Section 1.3.2)
3. Benign paroxysmal vertigo of childhood (listed in ICHD-2 under Section 1.3.3)

And the new category that was added is:

4. Benign paroxysmal torticollis

DIAGNOSIS OF MIGRAINE IN CHILDREN

Although the criteria are similar to those in adults, children have more bilateral migraines than do adults. Their headaches are also shorter, often lasting less than 1 hour, associated with vomiting, and followed by sleep, which is often restorative.

Cyclical Vomiting

This is a migraine variant that should be considered in young patients with frequent vomiting spells who have a family history of migraine. Episodes tend to be stereotyped in a given patient and are associated with pallor and lethargy; there is complete resolution of symptoms between attacks. It is a self-limited episodic disorder, but these children will likely develop typical migraine as they age. Secondary causes have to be ruled out first (i.e., gastrointestinal causes, increased intracranial pressure, etc.); then treatment can be initiated with sedatives and antiemetics. Triptans (off label) may also be considered if other treatments fail.

The ICHD-2 diagnostic criteria for cyclical vomiting are as follows:

Cyclical Vomiting
A. At least five attacks fulfilling criteria B and C
B. Episodic attacks, stereotypical in the individual patient, of intense nausea and vomiting lasting from 1 hour to 5 days
C. Vomiting during attacks occurs at least four times and hour for at least 1 hour
D. Symptom-free between attacks
E. Not attributed to another disorder

Abdominal Migraine

This is a childhood migraine variant (sometimes seen in adults) that is characterized by episodic midline abdominal pain, lasting 1 to 72 hours. Pain is associated with nausea, vomiting, and vasomotor symptoms. The child should return to normal between episodes and, just as in cyclical vomiting. Gastrointestinal disease should be ruled out. Migraine pain usually occurs years later.

The ICHD-2 diagnostic criteria for abdominal migraine are as follows:

Abdominal Migraine
A. At least five attacks fulfilling criteria B-D
B. Attacks of abdominal pain lasting 1 to 72 hours (untreated or unsuccessfully treated)
C. Abdominal pain has all of the following characteristics:
- Midline location, periumbilical or poorly localized
- Dull or "just sore" quality
- Moderate or severe intensity
D. During abdominal pain, at least two of the following:
- Anorexia
- Nausea
- Vomiting
- Pallor
E. Not attributed to another disorder

Benign Paroxysmal Vertigo of Childhood

This is a childhood migraine variant that is characterized by brief episodic attacks of vertigo that start suddenly and resolve spontaneously. The attacks may be associated with nystagmus and/or vomiting and may be associated with a unilateral throbbing headache. A child should be evaluated for secondary causes of vertigo as soon as possible as serious neurological conditions such as posterior fossa tumors can present in a similar way.

The ICHD-2 diagnostic criteria for paroxysmal vertigo of childhood are as follows:

Benign Paroxysmal Vertigo of Childhood

A. At least five attacks fulfilling criterion B

B. Multiple episodes of severe vertigo, occurring without warning and resolving spontaneously after minutes to hours

C. Normal neurological examination; audiometric and vestibular functions between attacks

D. Normal electroencephalogram

TREATMENT IN CHILDREN

Although the diagnosis of primary headaches in children is similar to that in adults, treatment is quite different, as only a few medications have been approved for use in adolescents and none have been approved for pediatric patients. We will describe treatments available for children suffering from migraine and TTH; for a more detailed diagnostic discussion of common primary headaches, see Chapter 1.

As in adults, an all-encompassing approach to treatment should also be taken for the pediatric patient. Identifying and avoiding triggers such as stress, lack of sleep, and exercise are extremely helpful in the treatment regimen. Maintaining a headache calendar or journal is very helpful for both the patient and the doctor. Depending on headache frequency, a decision can be made as to whether preventive medications should be used. In our experience, behavioral medicine services, including biofeedback training and keeping a calendar, are the most effective treatments for children, and there are no adverse effects.

TREATMENT OF CHILDHOOD MIGRAINE

Acute Treatment of Migraine*

The off-label use of over-the-counter nonsteroidal anti-inflammatory drugs (NSAIDs) is often helpful in children. If triptans are needed, all seven can be used (for details please see Chapter 1). The first triptan approved by the FDA for use in adolescents was almotriptan (Axert).

In an average-sized teenager, diphenhydramine 25 mg and naproxen 10 mg/kg are recommended. If the child is not better in 2 hours, diphenhydramine may be repeated with acetaminophen 15 mg/kg. If this regimen does not work, consider the use of triptans.

In an 8 to 12 year old child, NSAIDs (ibuprofen or naproxen) 10 mg/kg are recommended. If the child is not better in 2 hours, the NSAID can be repeated or acetaminophen 15 mg/kg can be tried. If that does not work, triptans can be considered: 20 mg

---

* Adapted from The Cleveland Clinic Manual of Headache Therapy.

sumatripan nasal spray, 5 mg Zomig nasal spray, or 2.5 or 5 mg zolmitriptan ZMT, an orange flavored, orally disintegrating tablet (ODT).

For nausea/vomiting, use ondasetron 2 to 4 mg ODT before starting above treatment. Promethazine (Phenergan) 12.5 mg liquid or tablet can be helpful and also slightly sedating.

Intravenous medications, which include diphenhydramine, ondansetron, magnesium, dihydroergotamine and valproic acid (in the form of intravenous Depacon), can be used, but these treatments are usually reserved for emergency departments. Also consider dopamine antagonists such as prochloroperazine in low doses.

Preventive Treatment of Migraine*

Initiation of a preventive medication should be considered in a pediatric patient with frequent headaches, or those poorly responsive to acute care treatment, for whom lifestyle modifications, stress management techniques, and especially biofeedback training have failed. Just as in adults, choosing a specific preventive medication will be individualized, depending on existing comorbidities.

The following can be tried:

Antihistamine/serotonin type 2 antagonist: cyproheptadine 4 to 12 mg/day
Antidepressant: amitriptyline 1 mg/kg/day
Anticonvulsants
Topiramate 50 to 150 mg/day
Gabapentin 300 to 1200 mg/day

Other medications that can be tried include valproic acid, preferably in the form of divalproex sodium ER (extended release), which should be avoided in girls due to increased risk of polycystic ovarian syndrome and in women of child bearing potential due to teratogenic effects on the fetal developing spinal cord; β-blockers (propranolol, atenolol); and calcium channel blockers (verapamil). Other categories of medication can also be tried.

CHILDHOOD TTH

TTHA in children is similar to that in adults and is described in detail in Chapter 1. In brief, it is characterized as bilateral, steady, mild to moderate headache without nausea which tends not to be disruptive to normal routines of daily living.

Acute Treatment of TTH*

Naproxen, at 10 mg/kg, can be used as long as its use does not exceed 2–3 days per week. If it does, the clinician needs to think about preventive medication (see Chapter 1 for discussion on preventive treatment of TTH in adults).

SUMMARY

Headache is a common, debilitating disorder that affects people of all ages.
The first step to successful treatment is a correct diagnosis.
Differentiating between a primary and a secondary headache is key, as headache could be a presenting symptom of a focal, systemic, or life-threatening disease.

Remember to use the SSNOOP mnemonic (see Chapters 1 and 2) to identify red
flags, the presence of which should prompt a thorough workup and referral
to a specialist.

ICHD-2 classification lists three types of primary headaches, numerous secondary
headaches, cranial neuralgias, and temporomandibular joint dysfunction.

ICHD-3 beta classification is now available. and a few differences have been
delineated here.

Behavioral therapy, including behavior modification, relaxation techniques, biofeedback training, and other non-pharmacological treatments, is just as important
for the treatment of primary headaches as are pharmacological interventions.

Triptans are the drugs of choice for the acute treatment of migraine if not
contraindicated.

One NSAID is approved for migraine in adults: diclofenac potassium for solution
(Cambia).

Special considerations should be given when evaluating female patients of child-
bearing potential, those who are pregnant, and those who are breastfeeding.

Migraine presents differently in the pediatric population, with more bilaterality
and shorter duration; every child with a new or changing headache should be
promptly evaluated to rule out organic pathology.

*Remember that you can refer your patient to a headache specialist at any point during
the course of your treatment.*

ACKNOWLEDGMENTS

The authors give special thanks to Roland McFarland for helpful comments on this
chapter.

SUGGESTED READING

Abu-Arefeh I, Razak S, Silvaraman B, Graham C. Prevalence of headache and migraine in
children and adolescents: a systematic review of population-based studies. Dev Med
Child Neurol 2010;52:1088–1097.

Bigal ME, Rapoport AM. Obesity and chronic daily headache. Curr Pain Headache Rep
2012; 16(1): 101–109.

Olesen J, Tfelt-Hansen P, Welch KMA, Goadsby PJ, Ramadan NM. *The Headaches*, 3rd ed.
Philadelphia, PA: Lippincott Williams and Wilkins; 2006.

Purdy A, Rapoport A, Tepper S, Sheftell F, editors. *Advanced therapy of headache*, 2nd ed.
Toronto, Canada: BC Decker; 2005.

Silberstein SD, Lipton RB, Dodick DW. *Wolff's headache*. New York, NY: Oxford University
Press; 2007.

Tepper SJ, Tepper DE. *The Cleveland Clinic manual of headache therapy*, 3rd ed. New York,
NY: Springer Science and Business Media; 2011.

The International Classification of Headache Disorders (ICHD) II. Cephalalgia 2004;
24(Suppl 1):1–160.

The International Classification of Headache Disorders (ICHD) 3rd edition (beta version).
Cephalalgia 2013;33:627–808.

SECTION TWO
CEREBROVASCULAR
DISORDERS

5 Transient Ischemic Attack

Comana Cioroiu and Olajide Williams

INTRODUCTION

The diagnosis of transient ischemic attack (TIA) may have inconsistent agreement even among stroke-trained neurologists, given its transient nature and the dependence on retrospective accounts for diagnosis. A new "tissue- based" definition of TIA was proposed in 2002 that defines *TIA* as "a brief episode of neurological dysfunction caused by focal brain or retinal ischemia, with clinical symptoms typically lasting less than one hour, and without evidence of acute infarction." Given the inherently transient nature of a TIA, it is important to distinguish this clinical entity from other diagnoses that may also present with temporary clinical symptoms. Up to 25% of patients admitted to the hospital with a diagnosis of TIA may have a final diagnosis of a TIA mimic. These can include migraine, seizure, neuropathy, syncope, metabolic disturbance, multiple sclerosis flare, and conversion disorder. Clinical characteristics more predictive of a TIA mimic include memory loss, headache, blurred vision, and a lack of a hemiparesis. Features such as the presence of aphasia, dysarthria, sensory loss, or elevated blood pressure have not been found to be predictive of either a mimic or true TIA; however, an exact time of onset, definite focal symptom, abnormal vascular finding, neurological sign, and an ability to lateralize or determine a stroke subtype may be more predictive of stroke (Table 5.1). The Recognition of Stroke in the Emergency Room (ROSIER) scale score, derived from both clinical history and neurological signs, may assist in recognizing a stroke in an emergency department setting (Table 5.2). It is equally important to recognize TIAs that may present as other neurological diagnoses such as limb shaking TIA in the setting of internal carotid occlusion, which is often misdiagnosed as a seizure.

RISK STRATIFICATION

The decision to admit or discharge a patient newly diagnosed with a TIA is often challenging. To address this, Johnston and colleagues combined the California score with the ABCD (age, blood pressure, clinical features, and duration) score to create and validate the ABCD2 score (Table 5.3). They proposed that those patients with a high-risk score would benefit most from immediate evaluation.

The ABCD2 score is now included in the diagnostic workup of TIA internationally in several countries. Nevertheless, there are limits to the predictive power of

Table 5.1 Distinguishing TIA from Mimics

Clinical Features Predictive of TIA	Clinical Features Predictive of TIA Mimic	Clinical Features Predictive of Neither
• Exact time of onset • Definitive focal symptoms (i.e., hemiparesis) • Abnormal vascular finding • Clear neurological syndrome (i.e., left MCA syndrome) • Ability to lateralize symptoms • Ability to determine a stroke subclassification	• Memory loss/cognitive impairment • Headache • Blurred vision • Lack of hemiparesis • Abnormal sign in another organ system	• Aphasia • Dysarthria • Sensory loss • Blood pressure

the ABCD2 score alone in assessing those at highest risk, and for these reasons the ABCD2 score should not be the sole factor used to determine which patients are best suited for immediate evaluation. Indeed, up to 24% of patients with recurrent strokes within 90 days may have a low score (between 0 and 3). Moreover, the score's utility is lower when used by nonspecialists who may not be as experienced with the neurological examination. The ABCD2 score does not provide insight into stroke mechanism such as large artery atherosclerotic disease causing focal stenosis or atrial fibrillation causing cardiac embolism. Large artery atherosclerosis has been found in several studies to be a stronger or as strong a predictor of stroke risk as an ABCD2 score greater than 5. Patients with an ABCD2 score less than 4 but with either carotid/intracranial stenosis of greater than 50% or a cardiac source of embolus were found to have an equal 90-day stroke risk as those with a score greater than 4. For these reasons among others, the ABCD2 score has been expanded to include those patients who have had a prior TIA within 1 week (ABCD3) and positive vascular imaging (defined as at least 50% stenosis on carotid or intracranial imaging).

Table 5.2 ROSIER Scale

Loss of consciousness or syncope?	Yes = −1 point	No = 0 points
Seizure activity?	Yes = −1	No = 0
Acute onset		
Asymmetric facial weakness?	Yes = +1	No = 0
Asymmetric arm weakness?	Yes = +1	No = 0
Asymmetric leg weakness?	Yes = +1	No = 0
Speech disturbance?	Yes = +1	No = 0
Visual field defect?	Yes = +1	No = 0
	Total= −2 to 5	
Stroke more likely with score >0.		

Table 5.3 ABCD2 Score

Patient Characteristic	Score
Age ≥60 years	1
Blood pressure ≥140/90 mm Hg	1
Clinical symptoms	
Focal weakness	2
Speech impairment without weakness	1
Duration of TIA	
≥60 minutes	2
10–59 minutes	1
Presence of diabetes mellitus	1
Two-day stroke risk	Total score
0%	0–1
1.3%	2–3
4.1%	4–5
8.1%	6–7

TRIAGING THE TIA PATIENT

All patients with TIA should be evaluated as soon as possible. In the United States, approximately 50% of TIA patients are hospitalized. The benefit of hospitalization includes earlier introduction of secondary stroke prevention therapy and easier access to thrombolysis in cases of stroke in the period immediately following TIA. Each hospital should develop a triage process for TIA patients, a TIA admission policy, and a protocol for early referral to specialist assessment clinics. Hospitalization for patients with TIA in the past 24 to 48 hours is reasonable. For TIAs occurring within 1 week of presentation, timely hospital referral for further evaluation is also reasonable and hospital admission is recommended in cases of crescendo TIAs, duration of symptoms greater than 1 hour, symptomatic carotid stenosis greater than 50%, known cardiac source of embolus, known hypercoagulable state, or a high-risk ABCD2 score. Patients who are not admitted should have rapid (within 12 hours) access to urgent assessment and investigation, which should include computed tomography (CT)/magnetic resonance imaging (MRI) of the brain, electrocardiogram (ECG), and carotid Doppler. If these studies are not done in the emergency department, patients should be assessed within 24 to 48 hours to determine the ischemic mechanism and to begin secondary prevention. It is important to keep in mind socioeconomic barriers when considering which patients to admit because some patients may not be reliable for outpatient follow-up for a variety of reasons. A newer model of TIA management includes the concept of a same-day rapid-access TIA clinic, with both diagnostic and treatment capabilities. Studies looking at cost have found these clinics to be both safe and more cost-effective than hospitalization. One such clinic in Paris reported a 90-day stroke rate in 1085 patients of 1.24%, compared with 5.96%, which would have been predicted by the ABCD2 score. Some emergency departments have developed TIA observation units with an accelerated diagnostic protocol for rapid evaluation and management of these patients, which have also been shown to improve both cost and length of stay.

DIAGNOSTIC WORKUP

The goals of diagnostic evaluation are to properly diagnose TIA and to help identify or exclude etiological factors for which intervention can reduce the risk of recurrence. Routine blood tests such as a complete blood cell count, blood chemistries, coagulation studies, and a fasting lipid panel are reasonable in the initial evaluation of TIA patients both to help exclude mimics such as hypoglycemia and to aid risk stratification (e.g., with low-density lipoprotein (LDL) values). Brain imaging with either CT or MRI, preferably with diffusion weighted imaging (DWI) sequences, is important for excluding alternative diagnoses, as well as differentiating TIA from an ischemic infarction with clinical resolution of symptoms. Although CT has benefits such as speed and cost-effectiveness, MRI has increasingly become the imaging study of choice due to its superior sensitivity in identifying infarction of all ages. Studies have shown that about 4% of patients with TIA have a new brain infarction seen on CT, whereas about 31% of TIA patients will have an associated brain infarction on MRI. In patients with TIA symptoms of less than 24-hour duration, it has been shown that approximately half will have evidence of restricted diffusion on MRI. Furthermore, imaging can provide important prognostic information, as infarcts seen on imaging are predictors of future stroke risk and associated with a higher frequency of cardiac and other vascular disorders and other vascular events. Factors associated with positive DWI lesions on MRI have been found to include duration of longer than 1 hour; symptoms of dysphasia, dysarthria, and motor weakness; the presence of atrial fibrillation; and carotid stenosis greater than or equal to 50%.

It is clear that the presence of large artery stenosis puts patients with TIA at a higher risk for stroke, thereby making the evaluation of both the intracranial and extracranial vasculature with either ultrasound, MR angiography (MRA), or CT angiography (CTA) essential. Determining the presence and degree of carotid stenosis is of some urgency since prompt surgical intervention is known to reduce stroke recurrence rate in patients with stroke or TIA in the setting of carotid stenosis greater than or equal to 70%. There is, however, no clear consensus on the best vascular imaging modality. Studies have found carotid Doppler to be 88% sensitive and 76% specific, and MRA of the neck to have a sensitivity of about 92% and specificity of 76% for carotid stenosis. CTA of the neck is also an excellent screening tool in assessing for carotid stenosis of greater than 70%, with one study demonstrating both a sensitivity and negative predictive value of 100% and a specificity of 63%. However, with regard to cost-effectiveness, carotid Doppler remains superior to CTA and MRA. Carotid Doppler and CTA of the neck have been shown to have good concordance rates, but there may be occasional discrepancy. Thus, when one test is suggestive, it is good practice to perform a second noninvasive confirmatory test. Contrast-enhanced MRI may also be pursued as a confirmatory test before surgery, as can the use of cerebral angiography.

The assessment of intracranial vasculature is slightly more controversial and should only be pursued when knowledge of intracranial stenosis will alter the management of the patient even though intracranial stenosis is an independent predictor of stroke at 7 days. Both transcranial Doppler (TCD) and MRA of the head have been shown to identify 50% to 99% of intracranial stenosis. Currently, there is a lack of evidence demonstrating any benefit of stenting or angioplasty for intracranial stenosis, and maximal medical management remains the standard of care for these patients.

Much of what we know about the cardiac evaluation of TIA patients is derived from the stroke literature. An ECG is recommended in routine workup, as it is cost-effective and can rapidly change management if an arrhythmia such as atrial fibrillation is discovered (as has been observed in about 2.3% of TIA patients with no prior diagnosis). Moreover, up to 68% of patients in one study were found to have atrial fibrillation more than 2 days after presenting with ischemic stroke, making an argument for prolonged cardiac monitoring, particularly in patients in whom no other embolic source has been found. In addition, up to 23% of cryptogenic patients monitored for 21 days were found to have atrial fibrillation. For these reasons, 21-day Holter monitoring is recommended in the evaluation of cryptogenic stroke. Echocardiography is useful for the detection of intracardiac thrombus, which, if found, can significantly alter management. Several studies have shown that in a significant number of stroke or TIA patients in whom a cardiac source of embolus is suspected (in some series up to 40%), transthoracic echocardiography (TTE) did not revealed the embolic source, whereas transesophageal echocardiography (TEE) did reveal the embolic source, demonstrating the need to proceed with TEE in patients in whom an embolic source is suspected. TEE is also more useful when the identification of conditions such as a patent foramen ovale, aortic arch atherosclerosis, and valvular disease will alter treatment.

MEDICAL MANAGEMENT AND SECONDARY STROKE PREVENTION

Very few studies exist looking at acute management of TIA alone, and therefore most medical treatment recommendations for TIA are extrapolated from data for acute ischemic stroke and TIA combined (see Chapter 6). Aspirin given early, particularly within 48 hours of symptoms, is beneficial and recommended, leading to approximately nine fewer deaths and nonfatal strokes per 1000 patients within the first 2 to 4 weeks, with an absolute risk reduction of about 0.9%. In patients who are unable to tolerate aspirin (81 mg or 325 mg daily), clopidogrel (75 mg/day) is also a reasonable option, and in some studies it has shown a marginal benefit over aspirin, particularly in patients with peripheral vascular disease. Aspirin plus dipyridamole can also be used as an alternative therapy for secondary stroke prevention in these patients. It is important to note that, unlike aspirin, neither clopidogrel nor the combination pill of aspirin plus dipyridamole has been studied in the acute setting. There is no evidence to support the practice of switching antiplatelet agents following ischemic stroke or TIA in the setting of aspirin use for secondary stroke prevention. Current guidelines also do not recommend the addition to aspirin to clopidogrel for secondary stroke prevention even though preliminary data suggest a possible benefit in certain cases.

In patients with known atrial fibrillation, the long-term use of warfarin for stroke prevention is well established. Patients with a contraindication to anticoagulation may receive aspirin as an alternative therapy. In the absence of atrial fibrillation, mechanical heart valves, and intracardiac thrombus, there is no proved role for routine anticoagulation of the TIA or stroke patient in the acute setting.

All patients with TIA need to be assessed and properly educated regarding secondary stroke prevention and modifiable risk factors. Aside from antiplatelet treatment, this includes proper management of comorbidities such as hypertension, hyperlipidemia, and diabetes. It is known that lowering blood pressure is associated with a stroke risk reduction of up to 30%. This remains true for any commonly used antihypertensive therapy, with few studies suggesting a possible benefit of diuretics or the combination of diuretics and angiotensin-converting enzyme inhibitors over the rest. In addition, current guidelines recommend the use of statin therapy in patients with stroke or TIA with evidence of atherosclerosis to a goal LDL reduction of 50% or target LDL of less than 70 mg/dL. However, there remains no clear data supporting the benefit of statin therapy in the very acute setting. Patients with diabetes should be counseled regarding the importance of strict glycemic control, and smoking cessation should be emphasized and supported. Healthy eating and physical activity are an important component of stroke risk reduction and should be strongly encouraged.

SURGICAL MANAGEMENT

The two landmark trials establishing the utility of endarterectomy for symptomatic carotid stenosis were the North American Symptomatic Carotid Endarterectomy Trial (NASCET) and the European Carotid Surgery Trial (ECST). The 1-month stroke risk in patients with symptomatic carotid stenosis treated medically was found to be about 26%, which was reduced to 9% after carotid endarterectomy (CEA), corresponding to an absolute risk reduction of about 12% to 17% over 2 to 3 years. Among those presenting with just TIA, the absolute risk reduction for ipsilateral stroke was about 15% within 5 years. When considering CEA, physicians must take note of the complication rate of surgeons at their own institution, which was preselected by NASCET investigators to include only surgeons with a rate less than 6%. CEA is currently recommended for all patients with recent TIA or ischemic stroke within the past 6 months and ipsilateral carotid stenosis of 70% to 99%, if the perioperative morbidity and mortality risk are estimated to be less than 6%. Given the high risk of recurrent stroke (about 1% per day) within the first couple of weeks after TIA in the setting of carotid stenosis, it is most prudent to intervene as early as possible, within 2 weeks if possible. Regarding the role of carotid stenting, the CREST trial suggested that symptomatic patients undergoing endarterectomy had a lower rate of stroke in the first 30 days than those who had stenting, and patients older than 70 years in the stent group were more likely to have adverse events than those undergoing CEA. Carotid stenting is now considered as an alternative to CEA in those symptomatic patients at average or low risk for complications associated with the intervention.

SUGGESTED READING

Amort M, Fluri F, Schäfer J, et al. Transient ischemic attack versus transient ischemic attack mimics: frequency, clinical characteristics and outcome. Cerebrovasc Dis 2011;32:57–64.

Brott TG, Hobson RW 2nd, Howard G, et al; CREST Investigators. Stenting versus endarterectomy for treatment of carotid-artery stenosis. N Engl J Med 2010;363:11–23.

Easton JD, Saver JL, Albers GW, et al; American Heart Association; American Stroke Association Stroke Council; Council on Cardiovascular Surgery and Anesthesia; Council on Cardiovascular Radiology and Intervention; Council on Cardiovascular Nursing; Interdisciplinary Council on Peripheral Vascular Disease. Definition and evaluation of transient ischemic attack: a scientific statement for healthcare professionals from the American Heart Association/American Stroke Association Stroke Council; Council on Cardiovascular Surgery and Anesthesia; Council on Cardiovascular Radiology and Intervention; Council on Cardiovascular Nursing; and the Interdisciplinary Council on Peripheral Vascular Disease. Stroke 2009;40:2276–2293.

Ferguson GG, Eliasziw M, Barr HW, et al. The North American Symptomatic Carotid Endarterectomy Trial: surgical results in 1415 patients. Stroke 1999;30:1751–1758.

Furie KL, Kasner SE, Adams RJ, et al; American Heart Association Stroke Council, Council on Cardiovascular Nursing, Council on Clinical Cardiology, and Interdisciplinary Council on Quality of Care and Outcomes Research. Guidelines for the prevention of stroke in patients with stroke or transient ischemic attack: a guideline for healthcare professionals from the American Heart Association/American Stroke Association. Stroke 2011;42:227–276.

Johnston SC, Albers GW, Gorelick PB, et al. National Stroke Association recommendations for systems of care for transient ischemic attack. Ann Neurol 2011;69:872–877.

Johnston SC, Nguyen-Huynh MN, Schwarz ME, et al. National Stroke Association guidelines for the management of transient ischemic attacks. Ann Neurol 2006;60:301–313.

Johnston SC, Rothwell PM, Nguyen-Huynh MN, et al. Validation and refinement of scores to predict very early stroke risk after transient ischaemic attack. Lancet 2007;369:283–292.

Nor AM, Davis J, Sen B, et al. The Recognition of Stroke in the Emergency Room (ROSIER) scale: development and validation of a stroke recognition instrument. Lancet Neurol 2005;4:727–734.

Sanders LM, Srikanth VK, Blacker DJ, et al. Performance of the ABCD2 score for stroke risk post TIA: meta-analysis and probability modeling. Neurology 2012;79:971–980.

6 Acute Ischemic Stroke

Joshua Z. Willey

INTRODUCTION

Acute ischemic stroke is one of the leading reasons for acute neurological consultation and a condition with a broad evidence base to guide treatment. Clinical features usually appear suddenly, and their manifestation reflects the function of the area of the brain under threat. Common stroke symptoms include sudden numbness or weakness of the face, arm, or leg, especially on one side of the body; sudden confusion; trouble speaking or comprehending; sudden trouble seeing in one or both eyes; sudden trouble walking; dizziness, loss of balance, or incoordination; and sudden severe headache with no known cause.

TREATMENT

Therapeutic approaches for acute ischemic stroke remain multifaceted, with treatment directed at (1) reducing cerebral injury from the initial stroke (thrombolysis and neuroprotection) and (2) reducing the risk of recurrent stroke. An additional important component of acute ischemic stroke treatment includes prevention of associated medical complications, which are the leading cause of stroke-related morbidity and mortality. Therapeutic approaches to acute stroke treatment are summarized in Table 6.1.

Intravenous Thrombolysis

The initial goal of the evaluation of any patient arriving at the emergency department with a focal neurological complaint is to evaluate eligibility for intravenous (IV) thrombolysis with recombinant tissue plasminogen activator (rtPA). Thrombolysis is predicated on the presence of an ischemic penumbra, defined as cerebral tissue that is injured by ischemia but viable if blood flow were to be restored. With dissolution of the thrombus responsible for the cerebral ischemia, blood flow would be restored and the final degree of cerebral injury would be reduced, thereby leading to an improved neurological outcome. Treatment with IV rtPA targets the coagulation cascade at the level of formation of thrombin, with the compound being most active in the presence of fibrin and when the thrombus is not as well organized. During active thrombosis, fibrinogen is activated by thrombin (or activated factor II), leading to the formation of fibrin and a subsequent clot. Plasminogen is a proenzyme released by the liver in a conformation that is resistant to activation by other enzymes. Plasminogen, however, binds to both thrombi and cell surfaces to adopt a more reactive moiety that can then be activated by additional enzymes. Endothelial cells release tPA in response to

Table 6.1 Therapeutic Approaches to Acute Stroke Treatment

Trial (Reference)	Time Window	Treatments Studied	Primary Outcome (S)	Effect Size
NINDS tPA trial (NEJM 1995;333:1581) Phase III	<3 hours from onset	rtPA 0.9 mg/kg versus placebo	3-month composite outcome of BI, NIHSS, mRS, and GOS	Favors intravenous rtPA (39% versus 26%)
ECASS III (NEJM 2008;359:1317)	3–4.5 hours from onset	rtPA 0.9 mg/kg versus placebo	mRS at 90 days	Favors intravenous rtPA (52.4% versus 45.2%)
PROACT-II (JAMA 1999;282:2003)	Within 6 hours of onset with angiographically documented MCA occlusion	9 mg intra-arterial prourokinase and heparin versus heparin	mRS at 90 days and recanalization	Favored intra-arterial urokinase (40% versus 25%) for mRS and recanalization (66% versus 18% recanalization)
IMS-III (NEJM 2013;368:893–903)	Within 3 hours who received IV rtPA	IV rtPA followed by intra-arterial therapy with any modality versus IV rtPA alone	mRS 0–2 at 90 days	No difference in functional outcome (40.8% with endovascular and 38.7% with IV rtPA alone)
SYNTHESIS-Expansion (NEJM 2013;368:904–913)	Within 4.5 hours from onset	IV rtPA alone versus intra-arterial alone with any modality	mRS 0–1 at 90 days	No difference in functional outcome (30.4% with endovascular alone and 34.8% with IV rtPA alone
MR-RESCUE (NEJM 2013;368:914–923)	Within 8 hours from onset	Mechanical embolectomy versus standard of care, stratified on penumbral pattern	Mean mRS at 90 days	No difference in functional outcome or mortality at 90 days or based on penumbral pattern

Table 6.1 Continued

Trial (Reference)	Time Window	Treatments Studied	Primary Outcome (S)	Effect Size
CAST (Lancet 1997;349:1641)	Within 48 hours of stroke	Aspirin 162 mg/day versus placebo	Death or dependence at 4 weeks	Favoring aspirin (3.3% versus 3.9% mortality, and 1.6% versus 2.1% recurrent stroke)
IST (Lancet 1997;349:1569)	As soon as possible	Heparin (5000 or 12,500 units twice daily) versus avoiding heparin. The latter group randomized to aspirin 300 mg/day or plaebo	Death within 14 days or death/dependency at 6 months	No difference in outcomes in heparin allocation. Aspirin with fewer recurrent strokes (2.8% versus 3.9%)
TOAST (JAMA 1998;279:1265)	Within 24 hours of stroke	Heparinoid versus placebo in noncardioembolic stroke	GOS and BI at 3 months	No differences in outcomes
HAEST (Lancet 2000;355:1205–1210)	Within 30 hours of stroke onset	Low-molecular-weight heparin versus aspirin in atrial fibrillation related stroke	Recurrent stroke at 14 days	No differences in outcomes (8.5% versus 7.5%, nonsignificant)
SCAST ((Lancet 2011;377:741–750)	Within 30 hours of stroke onset	Candesartan versus placebo	Composite of stroke, myocardial infarct, vascular death at 6 months; mRS at 6 months	No difference in composite outcome, trend to poorer functional outcome in candesartan group
Decompressive hemicraniectomy (Lancet Neurol 2007;6:215)	Within 48 hours of stroke onset	Hemicraniectomy in space occupying MCA infarction versus medical management	mRS favorable (0–4); mortality	Favoring hemicraniectomy (75% versus 24% for mRS; 78% versus 29% for mortality)

thrombi to activate plasmin from its plasminogen precursor. The activated plasmin enzyme acts on multiple plasma proteins but has its most relevant effect on fibrin, where it potentiates thrombolysis. Treatment with exogeneous tPA enhances the coagulation cascade's already present thrombolysis pathways, leading to dissolution of the clot.

Several previous trials have evaluated the efficacy of thrombolysis up to 6 hours from stroke onset without demonstrating a clinical benefit. Subsequent randomized clinical trials explored dosing and time targets for treatment with IV rtPA, with the landmark study being the National Institute of Neurological Disorders and Stroke (NINDS) tPA trial showing efficacy of 0.9 mg/kg rtPA when administered within 3 hours of acute ischemic stroke onset. The trial consisted of two parts, which, in summary, showed a clinical benefit at 3 months in terms of a global score of disability (odds ratio [OR] 1.7, 95% confidence interval [CI] 1.2 to 2.6). The clinical benefit, summarized by the number needed to treat to improve to a favorable functional outcome, is greatest within the first 90 minutes from stroke onset (NNT 3.6) and declines thereafter to 5.9 up to 270 minutes. One additional trial, the European Cooperative Acute Stroke Study III (ECASS-III), has investigated treating in the time window of 3 to 4.5 hours from onset with IV rtPA. Notably, this trial excluded participants (1) over the age of 80, (2) who had a prior clinical stroke and diabetes, (3) were taking any anticoagulants, or (4) had a National Institutes of Health Stroke Scale (NIHSS) score greater than 25. ECASS III demonstrated a more modest but still present benefit from IV rtPA in the 3- to 4.5-hour time window for improvement in disability (52.4% versus 45.2 %, OR 1.34, 95% CI 1.02 to 1.76). The largest trial completed to date on thrombolysis is the International Stroke Trial-3 (IST-3), which randomized patients up to 6 hours from stroke onset and included a sizeable proportion of patients over the age of 80. Overall, a clinical benefit was noted in all patients, regardless of age, from thrombolysis, although the study was underpowered to detect a difference between the 0- to 3-hour and 3- to 6-hour intervals. An accompanying meta-analysis supported the benefit of treatment from 0 to 3 hours but not an extension to the 3- to 6-hour time window.

The most dreaded complication stemming from thrombolysis is hemorrhage, for which several exclusion criteria have been established. Table 6.2 lists the important absolute and relative contraindications to treatment. Several of the relative contraindications are noteworthy to discuss, particularly the rapidly improving/mild deficit presentations and the international normalized ratio (INR) cutoffs; the former is the most common reason from exclusion of treatment after delayed arrival. Case series have pointed to a trend in poor outcomes in approximately 30% of mild stroke patients who are not treated, although results have remained mixed when comparing those treated with those untreated. This may in part reflect ambiguity as to what is a mild stroke—commonly used definitions are an NIHSS score of less than 3 and an NIHSS score of less than 5. Treating mild stroke patients or stroke mimics, on the other hand, is associated with a very low risk of hemorrhagic complications. The NINDS tPA trial only required a deficit that was measurable with the NIHSS score and excluded isolated facial weakness and isolated sensory loss. Case series have also pointed to a potential increase in hemorrhage risk among patients taking vitamin K antagonists regardless of the INR, although this has been difficult to tease apart from the higher hemorrhagic transformation risk in patients with a cardioembolic source. As of now, there is insufficient evidence to remove any of the exclusion criteria from treatment with IV rtPA.

Table 6.2 Relative and Absolute Exclusion Criteria for Administering Intravenous Tissue Plasminogen Activator Within 3 Hours of Acute Ischemic Stroke Onset

Absolute Contraindications to rtPA

Suspicion of SAH

Other stroke or trauma within 3 months

Arterial puncture at a noncompressible site within 7 days

Neurosurgery (spinal or intracranial) within the past 14 days

History of ICH

Sustained blood pressure >185/110 mm Hg

Aggressive drug therapy needed to control blood pressure

Intracranial tumor, arteriovenous malformation, or aneurysm

Active internal bleeding

Acute bleeding diathesis*: heparin received within the past 48 hours and PTT elevated; anticoagulant use with INR >1.7 or PT >15 seconds; platelet count <100,000; direct thrombin inhibitor or anti–factor Xa inhibitor use with elevated laboratory tests (PTT, INR, ecarin clotting time, anti–factor Xa levels)

Plasma glucose level <50 mg/dL

Computed tomorgraphy shows >⅓ hypodensity in the cerebral hemisphere

Relative contraindications to rtPA

Minor or rapidly improving symptoms

Seizure at stroke onset

Major surgery or serious trauma within 14 days

GI or GU hemorrhage within 21 days

Acute myocardial infarction within 3 months

GI, gastrointestinal; GU, genitourinary; ICH, intracranial hemorrhage; PTT, partial thromboplastin time; rtPA, recombinant tissue plasminogen activator; SAH, subarachnoid hemorrhage.

*Results of the coagulation profile and platelet count are not necessary before administering rtPA unless the patient is taking anticoagulant medications or there is a clinical suspicion for a bleeding diathesis.

Adapted from Jauch EC, Saver JL, Adams HP, et al. Guidelines for the early management of patients with acute ischemic stroke: a guideline for healthcare professionals from the American Heart Association/ American Stroke Association. Stroke 2013;44:870–947; table 10.

The decision on whether to treat with any of the relative exclusion criteria remains a case-by-case decision considering specifics regarding the patient's baseline and likelihood of disability based on the nature of the deficit.

The most dreaded complication from thrombolysis is hemorrhage, particularly intracerebral hemorrhage (ICH). Not all ICH is necessarily indicative of a poor outcome, particularly petechial blood within the bed of the infarct. Poor outcomes have been typically defined as blood seen on the head computed tomography (CT) with associated change in neurological status. There is no clear consensus as of yet on the best definition of symptomatic ICH, although a commonly adopted definition includes a decline in the NIHSS score of 4 or more points attributable to the ICH. The rates of ICH after treatment with IV rtPA remain consistently close to 6% in most clinical trials and case series. Several risk factors for symptomatic ICH have been identified, including blood pressure elevations, treatment beyond the allotted window, larger stroke sizes, and hyperglycemia. Whether hyperglycemia should be treated after acute ischemic stroke remains unknown. To avoid hemorrhagic complications after IV rtPA, physicians should adhere to a strict protocol after treatment, including avoiding antithrombotic agents for 24 hours and maintaining the blood pressure pretreatment below 185/110 mm Hg and post-treatment below 180/105 mm Hg. Blood pressure should be carefully monitored before and after thrombolysis based on predefined protocols, such as every 15 minutes for the 2 hours, followed by every 30 minutes for 6 hours, and hourly for the following 16 hours. Aggressive therapy should be instituted with IV labetalol pushes or continuous nicardipine infusion. An additional rare complication (<2%) with IV rtPA is angioedema, for which no identified risk factors are known but which is treated in a similar manner as with angiotensin-converting enzyme inhibitors.

Several additional difficulties remain with IV rtPA beyond the limitation of most patients not arriving at the emergency department in a timely manner, including failure to recanalize and reocclusion. Several promising adjuncts to treatment with IV rtPA remain in investigation, including the use of transcranial Doppler to enhance thrombolysis or expansion of the time window based on results of multimodality neuroimaging. These modalities remain experimental and have not yet been adopted into mainstream guidelines for acute ischemic stroke.

Intra-arterial Therapy

Treatment with intra-arterial modalities has gained significant attention and is being used more often as part of routine clinical care. There has been only one randomized controlled clinical trial for intra-arterial treatment modalities with published results, the Prolyse in Acute Cerebral Thromboembolism II (PROACT-II), along with several published studies without a control arm. Intra-arterial modalities are administered either as an adjunct to IV rtPA, termed bridging therapy, or at other times when patients are not eligible for IV thrombolysis. Bridging therapy was tested in two early-phase clinical trials, Interventional Management of Stroke (IMS) I and II with encouraging results; the phase III IMS III was halted early by the Data Safety Monitoring Board, however. The results of IMS III have not been published as of the writing of this chapter. These treatment modalities are reserved for patients with major arterial occlusions, principally M1 and M2 segments of the middle cerebral artery (MCA), top of the internal carotid artery (ICA), and basilar artery within 6 to 8 hours from stroke onset. Treatment for basilar thrombosis is frequently extended for up to 24 hours in basilar thrombosis given the high likelihood of mortality (close to 80%), although large case series have not necessarily shown improvements when extended beyond 9 hours.

Intra-arterial Thrombolytics

The PROACT-II study evaluated the efficacy and safety of 9 mg of intra-arterial prourokinase compared with IV heparin in patients with acute ischemic stroke due to large-vessel occlusion within 6 hours of onset. The clinical end point was a good clinical outcome at 3 months (modified Rankin Scale [mRS] 0 to 2), which was achieved in 40% compared with 25% in the non–endovascular treatment arm. Recanalization was associated with a good outcome and occurred in 66% compared with 18% in the non-treatment arm. Symptomatic ICH occurred at 10% in the prourokinase arm and 2% in the heparin arm. Based on PROACT-II, the American Heart Association has given a

Class 1B recommendation for intra-arterial thrombolysis for patients who are within 6 hours of stroke onset and who are otherwise not eligible for IV rtPA.

Mechanical Thrombectomy

A series of mechanical thrombectomy devices have emerged in the market, starting with the first-generation Merci® (concentric medical) devices, which have been approved by the U.S. Food and Drug Administration to remove thrombi from cerebral arteries. These devices are commonly used within 8 hours from stroke onset, with or without preceding IV rtPA or multimodality imaging. With each subsequent iteration of devices, recanalization rates have steadily improved with an associated improvement in clinical outcomes compared with historical controls, as well as a decline in device-related complications. The rates of symptomatic ICH remain higher than reported rates for IV rtPA or placebo but similar to those of PROACT-II.

Randomized Clinical Trials

The approach to clinical care of acute stroke patients changed with publication of the results of three randomized clinical trials in 2013. The Interventional Management of Stroke (IMS) III trial tested the hypothesis of whether bridging therapy, defined as intra-arterial therapy following IV rtPA, was superior to IV rtPA alone in improving 3 months outcomes. The Mechanical Retrieval and Recanalization of Stroke Clots Using Embolectomy (MR-RESCUE) investigators examined whether any specific penumbral pattern predicted a positive response to endovascular therapy, while the Local Versus Systemic Thrombolysis for Acute Ischemic Stroke (SYNTHESIS) examined whether intra-arterial therapy alone was superior to IV rtPA alone in acute ischemic stroke within 3 hours of onset. All three trials failed to show a clinical benefit for intra-arterial therapy; furthermore, MR-RESCUE failed to identify a favorable penumbral imaging profile for predicting a positive response to intra-arterial therapy. At this junction, intra-arterial therapy remains unproved as the standard of care and has a limited role in acute stroke therapy.

Antithrombotic Agents

Aspirin and Other Antiplatelet Agents

In patients otherwise ineligible for IV rtPA, the only proved therapy in the acute setting remains aspirin administered within 48 hours from ischemic stroke onset. In the Chinese Acute Stroke Trial (CAST) and IST, a minimum dose of 160 mg of aspirin was compared with a placebo, with the primary outcomes being morality and recurrent stroke at 2 weeks. Aspirin in both studies was associated with a modest but statistically significant reduction in recurrent stroke (1.6% versus 2.1% in CAST; 2.8% versus 3.9% in IST) with no effect on mortality or ICH. Other antiplatelet agents, including clopidogrel or aspirin/dipyridamole, have not been studied in the acute stroke setting.

Preliminary data suggest a possible benefit of the combination of aspirin and clopidogrel in certain acute stroke situations. A pilot trial examined aspirin and clopidogrel for a short period in combination and showed a significant reduction in neurological deterioration after the diagnosis of ischemic stroke or TIA. Similar trends toward reduction in recurrent stroke and TIA were observed in the larger Fast Assessment of stroke and Transient Ischemic Attack to Prevent Early Recurrence (FASTER) trial. The combination of aspirin and clopidogrel appeared more effective at reducing micro-embolic signals in patients with symptomatic large-artery atherosclerosis, although studies have been underpowered to detect a clinical benefit. These findings should be interpreted with caution given the long-term hemorrhagic risk of prolonged aspirin and clopidogrel combined for secondary stroke prevention. Comprehensive medical management of intracranial atherosclerosis in the Stenting and Aggressive Medical Management for Preventing Recurrent Stroke (SAMMPRIS) trial, including the com-bination of aspirin/clopidogrel, led to a lower than expected stroke rate at 30 days in the nonstenting arm. Until data from larger clinical trials are published, the combina-tion should be used only on a case-by-case basis with consideration of the potential harms.

Intravenous Heparin and Other Heparinoids

In previous years, IV heparin remained the mainstay of inpatient treatment of acute ischemic stroke. Several clinical trials, however, have established a lack of efficacy with various combinations of heparinoids for secondary stroke prevention in the acute set-ting. In the IST, subcutaneous heparin showed a modest clinical benefit against recur-rent stroke that was offset by an increase in hemorrhagic complications. Similar results were also seen in the Trial of ORG 10172 in Acute Stroke Treatment (TOAST) trial for all noncardioembolic strokes, as well as in the Heparin in Acute Embolic Stroke Trial (HAEST) in patients with atrial fibrillation–related acute ischemic strokes. At this point, heparinoids are not routinely recommended for acute ischemic stroke; treatment may be used for patients with a mechanical valve, as well as other highly thrombogenic conditions such as a cardiac mural thrombus. Intravenous heparin also remains commonly used in patients with acute cervicocephalic artery dissection, although case series indicate a modest, if at all present, benefit compared with anti-platelet agents and in dural sinus thrombosis.

Antihypertensive Therapy

The American Heart Association guidelines on acute ischemic stroke include allow-ing a blood pressure up to 220/120 mm Hg for patients not receiving thrombolysis unless there is evidence for end organ damage until hospital discharge; different tar-gets are recommended for patients receiving IV rtPA as outlined earlier. Several phase II studies have investigated the possible benefit of starting antihypertensive agents early in the course of stroke, with overall results pointing to acceptable safety. In the Scandinavian Candesartan Acute Stroke Trial (SCAST), candesartan was compared with placebo in acute stroke patients treated within 30 hours from stroke onset. There was no reduction in the end points of stroke, myocardial infarction, or death, although there was a statistical trend toward neurological worsening in the patients treated with candesartan. Acute blood pressure lowering should be considered in patients with evi-dence of hemorrhagic transformation, as well as other medical complications such as congestive heart failure or myocardial ischemia.

Statins

The use of statins for primary and secondary ischemic stroke prevention has increased substantially in the past several years. Statin medications are extremely effective at reducing LDL cholesterol and are in general very well tolerated. Several potential mechanisms of action on how statins may be protective against stroke have been postulated since the effect appears to be independent of LDL levels and include endothelial stabilization and reduction of inflammation. Case series have consistently shown that patients who are taking a statin before their stroke are more likely to have a milder deficit and better outcome, while others have shown that withdrawing statins is associated with a poorer outcome. In stroke due to intracranial atherosclerosis, the SAMMPRIS trial established that aggressive risk factor control within 30 days, which included treatment with a statin, was effective at reducing the risk of stroke at 30 days compared with older literature. The Stroke Prevention by Aggressive Reduction of Cholesterol Levels (SPARCL) trial was the landmark study of secondary stroke prevention that established the efficacy of statins in reducing the risk of recurrent stroke. The effect on outcomes was mostly driven by a reduction in the risk of ischemic stroke that was not offset by a significant increase in the risk of ICH. SPARCL, however, does not address the efficacy of statins in the acute ischemic stroke setting as the study enrolled at least 30 days after the initial stroke symptom and the LDL cholesteroal level had to be greater than 100 mg/dL. In the FASTER trial, patients were randomized to placebo versus 40 mg simvastatin acutely, in addition to dual antiplatelet agents, with statins not showing any clinical efficacy. Quality of care stroke metrics at many countries nonetheless include discharge on a statin if the LDL cholesterol level is greater than 100 mg/dL with an ischemic stroke. Until randomized clinical trials are completed, patients should remain on statins if they were prescribed before the stroke. A high-dose statin could be considered in all ischemic stroke patients with LDL greater than 100 mg/dL or an atherosclerotic stroke subtype as soon as dysphagia has been assessed. Whether one statin should be considered over others and what dose should be used remain unknown.

Surgical Therapy

Hemicraniectomy

Malignant MCA infarctions, defined as infarction with associated cerebral edema and herniation, may carry a mortality close to 75%. Pooled analyses from three hemicraniectomy trials have shown a significant mortality benefit of early (within 48 hours) decompressive surgery, as well as reduction in severe disability/death (75% versus 24%). These trials included patients younger than 60 with greater than 50% involvement of MCA territory, a score of 1 on the NIHSS 1a item, and the absence of bilateral pupillary involvement. The reduction in mild disability was more modest, while sidedness of the infarction did not influence outcomes. Early hemicraniectomy should be offered to patients with malignant MCA infarction after a careful discussion with family regarding the potential benefits of treatment.

Carotid Endarterectomy/Revascularization

The North American Symptomatic Carotid Endarterectomy Trial (NASCET) and other trials have established a clear benefit of carotid endarterectomy in patients with nondisabling ischemic stroke or TIA and greater than 70% stenosis. Patients undergoing CEA had a risk of recurrent stroke reduced from 26% to 9% at 2 years, with an NNT of 6. The trial enrolled up to 6 months from the initial event, although subanalyses identified that patients treated within 2 weeks of stroke onset had a greater clinical benefit. These data have been confirmed in epidemiological studies establishing a risk of close to 1% per day of stroke for the first 2 weeks after a symptomatic ICA stenosis is identified. Unless there are clear medical contraindications, carotid revascularization should be considered within 2 weeks of incident ischemic stroke or TIA. Carotid endarterectomy and stenting are overall equivalent at reducing the risk of stroke, myocardial infarction, or death, although two recent trials both pointed to a lower 30-day risk of stroke among patients undergoing endarterectomy.

Intracranial Stenting

The SAMMPRIS trial randomized patients with symptomatic intracranial stenosis greater than 70% to best medical therapy versus best medical therapy and intracranial stenting with the Wingspan device. Participants in the trial had to be within 30 days of ischemic stroke onset, with a significant proportion treated within 7 days or while still in the hospital. The study was stopped early by the Data Safety Monitoring Board due a near doubling of the stroke risk in the stenting arm (14.7% versus 5.8%). Stenting is not currently recommended as routine treatment for patients with symptomatic intracranial atherosclerosis.

Prevention of Medical Complications

In-hospital medical complications are the primary source of morbidity and mortality after ischemic stroke and TIA. Pulmonary emboli, urinary tract infection, and pneumonia are some of the most common, and preventive treatment is available. Unless any hemorrhagic contraindications are present, all ischemic stroke patients should be placed on daily deep venous thrombosis prophylaxis with a heparinoid agent; daily low-molecular-weight heparin may be more effective than unfractionated heparin but can only be used in patients with a normal creatinine clearance. Compression stockings appear to be ineffective at reducing the risk of deep venous thrombosis. Aspiration pneumonia may be reduced by adherence to specific stroke-related protocols, including performing a dysphagia screen before any oral intake, maintaining the head of the bed above 30 degrees, and ensuring good oral hygiene. Urinary tract infections are preventable with avoidance of the use of indwelling catheters. Early mobilization and rehabilitation are additional treatment modalities that may help in preventing the aforementioned complications. A comprehensive approach to prevention of medical complications with adherence to established protocols are a hallmark of stroke units, one of the few interventions that reduce long-term mortality after stroke.

SUGGESTED READING

Jauch EC, Saver JL, Adams HP, et al. Guidelines for the early management of adults with ischemic stroke: a guideline from the American Heart Association/American Stroke Association Stroke Council, Clinical Cardiology Council, Cardiovascular Radiology and Intervention Council, and the Atherosclerotic Peripheral Vascular Disease and Quality of Care Outcomes in Research Interdisciplinary Working Groups: the American Academy of Neurology affirms the value of this guideline as an educational tool for neurologists. Stroke 2013;44:870–947.

SUGGESTED READING

Amarenco P, Bogousslavsky J, Callahan A 3rd, et al. High-dose atorvastatin after stroke or transient ischemic attack. N Engl J Med 2006;355:549–559.

Benavente OR, Hart RG, McClure LA, et al. Effects of clopidogrel added to aspirin in patients with recent lacunar stroke. N Engl J Med 2012;367:817–825.

Broderick JP, Palesch YY, Demchuk AM, et al. Endovascular therapy after intravenous tPA versus tPA alone for stroke. N Engl J Med 2013;368:893–903.

Chimowitz MI, Lynn MJ, Derdeyn CP, et al. Stenting versus aggressive medical therapy for intracranial arterial stenosis. N Engl J Med 2011;365:993–1003.

Chimowitz MI. Endovascular treatment for acute ischemic stroke—still unproven. N Engl J Med 2013;368:952–955.

De Keyser J, Gdovinova Z, Uyttenboogaart M, Vroomen PC, Luijckx GJ. Intravenous alteplase for stroke: beyond the guidelines and in particular clinical situations. Stroke 2007;38:2612–2618.

Furie KL, Kasner SE, Adams RJ, et al; on behalf of the American Heart Association Stroke Council, Council on Cardiovascular Nursing, Council on Clinical Cardiology, and Interdisciplinary Council on Quality of Care and Outcomes Research. Guidelines for the prevention of stroke in patients with stroke or transient ischemic attack: a guideline for healthcare professionals from the American Heart Association/American Stroke Association. Stroke 2011;42:227–276.

Huttner HB, Schwab S. Malignant middle cerebral artery infarction: clinical characteristics, treatment strategies, and future perspectives. Lancet Neurol 2009;8:949–958.

Sandercock PAG, Gibson LM, Liu M. Anticoagulants for preventing recurrence following presumed non-cardioembolic ischaemic stroke or transient ischaemic attack [update of Cochrane Database Syst Rev. 2003;(1):CD000248]. Cochrane Database Syst Rev 2009;(2):CD000248.

7   Intracerebral Hemorrhage

Aaron Sylvan Lord and Olajide Williams

INTRODUCTION

The clinical manifestations of intracerebral hemorrhage (ICH) are highly variable and depend on the location of the hemorrhage and the amount of brain tissue injured. Symptoms appear suddenly and can progress rapidly (see Chapter 6). They include alterations in the level of consciousness, nausea and vomiting, headache, seizures, and focal neurological deficits. Patients with large hemorrhages often exhibit sudden onset of focal neurological signs, although smaller, more strategically located hemorrhages can have similar presentations. Headache and vomiting are typically seen with raised intracranial pressure (ICP), along with decreased level of consciousness. Indeed, some patients slip into coma before the hemorrhage is discovered. Seizures may also occur, often in the first 24 to 48 hours of onset.

PREHOSPITAL MANAGEMENT

The prehospital management of ICH is limited. Even when a stroke is recognized clinically, neuroimaging is required to distinguish between a hemorrhagic and an ischemic stroke. Therefore, many of the treatments started in the emergency department (ED) cannot be started in the field. Standard assessment of airway, breathing, and circulation (ABCs) is appropriate, and protection of the airway with endotracheal intubation may be necessary for severe cases. Fingerstick blood glucose should be checked as hypoglycemia and hyperglycemia may cause focal neurological deficits. Except for extreme blood pressure elevations beyond a systolic of 220 mm Hg, blood pressure should not be lowered as this may be harmful if the stroke is ischemic. Patients should be transported at 30 degrees to reduce aspiration risk and to minimize ICP. Transport should proceed to an ED capable of dealing with acute stroke emergencies. Every effort should be taken to obtain a history and medication list and to prenotify the receiving hospital of the patient's pending arrival so that the staff is ready to act quickly.

EMERGENCY DEPARTMENT

Initial Assessment

Patients should initially be assessed for ABCs with special attention paid to whether the patient has sufficient control over oral and pharyngeal muscles to maintain airway integrity. Should intubation be necessary, nondepolarizing agents (*cis*-atracurim, vecuronium) should be considered before succinylcholine, as there is a theoretical side effect of increased ICP with this agent. Additionally, lidocaine can be used as an adjuvant to ameliorate the theoretical increase in ICP. Patients with ICH tend to have central hyperventilation as opposed to hypoventilation, so intubation due to diminished respiratory drive is rare unless the patient is acutely herniating. Hypotension is rare after ICH but, when present, is often due to neurocardiogenic stunning (tako-tsubo cardiomyopathy), and inotropic support might be necessary in addition to vasopressors. Hypertension is much more common than hypotension after ICH and its management is addressed here.

After initial assessment of ABCs, a neurologist should immediately assess the patient. Basic laboratory tests including basic metabolic panel, coagulation tests, and complete blood cell count should be obtained immediately, ideally during the rapid establishment of an intravenous (IV) line. An 18-gauge catheter in the antecubital position is preferred in case computed tomography (CT) angiography needs to be performed. If a smaller IV line has been successfully placed, time should not be spent trying to place an 18-gauge until after noncontrast head CT is performed.

Acute Neuroimaging

The most important test in the ED is noncontrast head CT. This is the fastest test that will distinguish between ischemic and hemorrhagic infarction or other lesions. By the time CT is performed, most acute intracranial blood will be hyperdense. Once a hemorrhage is identified, it is important to distinguish between types of intracranial hemorrhage. This chapter focuses on management of intraparenchymal, hemorrhagic infarction; additional chapters will focus on other types of hemorrhage. However, if an intraparenchymal hemorrhage is identified along with subarachnoid blood, one must consider an aneurysmal source as subarachnoid blood is rare in spontaneous ICH. Additionally, the presence of subdural blood in addition to ICH might signify a traumatic etiology. Also, a large hypodensity in a vascular territory surrounding the ICH might suggest hemorrhagic conversion of an ischemic stroke. After a quick but thorough review of the CT has been made, appropriate treatment and further diagnostic measures can be pursued safely.

Once the diagnosis of spontaneous ICH has been made, one can consider performing CT angiography (CTA) of the head for two reasons: (1) to evaluate for aneurysms and other vascular malformations and (2) to evaluate for a "spot sign." While digital-subtraction angiography remains the gold standard for diagnosis of arteriovascular malformations (AVMs), acute knowledge of a large AVM might influence short-term management, especially if an intranidal aneurysm is present. However, in patients with long-standing hypertension and deep hemorrhages or in elderly patients with lobar hemorrhages, angiography might not be necessary for diagnostic purposes given low pretest probabilities of abnormal findings. The additional benefit of acute vascular imaging in ICH is for evaluation of the spot sign, which represents extravasation of CT contrast agent out of the vessel into the parenchyma. The presence of this "spot" of contrast within the hemorrhage increases the risk of hematoma expansion. In one study, 77% of patients with the sign had hematoma expansion compared with only 4% of those without it. Further studies are needed to determine the generalizability of these data, although the potential to identify patients at risk of hematoma expansion would be useful.

It is important to note that when performing all of the various items cited in the preceding Initial Assessment and Neuroimaging sections, they should NOT be performed in a rigid "sequence." Rather, they should be occurring in "parallel" so as to not delay care, whether it is tissue plasminogen activator (tPA) for ischemic stroke or blood pressure reduction and reversal of coagulopathy for hemorrhagic stroke. While the clinician is drawing blood, mental status questions can be asked; histories and even some examination elements can be performed on the way to the CT scanner. While the patient is alone in the CT scanner, further history and medication lists can be obtained from family (if present) or the medical record reviewed for prior history that might affect current treatment (medication lists, known coagulation disorders, known AVMs, liver disease, prior ICH, etc.).

INTENSIVE CARE UNIT AND HOSPITAL MANAGEMENT

Once the diagnosis of ICH is made, every effort should be made to manage the patient in an intensive care unit setting, preferably one with neurocritical care experience. The exceptions are patients with either small, minimally symptomatic hemorrhages or stable patients with hemorrhages that are many days old who can be cared for in a stroke unit with close observation. No matter where the patient is located, there should be no delay in instituting the following essential treatments to reduce hematoma expansion: blood pressure control and reversal of coagulopathy or thrombocytopenia.

Blood Pressure Control

Acute severe elevations in systemic blood pressure (SBP) often accompany ICH. The evidence that treating systemic hypertension either prevents hematoma expansion or improves functional outcomes is weak and an ongoing area of research. However, most guidelines recommend treating severe elevations in SBP, as observational data exist linking systolic hypertension to poor outcomes. The American Heart Association/American Stroke Association (AHA/ASA) 2010 Guidelines for the Management of Spontaneous Intracerebral Hemorrhage recommend treatment of SBPs greater than 180 mm hg with IV agents. Table 7.1 provides initial doses and titration of three commonly used agents. However, SBP should not be reduced by more than 15% to 30% in the first 24 hours. The use of a continuous IV infusion agent with a short half-life is recommended to allow for optimum titration. Placement of an arterial line for continuous blood pressure management is often helpful.

Based on evidence from the Intensive Blood Pressure Reduction in Acute Cerebral Haemorrhage Trial (INTERACT), some authors recommend treating to an SBP goal of less than 140 mm Hg. The INTERACT demonstrated that patients randomized to SBP of less than 140 mm Hg had a trend toward less hematoma expansion compared with SBP less than 180 mm Hg. Additionally, the Antihypertensive Treatment of Acute Cerebral Hemorrhage (ATACH) trial demonstrated safety of treating to SBP less than 140 mm Hg. A follow-up study, ATACH-II, is currently evaluating the efficacy of different SBP targets.

Table 7.1 Initial Management of ICH

Initial Triage and Diagnostic Workup

Initial assessment of airway, breathing, and circulation

  A. Intubate only if not protecting airway; do not "prophylactically" intubate

  B. If intubating, avoid succinylcholine as theoretically can increase ICP

Place 18-gauge IV line in antecubital position

Initial blood tests

  A. CBC, prothrombin time/INR, partial thromboplastin time, basic metabolic panel, type/screen

  B. Send to STAT lab in special "stroke" bag or via protocol

Obtain brief history and physical (on way to CT scanner)

  A. Time of onset

  B. Prior neurological deficits

  C. Risk factors for hemorrhage (AVM, hypertension, dementia/age, coagulopathy)

  D. Medications (anticoagulants, antiplatelets)

Neuroimaging

  A. Noncontrast head CT

  B. Consider CT angiogram of head to determine "spot sign" and to detect for possible aneurysm/other vascular malformation

  C. Measure size of bleed using ABC/2 method

  D. If current or pending herniation, call neurosurgery immediately

Initial Management After Diagnosis of ICH

Blood pressure management

  A. Definitely treat to maintain SBP <180 mm Hg

  B. Consider treating to maintain SBP <140 mm Hg

  C. Do not reduce SBP by more than 15%–30% over first 24 hours

  D. Eventual arterial line placement

  E. Use only intravenous agents

    1. Labetalol

      a. Bolus: 10–20 mg IV push; followed by

      b. Drip: 1–2 mg/min, titrate by 1 mg/min every 5 minutes. Soft max 6 mg/min

    2. Nicardipine

      a. Bolus: not recommended

      b. Drip: 3–5mg/hr, titrate by 2.5 mg every 5–10 minutes. Soft max 15 mg/hr

    3. Esmolol

      a. Bolus: 500 mcg/kg IV push; followed by

      b. Drip: 50 mcg/kg/min, titrate by 25 mcg/kg/min every 5 minutes. Soft max 300 mcg/kg/min

Correct coagulopathies (for all medication-related coagulopathies, first step is to stop agent)

  A. Coumadin

    1. Give FFP or PCCs until INR <1.5

      a. If using 3-factor PCC, also give 1–2 units of FFP to replace factor VII

      b. Do not use activated factor VIIa to replace factor VII in 3-factor PCC

    2. Vitamin K

(continued)

Table 7.1 Continued

71

Intracerebral Hemorrhage

B. Low-molecular-weight heparins (enoxaparin, dalteparin, tinzaparin, fondaparinux)
   a. Protamine sulfate
   b. Consider activated factor VII

C. Dabigatran
   a. Activated oral charcoal if recent ingestion (<3 hours)
   b. Hemodialysis or hemoperfusion (with activated charcoal)
   c. No role for FFP
   d. Activated factor VIIa has unclear but potential benefit
   e. Four-factor PCC has possible benefit, 3-factor PCC has unclear but potential benefit

D. Rivoraxaban/apixaban
   a. Activated oral charcoal if recent ingestion (<3 hours)
   b. Hemoperfusion (with activated charcoal) has possible benefit; no role for hemodialysis
   c. No role for FFP
   d. Activated factor VIIa has unclear but potential benefit
   e. Four-factor PCC has possible benefit, 3-factor PCC has unclear but potential benefit

E. Liver disease/factor deficiency
   1. Replace factors as needed until INR <1.5

Thrombocytopenia/platelet dysfunction
A. If platelets <100, transfuse platelets until >50 (usually 1–2 units)
B. If CKD/ESRD, consider 3 mcg/kg DDAVP to reverse qualitative platelet dysfunction
C. If on aspirin or Plavix, consider platelet transfusion (1–2 units) ± 3 mcg/kg DDAVP

No evidence exists for benefit of recombinant factor VII in ICH. Do not use.

Reversal of Coagulopathy

Table 7.1 includes a list of steps needed to reverse each type of coagulopathy. Table 7.2 includes the dosing for commonly used coagulopathy reversal agents. Patients receiving vitamin K antagonists, such as warfarin, should have their warfarin stopped immediately. Fresh frozen plasma (FFP) should be administered promptly to reduce the international normalized ratio (INR) to less than 1.5. The optimal dosing of FFP is unclear, but patients with therapeutic INRs in the range of 2 to 3 should receive on the order of 4 to 6 units FFP. Continue to check INRs and give FFP until the INR is less than 1.5. Many centers have transitioned to use of prothrombin complex concentrates (PCCs) in lieu of FFP, as studies have demonstrated a more timely reduction in INR along with fewer side effects. PCCs are concentrated forms of the unactivated vitamin K–dependent coagulation factors and are available in either three-factor (factors II, IX, and X [Profilnine SD and Bebulin VH]) or four-factor (factors II, VII, IX, and X [Octaplex and Beriplex]) products. The four-factor products are preferred and are in use in Europe. Only the three-factor products (Profilnine SD and Bebulin VH)

Table 7.2 Dosing of Commonly Used Coagulopathy Reversal Agents

Agent	Dosing	Helpful Hints
Vitamin K	10 mg IV push bolus/30 minutes STAT and then daily for a total of 3 doses	• Infusion over 30 minutes significantly reduces risk of anaphylactoid reaction • DO NOT GIVE IM/SQ/PO
Protamine sulfate	Heparin: 1 mg/100 units given in previous 2–3 hours Enoxaparin: 1 mg/mg given in previous 8 hours Dalteparin/tinzaparin: 1 mg/100 units given in previous 8 hours	• Full reversal of UFH • 60%–80% reversal of LMWH • No reversal of fondaparinux
Platelets	1 unit (apheresis unit, same as 6 whole blood units)	• Each unit raises count by 30 • Goal in ICH is platelets >100 • Use is controversial if indication is qualitative platelet dysfunction (aspirin, Plavix)
FFP	10–30 mL/kg (1 unit = 250 mL)	• Goal INR <1.5 • Need extremely large volumes • Long time of administration/thawing
PCC	25–50 units/kg IV	• Goal INR <1.5 • Small volumes, infused over 10–30 minutes • Contraindicated if history of Heparin Induced Thrombocytopenia (HIT) • Also give 1–2 units of FFP if using 3-factor PCC
Activated factor VIIa	70–90 mcg/mg	• High risk of thrombosis (5%–10%) • Only restores factor VIIa • Did not improve outcomes in FAST Trial (in patients without coagulopathy, however)
Desmopressin (DDAVP)	0.3 mcg/kg	• Use is controversial • Risk of iatrogenic hyponatremia

Adapted from American Hematological Association 2011 Clinical Practice Guide on Anticoagulant Dosing and Management of Anticoagulant-Associated Bleeding Complications in Adults.

are available in the United States at this time, and their use should be supplemented with low-dose FFP (1 to 2 units). A four-factor product with unactivated factors II, IX, and X and activated factor VII is available in the United States (FEIBA NF), but concern remains about potential thrombotic complications with its use. A protocol should be developed for the use of these agents for the treatment of life-threatening Warfarin-related hemorrhages (such as ICH).

Patients receiving heparin or low-molecular-weight heparin should receive the reversal regimen given in Table 7.1 as recommended by the American Hematological Society. Patients receiving new oral anticoagulants (direct thrombin inhibitors and factor Xa inhibitors) should receive the therapies listed in the table based on May 2012 guidance from the Thrombosis and Hemostasis Summit of North America. For patients with factor-specific coagulopathies, deficient factors should be replaced. Patients with end-stage liver disease and coagulopathy should receive FFP until INR is less than 1.5. Recombinant activated factor VII can be considered (70 to 90 mcg/kg) for severe bleeds, although its administration will artificially lower the measured INR. Patients with other rare types of bleeding disorders should receive prompt hematological consultation for the best strategy to achieve hemostasis.

Reversal of Thrombocytopenia and Platelet Disorders

Patients who present with thrombocytopenia (platelets less than 100) should receive platelet transfusion to bring their platelets levels above 100. One to 2 units of platelets is usually sufficient, but repeat counts should be obtained to ensure proper levels. Controversy exists over the transfusion of platelets and/or use of DDAVP in patients with qualitative platelet dysfunction (aspirin, Plavix, end-stage renal disease) but both are options.

Additional Neuroimaging

After the initial diagnostic CT and/or CTA, additional noncontrast head CTs may be of use. A follow-up CT, usually 8 to 12 hours after initial scan, can be helpful in establishing clot stability or diagnosing hematoma expansion. If the follow-up CT shows expansion, an additional CT 8 to 12 hours later should be obtained to assess for stability.

For patients with ICH without a history of advanced age or hypertension, additional neuroimaging may help determine the cause of the bleed. CTA is sensitive in detecting AVMs and aneurysms of up to 2 mm in diameter, although it may not be as sensitive as conventional angiography for small aneurysms or small malformations. MRI within the first 30 days of ictus has recently been demonstrated to increased diagnostic yield with results that often change management and so should be considered. MRI is useful in detecting brain tumors, including metastases and hemorrhagic conversion of ischemic infarcts, and is the only modality that can detect old hemorrhages, which can aid in the diagnosis of amyloid angiopathy. Patients with long-standing hypertension or known amyloid angiopathy do not need additional imaging if the ICH conforms to their known illness, unless there is clinical suspicion for another etiology.

Surgical Treatment Options

In general, the benefit of surgery in ICH patients as a whole is limited. The best evidence for the utility of surgery after ICH arises from the Surgical Treatment for Ischemic Heart Failure (STICH) Trial, in which 1033 ICH patients were randomized to either early surgery or medical management. The study failed to demonstrate an overall benefit to surgery, although in a prespecified subgroup analysis, those with hematomas within 1 cm of the cortical surface did show a benefit from early surgery. Patients with large (>3 cm diameter) or brainstem-compressing cerebellar hemorrhages have been excluded from trials due to their severe nature and should receive immediate, life-saving decompression. Also, patients presenting with uncal or brainstem herniation from lobar hemorrhages should receive life-saving decompression via hemicraniectomy. Studies evaluating the use of less invasive surgical techniques for hematoma removal (Minimally Invasive Surgery plus rt-PA for ICH Evacuation [MISTIE]) are ongoing.

The use of ICP measurement via a fiberoptic parenchymal monitor or a ventricular catheter is unclear. Patients with suspected, symptomatic intracranial hypertension from hydrocephalus or intraventricular hemorrhage will likely benefit from cerebrospinal fluid diversion by means of an external ventricular drain (EVD). Data for ICP monitoring in ICH are minimal, and the AHA/ASA provide guidelines based on the traumatic brain injury literature: patients with a Glasgow Coma Scale score of 8 or less, those with clinical evidence of transtentorial herniation, or those with significant IVH or hydrocephalus should be considered for ICP monitoring and treatment.

For those patients with significant IVH, an EVD can be placed, but drainage is often complicated by clot burden in the catheter. Instillation of intraventricular tPA has been demonstrated to be safe in the Clot Lysis: Evaluating Accelerated Resolution of Hemorrhage with rt-PA (CLEAR)-IVH trial, but its efficacy in improving patient outcomes is still under investigation.

PREVENTION AND TREATMENT OF MEDICAL COMPLICATIONS

Seizures/Electroencephalographic Monitoring: Seizures are common after ICH with many occurring at ictus. If a seizure is suspected clinically, patients should be loaded with an antiepileptic drug (AED) to prevent further localization-related seizures (e.g., but not limited to fos-phenytoin and levetiracetam). There is no evidence to support the prophylactic use of AEDs, and some studies have demonstrated an association with prophylactic AED use and worsened outcomes. For patients with poor mental status or coma, continuous electroencephalographic monitoring should be performed to rule out nonconvulse seizures, as the incidence may be as high as 20% in these patients.

Deep Vein Thrombosis and Prophylaxis: The incidence of deep vein thrombosis after ICH is high. Intermittent pneumatic compression devices should be used throughout the duration of the hospital stay until the patient is fully ambulatory, as this has been shown to decrease the incidence from around 15% to 4% compared with just compression stockings. For spontaneous ICH without a clear source of bleeding, the AHA recommends consideration of low-dose heparin or low-molecular-weight heparin after the bleed is determined to be stable on the basis of serial CT scans.

Hyperglycemia: While hyperglycemia on admission has been associated with worse outcomes after ICH, data from general critical care literature, especially the Normoglycemia in Intensive Care Evaluation and Survival Using Glucose Algorithm Regulation (NICE-SUGAR) trial, have demonstrated excess mortality due to tight glycemic control (80 to 110 mg/dL).

Treatment of Fever: Fever within the first 72 hours of admission is an independent risk factor for poor outcome, but treatment of fever has not been studied in ICH patients. In general, patients should receive acetaminophen to treat fevers. Many centers are now using therapeutic temperature modulation to treat fever or even perform hypothermia, but this has not been systematically studied.

SECONDARY PREVENTION

The prevention of recurrent ICH is dependent on its initial cause. For patient with ICH secondary to hypertension, the patient must achieve good blood pressure control with a goal of normotension (blood pressure 120/70 mm Hg). While this effort will be made in conjunction with a stroke physician, good primary care follow-up is a key element in secondary ICH prevention.

Patients with ICH who were receiving antiplatelet medications can generally restart these medications after the acute ICH period (usually after 1 week). The question of restarting anticoagulation is more complicated. For those patients on anticoagulation for atrial fibrillation, data suggest they should not be restarted on warfarin if the location of the initial ICH was lobar due to the high rate of recurrence. If the ICH was in a deep location, it is probably safe to restart anticoagulation after the acute period. Risk factors for recurrent ICH other than resuming anticoagulation include risk factors for amyloid angiopathy: presence of multiple microbleeds on MRI, lobar location of ICH, old age, and apolipoprotein E ε2 or ε4 alleles.

REHABILITATION

Patients with ICH have an unclear and variable trajectory of recovery, which can be difficult for patients, families, and providers. Improvements are usually greatest and fastest in the first few weeks but can continue for months and even years. All patients with deficits after stroke should receive rehabilitation to the extent that they can participate. Efforts should be made to not only increase motor and cognitive functioning but also prevent contractures, treat poststroke pain, manage spasticity, and train on assistive devices to increase mobility and independence. Almost half of all ICH patients will continue to have some sort of dependency even after recovery, so efforts should be made early to arrange the needed care.

SUGGESTED READING

Cushman M, Lim W, Zakai NA. Clinical practice guide on anticoagulant dosing and management of anticoagulant-associated bleeding complications in adults. American Society of Hematology. 2011. See http://www.hematology.org/Practice/Guidelines/7243.aspx

Diedler J, Skyora M, Hacke W. Critical care of the patient with acute stroke. In: Mohr JP, Wolf PA, Grotta JC, et al, editors. Stroke: pathophysiology, diagnosis, and management. Philadelphia, PA: Elsevier Saunders; 2011.

Kaatz S, Kouides PA, Garcia DA, et al. Guidance on the emergent reversal of oral thrombin and factor Xa inhibitors. Am J Hematol 2012;87(Suppl 1):S141–S145.

Mendelow AD, Gregson BA, Fernandes HM, et al. Early surgery versus initial conservative treatment in patients with spontaneous supratentorial intracerebral haematomas in the International Surgical Trial in Intracerebral Haemorrhage (STICH): a randomised trial. Lancet 2005;365:387–397.

Morgenstern LB, Hemphill JC 3rd, Anderson C, et al. Guidelines for the management of spontaneous intracerebral hemorrhage: a guideline for healthcare professionals from the American Heart Association/American Stroke Association. Stroke 2010;41:2108–2129.

8 Aneurysmal Subarachnoid Hemorrhage

Sachin Agarwal and Neha Dangayach

INTRODUCTION

Aneurysmal subarachnoid hemorrhage (SAH) is an acute cerebrovascular event due to rupture of aneurysms around the circle of Willis in the brain. The average case-fatality rate for subarachnoid hemorrhage is 51%, with approximately one-third of survivors needing lifelong care. Most deaths occur within 2 weeks after the ictus, with 10% occurring before the patient receives medical attention and 25% within 24 hours after the event. The most common presenting complaint in 80% of SAH patients is a sudden severe headache immediately reaching maximal intensity ("thunderclap headache"). This headache may be associated with other red flag signs such as nausea and vomiting, neck stiffness, and focal neurological deficits, although it is important to recognize that neurological examination results may be normal. A sentinel headache is present in 10% to 43% patients. This sentinel headache may occur about 2 to 8 weeks before the SAH and increases the odds of early rebleeding by 10-fold. Aneurysmal rupture typically tends to occur during physical exertion or stress. SAH is a life-threatening medical emergency that requires a high level of suspicion in patients with sudden onset of severe headache with no known reason. Seizures may occur in the first 24 hours of a SAH, particularly in patients with anterior communicating or middle cerebral artery aneurysms with an associated intraparenchymal bleed. The sensitivity of a noncontrast head computer tomography (CT) remains nearly 100% in the first 72 hours following a bleed but declines sharply after 5 to 7 days. Thus, the presence of xanthochromia on lumbar puncture should be used to diagnose patients with a delayed presentation or in CT negative patients. Magnetic resonance imaging (MRI) with fluid attenuated inversion recovery (FLAIR), diffusion weighted imaging, gradient recalled-echo, and proton density sequences may also be helpful in these cases. Once the SAH is diagnosed; grading scales (Tables 8.1 and 8.2) may be used to predict mortality as well as their future risk of vasospasm. The diagnostic algorithm after the SAH is suspected (Figure 8.1) should be followed as rapidly as possible.

CT angiography (CTA) can be used to detect aneurysm, but the gold standard continues to be conventional digital subtraction angiography (DSA). Aneurysms of less than 3 mm can be missed on CTA. MR angiography (MRA) has a less important role due to logistical constraints, cost, and poorer vascular definition compared with CTA. In patients with initial negative DSA, a repeat DSA, delayed by a week

Table 8.1 Risk of Perioperative Mortality based on Hunt-Hess Grades

Grade	Criteria	Index of Perioperative Mortality (%)
0	Aneurysm is not ruptured	0–5
I	Asymptomatic or with minimum headache and slight nuchal rigidity	0–5
II	Moderate to severe headache, nuchal rigidity, but no neurological deficit other than cranial nerve palsy	2–10
III	Somnolence, confusion, medium focal deficits	10–15
IV	Stupor, hemiparesis medium or severe, possible early decerebrate rigidity, vegetative disturbances	60–70
V	Deep coma, decerebrate rigidity, moribund appearance	70–100

should be strongly considered. CTA may not be able to identify all the characteristics of an aneurysm that aid decisions regarding the optimal method to use for treatment such as endovascular treatment versus surgical clipping. Therefore, if an aneurysm is not detected on noninvasive vascular imaging, then three-dimensional DSA is recommended. A step by step guide for the clinical management of Subarachnoid Hemorrhage is provided in the Appendix.

SURGICAL AND ENDOVASCULAR TREATMENT

The International Subarachnoid Aneurysm Trial (ISAT) is the single multicenter randomized clinical trial (RCT) of 2143 patients comparing surgical and endovascular repair of

Table 8.2 Risk of Vasospasm Based on the Fisher and Modified Fisher Grades

Grade	Criteria	Patients, %	Percent Within Grade With Symptomatic Vasospasm
Modified Fisher Scale			
1	Minimal/thin SAH, no IVH in both lateral ventricles	21.6	24
2	Minimal/thin SAH, *with* IVH in both lateral ventricles	10.8	33
3	Thick SAH,* no IVH in both lateral ventricles	33.9	33
4	Thick SAH,* *with* IVH in both lateral ventricles	33.7	40
Fisher Scale			
1	No blood	8.1	21
2	Diffuse thin blood	10.9	25
3	Thick SAH present	67.7	37
4	ICH/IVH with either no or only diffuse SAH	13.3	31

*Completely filling ≥1 cistern or fissure.

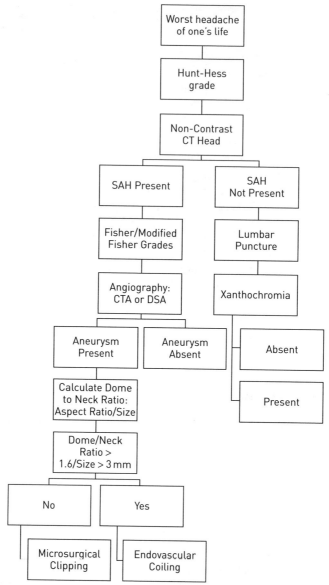

FIGURE 8.1

Clinical algorithm for suspected subarachnoid hemorrhage.

intracranial aneurysms. At 1 year from randomization, the endovascular arm performed better than the surgical arm due to a decrease in the rate of disability in that arm (16% in the endovascular arm versus 22% in the surgical arm). However, the incidence of late rebleeding was higher in the endovascular arm (2.9% versus 0.9%). Endovascular coiling can be offered to patients whose aneurysms are suitable for either endovascular or surgical repair. The neck diameter, dome size, and size of the aneurysm are important factors when considering endovascular repair. Although high-porosity stents improve the rate of aneurysm occlusion, the risk of complications may increase since these patients will require dual antiplatelets after the procedure to prevent thromboembolic events. Low-porosity flow-diverting stents with or without coils can be used for dissecting aneurysms.

Rebleeding

During the interval between the onset of SAH symptoms and the obliteration of aneurysm, blood pressure should be controlled with a short-acting agent to carefully balance the risk of stroke, hypertension-related rebleeding, and maintenance of cerebral perfusion pressure. The magnitude of blood pressure control to reduce the risk of rebleeding has not been established, but a decrease in systolic blood pressure to less than 160 mm Hg is a reasonable goal. Nicardipine offers an alternative to labetalol and sodium nitroprusside and appears to provide smoother blood pressure control compared with labetalol due to fewer dose adjustments. Nicardipine also does not adversely affect regional brain tissue oxygen. Clevidipine, a very short-acting calcium channel blocker, is another option for the acute control of hypertension, but data for SAH are lacking to support its use in this setting at this time. Early aneurysm repair remains the most effective way to prevent rebleeding. The administration of a short course of antifibrinolytic therapy before "early" aneurysm repair (begun at diagnosis and continued up to the point at which the aneurysm is secured or at 72 hours post-ictus, whichever is shorter) may be considered. This is based on the results from one RCT and case-control studies with 428 patients showing lower rebleeding rate when this treatment was given for short time before "early" repair. Delayed (more than 48 hours after the ictus) or prolonged (longer than 3 days) administration of antifibrinolytic therapy exposes patients to side effects, including cerebral ischemia, and should be avoided. Due to the increased incidence of DVT in SAH patients, antifibrinolytic therapy is relatively contraindicated in patients with risk factors for thromboembolic complications.

Seizures and Prophylactic Anticonvulsant Use

Seizure-like movements have been reported in about 26% of patients; but it is unclear whether these movements are true seizures or posturing. There are no RCTs guiding the decision to use seizure prophylaxis in SAH. Clinical seizures may occur in 1% to 18% of SAH patients. Delayed seizures may occur in 3% to 7% of patients. Risk factors for development of early seizures include age older than 65, aneurysm in the middle cerebral artery, thickness of SAH clot, presence of intracerebral hematoma, rebleeding, infarction, poor neurological grade, and a history of hypertension. In the ISAT study, patients treated with endovascular coiling were found to have a lower incidence of seizures. In two large retrospective studies, nonconvulsive status epilepticus was found in 10% to 20% of patients and was a predictor of poor outcome. In certain cases, continuous electroencephalogram (EEG) may be required to identify subclinical seizures. The current recommendations suggest that prophylactic anticonvulsant therapy may be used in the early posthemorrhagic period for 3 to 7 days, although the routine prophylactic use of long-term anticonvulsant therapy is not recommended.

Hydrocephalus

One-third of patients admitted with aneurysmal SAH require temporary or permanent cerebrospinal fluid (CSF) diversion. The incidence of chronic post-SAH hydrocephalus requiring shunt surgery is 15% to 20%. The method of aneurysmal repair does not significantly affect the development of chronic hydrocephalus. If neither a hematoma with compressive mass effect nor an obstructive element exists, CSF drainage with serial lumbar puncture is a reasonable alternative to ventricular drainage. Preoperative ventriculostomy is not associated with an increased risk of aneurysm rebleeding. Long-term outcomes in patients with a poor grade who improve after the placement of an external ventricular drain (EVD) are similar to patients with good-grade hemorrhages. Microsurgical management such as lamina terminalis fenestration may diminish the incidence of shunt-dependent hydrocephalus and, when combined with extensive cisternal blood cleansing, may reduce the incidence of stroke and poor outcomes in high-grade SAH. Permanent CSF diversion may be independently predicted by the presence of hyperglycemia at admission, findings on the admission CT scan (Fisher grade IV intraventricular hemorrhage and bicaudate index ≥ 0.20), and development of nosocomial meningitis. Compared with rapid weaning, gradual multistep weaning of EVDs provides no added advantage to patients in preventing the need for long-term shunt placement or reducing hospital stay.

Vasospasm and Delayed Cerebral Ischemia

Vasospasm refers to the narrowing of blood vessels as seen on vascular imaging studies. It is of paramount importance in the SAH patient because it can become symptomatic in about 50% of patients and lead to ischemia and brain tissue infarction. Patients with aneurysmal SAH may develop vasospasm as early as day 4, peaking around days 7 to 10, and continue to remain at risk for patients for up to 21 days following aneurysmal rupture. Current guidelines for treating vasospasm recommend the use of oral nimodipine, maintenance of euvolemia, treatment with triple-H therapy (hemodynamic augmentation therapy [hypervolemia, hypertension, and hemodilution]) in an intensive care setting, and/or endovascular therapy with vasodilators and angioplasty balloons, although good evidence from controlled trials to support these therapies is lacking. Trancranial Doppler studies are a reasonable way to monitor for the development of vasospasm. Prophylactic hypervolemia and prophylactic angioplasty are currently not recommended. A single case-control study supported the use of lumbar drains for the prevention of delayed cerebral ischemia. A recent meta-analysis of intrathecal thrombolytic infusion showed reduction in angiographic vasospasm, chronic hydrocephalus, and delayed neurological deficits. However, there is a lack of conclusive evidence to support the recommendation of intrathecal thrombolysis at this time. The use of statins in the prevention of vasospasm remains experimental.

MANAGEMENT OF MEDICAL COMPLICATIONS

Cardiac Complications

Cardiac injury is incrementally worse with increasing severity of SAH grades and is associated with persistent QTc prolongation and ventricular arrhythmias. Bradycardia, relative tachycardia, and nonspecific ST- and T-wave abnormalities are strongly and independently associated with 3-month mortality after SAH. Baseline cardiac assessment with serial enzymes, electrocardiography, and echocardiography is recommended, especially in patients with evidence of myocardial dysfunction. An elevated level of troponin is a good indicator of left ventricular dysfunction. Although regional wall motion abnormalities and depressed ejection fraction persist to some degree, cardiac dysfunction is generally reversible and should not preclude these patients from undergoing operative interventions or becoming heart donors. Clinical management may require more aggressive hemodynamic monitoring until cardiac function returns to normal. Standard management of heart failure is indicated, although cerebral perfusion pressure should be monitored and maintained.

Pulmonary Complications

Patients with pulmonary complications after SAH have a higher incidence of symptomatic vasospasm than do patients without pulmonary complications. Oxygenation abnormalities after SAH are frequently the result of noncardiogenic and hydrostatic causes and contribute to an increased length of hospital stay.

Hematological Complications

Anemia after SAH is strongly related to surgery, likely through greater blood loss and greater systemic inflammatory response on admission. Both anemia and transfusion are predictive of adverse outcomes in patients with SAH. Appropriate transfusion thresholds may vary depending on the presence or absence of clinical vasospasm. The use of packed red blood cell (PRBC) transfusion to treat anemia may be reasonable in patients with SAH who are at risk of cerebral ischemia, but whether transfusion is beneficial in mitigating the ischemia itself cannot be determined from the available data. Studies have shown that lower hemoglobin levels are associated with worse outcomes regardless of SAH severity or the development of vasospasm. The association is somewhat stronger among patients with more severe SAH. Furthermore, SAH patients with higher initial and mean hemoglobin values are associated with improved outcomes at discharge and 3 months. In a microdialysis-based study, the transfusion of PRBCs to anemic patients with SAH resulted in a significant increase in cerebral oxygen delivery without lowering global CBF. This was associated with reduced oxygen extraction fraction, which may improve tolerance of vulnerable brain regions to further impairments of CBF. Therefore, the American Neurocritical Care Society strongly recommends maintaining hemoglobin concentration above 8 to 10 g/dL.

Hypothalamic Dysfunction

Hypothalamic dysfunction should be considered in patients who are unresponsive to vasopressors. After SAH, almost two-thirds of the patients have been reported to meet the preestablished criteria for relative adrenal insufficiency. Administration of high-dose corticosteroids is not currently recommended in acute SAH; however, hormonal replacement with stress-dose corticosteroids for patients with vasospasm and unresponsiveness may be considered.

Fever

Refractory fever during the first 10 days after SAH is predicted by poor Hunt-Hess grade and the presence of intraventricular hemorrhage. Fever is associated with increased mortality, increased length of stay, depressed consciousness, and more functional and cognitive disability among survivors. Infectious causes of fever should always be sought and treated. Aggressive control of fever with standard or advanced temperature-modulating systems is reasonable in the acute phase of SAH. Treatment with an air-circulating cooling blanket may not be beneficial, and first-line agents should include traditional antipyretic medications such as acetaminophen and ibuprofen. Low-dose diclofenac infusion may be superior to intermittent non-steroidal anti-inflammatory medication dosing for temperature control. Noninvasive cooling devices such as the Arctic Sun and catheter-based cooling systems are superior to conventional cooling-blanket therapy for controlling fever. All patients should be monitored and treated for shivering with simple and reliable tools such as The Bedside Shivering Assessment Scale.

Hyperglycemia

An elevated admission plasma glucose level is extremely frequent in poor-grade patients with SAH and is associated with poor clinical outcomes. The degree of hyperglycemia correlates with the clinical and radiological extents of the initial injury. Insulin administration following SAH for the treatment of hyperglycaemia is feasible and safe. However, acute reductions in serum glucose, even to levels within the normal range, may be associated with brain energy metabolic crises and lactate-pyruvate ratio (LPR) elevation in poor-grade SAH patients. For example, a blood glucose target of 180 mg/dL or less resulted in lower mortality than did a target of 81 to 108 mg/dL. Current recommendations advocate that serum glucose should be maintained below 200 mg/dL, and hypoglycemia (serum glucose <80 mg/dL) should be avoided.

Hyponatremia

Hyponatremia may be more common than hypernatremia after SAH and is independently associated with poor outcomes. It is unclear whether the cause of hyponatremia is a syndrome of inappropriate secretion of antidiuretic hormone (SIADH) or cerebral salt wasting syndrome (CSWS) or both. Regardless of the clinical diagnosis of SIADH or CSWS, free water intake via intravenous and enteral routes should be limited. Inhibition of natriuresis with fludrocortisone can effectively reduce the sodium and water intake and prevent hyponatremia. Hypertonic (3%) sodium chloride/acetate can be administered to patients with mild hyponatremia in the setting of symptomatic vasospasm following SAH. Intermittent dosing of vasopressin receptor antagonists like intravenous conivaptan or oral tolvaptan may be effective in increasing free water excretion and correcting hyponatremia; however, extreme caution to avoid hypovolemia is needed if these agents are used for the treatment of hyponatremia.

Deep Vein Thrombosis

Measures to prevent deep venous thrombosis (DVT) should be used in all SAH patients. While pharmacological prophylaxis lowers the prevalence of symptomatic DVTs, the number of asymptomatic DVTs remains significant, particularly in patients with higher Hunt-Hess grades. Routine venous Doppler ultrasonography is an efficient, noninvasive means of identifying DVT as a screening modality in both symptomatic and asymptomatic patients. Sequential compression devices should be routinely used in all SAH patients, while the use of low-molecular-weight heparin or unfractionated heparin for prophylaxis should be withheld in patients with unprotected aneurysms and those who are expected to undergo surgery, for at least 24 hours before and after intracranial procedures.

SUGGESTED READING

Guidelines for the management of aneurysmal subarachnoid hemorrhage: a guideline for healthcare professionals from the American Heart Association/American Stroke Association. Stroke 2012;43:1711–1737.

Critical care management of patients following aneurysmal subarachnoid hemorrhage: recommendations from the Neurocritical Care Society's Multidisciplinary Consensus Conference. Neurocrit Care 2011;15:211–240.

Suarez JI, Tarr RW, Selman WR. Aneurysmal subarachnoid hemorrhage. N Engl J Med 2006;354:387–396.

Edlow JA, Caplan LR. Avoiding pitfalls in the diagnosis of subarachnoid hemorrhage. N Engl J Med 2000;342:29–36.

Frontera JA, Claassen J, Schmidt JM, et al. Prediction of symptomatic vasospasm after subarachnoid hemorrhage: the Modified Fisher Scale. Neurosurgery 2006;59:21–27.

Appendix
Subarachnoid Hemorrhage
Steps in Management

- Admit to an ICU
- Keep head of bed at 30 degrees *always*
- Increased ICP management: mannitol 1 g/kg or hypertonics 23.4%
- Head CT and CTA on admission to neurointensive care unit, if none prior
- Consider Amicar (aminocaproic acid) if significant SAH (Hunt-Hess ≥3) or anticipate delay in treatment
  - 4 g IV bolus over 60 minutes, then 1 g/hr, stop 4 hours before angiography planned
  - Contraindicated or caution in patients with coronary artery disease, stroke, pulmonary embolism, thrombosis, or vasospasm
- Levetiracetam or fosphenytoin 20 mg/kg IV ×1 STAT (loading dose)
- Place an arterial line
- Contact neurosurgery to arrange angiogram and possible EVD/ICP monitor if evidence of hydrocephalus or GCS score <8.
- Short-acting, low-dose sedation/analgesia as needed (e.g., acetaminophen, fentanyl, dexmedetomidine, propofol)
- Avoid NSAIDs, aspirin, and antiplatelets before surgery
- Diet: usually nil per mouth (NPO) for angiogram; place Duotube if necessary for oral medications
- IV: normal saline at 1.0 to 1.5 mL/kg/hr ± KCl (potassium chloride)
- Goal systolic blood pressure (SBP) <160 mm Hg, use nicardipine or labetalol drip as needed to maintain SBP <160 mm Hg
- Nimodipine standing orders for all SAH patients for 21 days
  - Nimodipine 60 mg orally/duotube every 4 hours for SBP >140 mm Hg
  - Nimodipine 30 mg orally/duotube every 4 hours for SBP 120–140 mm Hg
- Labs: complete blood count, basic metabolic profile, magnesium level, phosphate level, ionized calcium, liver function testss, coagulation profile, serial troponins, ß- human chorionic gonadotropin in young women, type and hold, urine analysis, urine toxicology
- Pan cultures (cultures, blood, urine, sputum, stool, cerebrospinal fluid as needed)
- Electrocardiogram
- Chest radiograph
- Transthoracic echocardiogram, portable

- If aneurysm protected, allow patient to autoregulate up to SBP 200 mm Hg 24 hours post clipping
- No subcutaneous heparin (e.g., Henoxiparin) until 24 hours post procedure (i.e., craniotomy)
- Maintain compressions systems (e.g., Venodynes) at all times
- Gastrointestinal prophylaxis: famotidine 20 mg/day orally
- Nicotine patch 14 to 21 mg/day (as needed)
- Ondansetron 4 mg IV every 6 hours as needed
- Acetoaminophen 650 mg orally/duotube/per rectum every 4 hours as needed for pain/fever
- Aggressive bowel regimen: senna 2 tabs orally/duotube at bedtime and/or docusate 100 mg orally/duotube 3 times daily
- Maintain normal pH, P_{CO_2} (end-tidal CO_2 goal of 33–38 mm Hg), Pa_{O_2} ≥80 mm Hg
- Aggressive glucose, seizure, and fever control during vasospasm period
- Daily transcranial Doppler examinations to evaluate for vasospasm using Lindegaard ratio for 14 days post SAH

9 Subdural and Epidural Hemorrhage

Christopher P. Kellner, Brendan F. Scully, and E. Sander Connolly, Jr.

INTRODUCTION

Epidural and subdural hemorrhages (EDH and SDH, respectively) are characterized by bleeding in the potential spaces surrounding the dura mater encasing the brain and spinal cord. Both most commonly occur after head trauma and are serious, life-threatening conditions. Prompt recognition and management are essential for maximizing the possibility of a good outcome.

EPIDURAL HEMORRHAGE

An *epidural hemorrhage* is defined as blood in the potential space between the skull and the dura mater. It occurs in approximately 2% of all head traumas and approximately 10% to 15% of severe head injuries. The temporoparietal region is the most common location (75%), most often after a fracture of the squamous temporal bone and laceration of the middle meningeal artery. Other common locations for EDH include the anterior cranial fossa, parasagittal sinuses, and posterior fossa. Approximately 80% of EDHs are secondary to arterial bleeding. EDH occurs most often in adolescents and young adults and is rare in children younger than 2 years and persons older than age 50.

Head trauma is the most common etiology of EDH, with skull fractures in 75% to 90% of cases. The classic presentation is loss of consciousness after a traumatic event, followed by a "lucid interval" in which the person is asymptomatic and then undergoes deterioration with varying symptoms from headache, confusion, and seizures leading to coma and death. However, it only occurs 20% to 47% of the time, and there is variation in the clinical presentation. The lucid interval can last for several minutes to several days depending on the extent of the bleeding. The inciting traumatic event might be minor trauma, and loss of consciousness does not always occur. Alternatively, in approximately one-third of EDHs, the trauma can be more severe, with accompanying lesions including contusion, intracerebral hemorrhage, or SDH. Over time, unchecked hematoma expansion leads to increased intracranial pressure (ICP), producing classic clinical signs, such as Kernohan's notch (ipsilateral paresis from compression of the contralateral cerebral peduncle against the tentorial edge) or Cushing's reflex (hypertension, bradycardia, and respiratory depression). The mass effect on the deep brain structures can be fatal if not treated emergently with surgery.

ACUTE SUBDURAL HEMORRHAGE

SDH is defined as a collection of blood between the dura and arachnoid mater. It is typically caused by venous bleeding (usually ruptured bridging veins) and can occur with minor or no direct trauma to the skull, especially in the elderly, chronic alcohol abusers, and those receiving anticoagulant medications. It does not require skull fracture, but linear acceleration of the brain inside leads to rupture of the bridging vessels between the dura and arachnoid membranes. SDH is more common in the elderly than in younger patients, as cerebral atrophy places patients at higher risk. As the brain atrophies, tension increases on bridging veins, making them more likely to tear secondary to head trauma. Commonly, a membrane forms that recruits friable neovascularization that is more likely to bleed than normal vessels, leading to recurrent hemorrhages.

Approximately 50% of acute SDH are comatose from the time of injury. Small SDHs may be asymptomatic, while larger hemorrhages can manifest with hemiparesis and coma. Although a lucid interval can occur, most patients are symptomatic from the moment of injury. The initial signs and symptoms are commonly unilateral headache and enlarged pupil on the ipsilateral side, with drowsiness or altered mental status.

CHRONIC SUBDURAL HEMORRHAGE

An SDH is considered chronic when it is recognized more than 2 weeks after the initial event. In approximately half of cases, no event is recalled. In these cases, chronicity is determined by duration of symptoms and characteristic findings on imaging. Cerebral atrophy is the most important factor predisposing to chronic SDHs; therefore, this condition is most commonly seen in the elderly and chronic alcoholics. The atrophic brain allows expansion of the hematoma without the development of intracranial hypertension, with milder symptoms that manifest several days to weeks after the event. These symptoms are typically global and insidious, including headache, dizziness, cognitive changes, and personality changes.

PREHOSPITAL MANAGEMENT

The prehospital management of traumatic brain injury is limited. In the field, standard assessment of airway, breathing, and circulation is necessary, and endotracheal intubation is preferred if there is any question of declining mental status. Fingerstick blood glucose should be checked as hypoglycemia may contribute the altered mental status while hyperglycemia may negatively impact neurological outcome. Patients should be transported with the head of the bed at 30 degrees to reduce aspiration risk and to minimize ICP. Transport should proceed to a center with the capabilities to intervene surgically if necessary. Every effort should be taken to obtain a history and medication list, especially if the patient takes anticoagulants, and to notify the receiving hospital of the patient's pending arrival so that the patient can be taken to imaging and the operating room as quickly as possible.

EMERGENCY DEPARTMENT

Initial Assessment: The Primary and Secondary Surveys

Patients with suspected traumatic brain injury and/or hemorrhage should be assessed for airway, breathing, circulation, disability (Glasgow Coma Scale [GCS] score, pupillary reflexes, localizing neurological signs), and exposure (wounds, deformities, other gross abnormalities) immediately on arrival. The secondary survey is a more detailed neurological examination and history often performed by the neurologist or neurosurgeon seeing the trauma consult. Obtaining a rapid computed tomography (CT) of the head without contrast is paramount and should not be delayed for any reason. This will confirm the presence of extra-axial blood, which then leads to the initiation of rapid techniques and interventions to lower ICP.

Acute Neuroimaging

Epidural Hematoma

An EDH is often easily distinguished from an SDH by a number of defining characteristics. The EDH is biconvex rather than concave, sharply demarcated, and hyperdense and respects suture lines. It is often located in the temporoparietal region, deep to the middle meningeal artery (Figure 9.1A). Depending on hematoma size, there may be radiographic signs of herniation such as midline shift, subfalcine herniation, or uncal herniation. When the blood is hyperacute or if the patient is taking anticoagulant medications, there may be a "swirl sign," which is evidence of the presence of unclotted blood in the hematoma. It is important to look for a fracture on the CT by examining the bone under the appropriate windowing (Figure 9.1B).

Acute Subdural Hematoma

Acute SDH, like EDH, is an extra-axial hyperdense lesion often causing mass effect on the underlying cortex (Figure 9.2). Unlike EDH, the lesion is concave and can cross

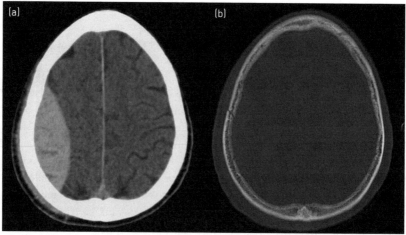

FIGURE 9.1

CT scan: (a) Temporoparietal Right Epidural Hematoma and (b) Associated bone fracture.

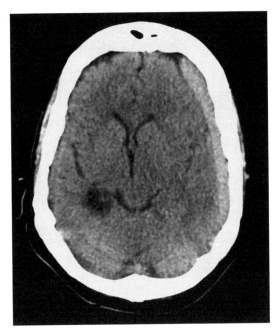

FIGURE 9.2
CT scan: Left Acute Subdural Hematoma.

suture lines. More than 85% of SDHs are unilateral. These lesions are associated with fractures less frequently than EDH. Other accompanying brain injury, however, occurs as frequently as 50% of the time, including EDH, intracerebral hemorrhage, and contusion. As in EDH, a swirl sign can represent hyperacuity or result from an anticoagulative state.

Chronic Subdural Hematoma

The density of the subdural blood decreases over time at a rate of 1.5 Hounsfield units/day. It becomes isodense to brain at approximately 2 weeks after the initial injury, and this is the time at which it is identified as a subacute to chronic SDH. Contrast is rarely used but may aid in diagnosis if there is any suspicion of an empyema or if it is difficult to differentiate an isodense hematoma from adjacent brain, because cortical vessels will delineate the two. Other helpful techniques for pinpointing the cortical edge include identifying the termination of cerebrospinal fluid (CSF)-filled sulci, looking for sulcal distortion and midline shift from mass effect, and identifying a potentially thickened cortex. Over time, the density of the collection approaches that of CSF. The presence of membranes has been correlated with an increased risk of rebleeding and is important to recognize on CT because it has important implications for surgical management (Figure 9.3).

Emergent Management

Once the diagnosis of a symptomatic extra-axial bleed is made by clinical presentation and imaging, it is crucial to perform emergent maneuvers to decrease ICP. These

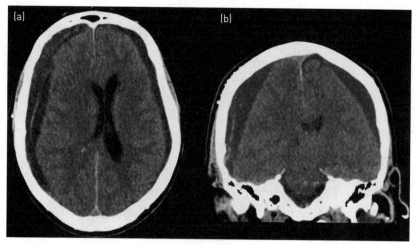

FIGURE 9.3

CT scan: Bilateral Chronic Subdural Hematoma.

include elevating the head of the bed, positioning the head midline so as to not compress either jugular vein, and maintaining physiological parameters within the appropriate range. Specific physiological guidelines are outlined in the third edition of the *Guidelines for the Management of Severe Traumatic Brain Injury* and are outlined here:

1. Mean arterial pressure >70 mm Hg
2. Cerebral perfusion pressure >60 mm Hg
3. O_2 saturation >93%
4. Pao_2 95–100 mm Hg
5. ICP >20 mm Hg
6. Serum Na 135–145 mEq
7. Euthermia
8. Eucapnia

Because the Pco_2 and O_2 saturation must be well controlled, all patients with severe head injury should be intubated. If the patient has or develops a focal neurological finding, hyperventilation to $Paco_2$ 30 to 32 mm Hg, increased sedation, and administration of 1 g/kg mannitol are recommended, although these should no longer be given empirically.

Second, once it has been established that a cerebral bleed is present, all anticoagulation and antiplatelet agents must be reversed. If the patient has recently taken aspirin or nonsteroidal anti-inflammatory drugs, both DDAVP and platelets are given. More details on correction of anticoagulation in brain hemorrhage can be found under the appropriate heading later in this chapter.

SURGICAL OPTIONS

Until recently, clear criteria for the surgical management of extra-axial hematomas did not exist and most often depended on surgeon preference. Guidelines for the surgical evaluation of acute EDH and acute SDH were developed in 2006 by the Congress of Neurological Surgeons and the Brain Trauma Foundation and presented in the "Guidelines for the Surgical Management of Traumatic Brain Injury" based on a review of the literature from 1975 to 2001. Criteria for the surgical evacuation of an EDH are predominantly based on size with the following indications:

1. An EDH >30 cm³—patient should be taken to the operating room immediately
2. An EDH < 30 cm³, <15 mm thick, <5 mm of midline shift, and GCS score >8 without focal deficit—can be managed nonoperatively

It is important to remain wary of inferior parietal and temporal hematomas because uncal herniation can lead to rapid brainstem compression with a smaller hematoma and lower ICP.

The indications to operative on a patient with an SDH also rely on the size of the hemorrhage and the patient's examination. Indications for surgery include the following:

1. An SDH >10 mm thick or with >5-mm midline shift
2. All patients with GCS score <9 should undergo ICP monitoring.
3. If the SDH is <10 mm thick, the midline shift <5 mm, and the GCS score <9, the patient should undergo surgical evacuation if neurological decline ≥2 GCS points, the pupils are anisocoric or fixed and dilated, or ICP is >20 mm Hg.

The indications for a chronic subdural evacuation are far less clearly defined. An early study by Cushing in 1925 advocated craniotomy and membrane resection. In the 1960s, multiple studies advocating burr-hole drainage of chronic SDHs showed improved results over the conventional craniotomy technique. In burr-hole drainage, irrigation is still possible, but the membrane cannot be resected. Twist drill drainage was then developed, which permits only the release of the chronic SDH fluid and is not accompanied by membrane resection or irrigation. Recently, the SEPS (Subdural Evacuation Port System by Medtronic) drainage kit has made bedside, twist drill evacuation with a closed drainage system an effective, low-cost, and low-risk alternative to craniotomy or burr holes. In this system, a bolt is placed at the bedside, membranes are perforated, and the bolt is connected to a suction bulb for light, continuous, self-suction. Burr-hole drainage, twist drill drainage, and SEPS drainage are not options in acute SDH because the clot is too thick for effective drainage.

INTENSIVE CARE UNIT AND HOSPITAL MANAGEMENT

Blood Pressure Control

A delicate balance exists between maintaining blood pressure to perfuse potentially injured brain parenchyma and incurring rebleeding. Prior to surgical evacuation, while mass effect and decreased cerebral perfusion pressure remain an issue, hypertension is tolerated assuming that the elevated pressure is effectively perfusing over an elevated ICP. An arterial line should be placed to allow for optimal assessment and monitoring of blood pressure. Intravenous antihypertensive agents, preferably medications with short half-lives such as labetolol or esmolol, should be used, and large fluctuations and dramatic reduction of blood pressure should be avoided. The head of the bed should be elevated to at least 30 degrees to reduce ICP as well as aspiration risk. If the patient is intubated, hyperventilation can also reduce ICP, and osmotic diuresis with mannitol is also an option. Glucocorticoids should be avoided because they may increase mortality in head trauma. After surgical evacuation, the blood pressure should be more tightly controlled with systolic pressures less than 140 mm Hg given the high concern for recurrence in the first 24 to 48 hours after surgery.

Reversal of Coagulopathy

Patients who present with SDH are often on anticoagulant medications from other comorbidities, and it is necessary to reverse the anticoagulation as urgently as possible, especially if the patient will be headed to surgery. EDH patients tend to be younger than SDH patients, and generally are not on anticoagulant medications to the degree seen in the SDH population. However, medications are only one of many causes of coagulopathy, and a full workup to evaluate and determine the cause of coagulopathy should be undertaken immediately on presentation.

The first step is to stop any current anticoagulant medications. A laboratory workup, including prothrombin time, partial thromboplastin time, and platelet count, should be sent. A type and screen should also be drawn in case blood products are needed. If possible, history of medication use, history of bleeding disorders, liver and renal disease, or alcohol abuse should be elicited from the patient or family members.

For patients receiving vitamin K antagonists such as warfarin, the goal should be to reduce the INR to a normal value, generally less than 1.3. Vitamin K can be given intravenously to patients on warfarin although correction will not occur immediatley. Fresh frozen plasma and unactivated prothrombin complex concentrates should be used to quickly correct an elevated INR. Proper amounts of products can be determined from the patient's INR and body weight, but generally, 4 to 6 units of fresh frozen plasma is needed to bring an INR in the range of 2 to 3 to less than 1.5. Laboratory values should be checked after administration to evaluate the degree of reversal and determine if more products are needed. Values should be followed serially.

For patients receiving heparin or low-molecular-weight heparin, protamine sulfate can be given to reverse a elevated partial thromboplastin time. Activated factor VII is an option. If patients are on new anticoagulant medications, activated charcoal can be given if ingestion occurred within the past 3 hours. Other therapies can be given based on the May 2012 guidance from the Thrombosis and Hemostasis Summit of North America. If patients have specific factor deficiencies or liver disease, those factors should be replaced as necessary.

In thrombocytopenic patients, platelet infusions should be given to increase the platelet count to greater than 100,000. Platelets and desmopression should be administered if antiplatelet agents (aspirin or plavix) were taken within 3 days or if platelet dysfunction (end-stage renal disease or uremia) is suspected.

Additional Neuroimaging

A postoperative CT is obtained immediately after evacuation if the patient will remain intubated and an exam cannot be immediately obtained. Evidence supports leaving drains in place for 1 to 2 days after evacuation of any kind, since recurrence rates are significant. A CT should be performed shortly after drain removal to screen for spontaneous recurrence. In addition to these two scans, there should be a low threshold for further scans in the setting of an examination change, again given the high concern for recurrence of the original hemorrhage.

Prevention and Treatment of Secondary Complications

Given the high morbidity of traumatic brain injury, intensive care, monitoring, and the prevention of secondary complications play an important role in the patient's comprehensive recovery plan. Details of intensive care unit management in neurological disease will not be covered in this book. The major factor impacting outcome in the postoperative course is recurrence, which is minimized by leaving drains in place 24 to 48 hours following the operation, restarting anticoagulation and antiplatelet medications in a delayed fashion, and preventing further trauma.

SECONDARY PREVENTION

The pillars of secondary prevention are prevention of further trauma, close follow-up, and appropriate reinitiation of anticoagulation medications. Elderly patients who are a fall risk are placed under close supervision and rehabilitation is emphasized. Anticoagulation is restarted as early as possible, weighing the indication for anticoagulation with the risk of further trauma and recurrence. There is no good evidence to guide restarting anticoagulation medication following SDH evacuation; 1 to 2 weeks is standard at our institution.

SUGGESTED READING

Brain Trauma Foundation, American Association of Neurological Surgeons, Congress of Neurological Surgeons. Guidelines for the management of severe traumatic brain injury. J. Neurotrauma 2007;24(Suppl 1):S1–106.

Markwalder TM. Chronic subdural hematomas: a review. J Neurosurg 1981;54:637–645.

Ringl H, Stiassny F, Schima W, et al. Intracranial hematomas at a glance: advanced visualization for fast and easy detection. Radiology 2013;267:522–530.

Safain M, Roguski M, Antoniou A, et al. A single center's experience with the bedside subdural evacuating port system: a useful alternative to traditional methods for chronic subdural hematoma evacuation. J Neurosurg 2013;118:694–700.

Santarius T, Kirkpatrick PJ, Ganesan D, et al. Use of drains versus no drains after burr-hole evacuation of chronic subdural haematoma: a randomised controlled trial. Lancet 2009;374:1067–1073.

Talving P, Benfield R, Hadjizacharia P, et al. Coagulopathy in severe traumatic brain injury: a prospective study. J Trauma 2009;66:55–61; discussion 61–62.

10 Cerebral Venous Thrombosis

Marco A. Gonzalez Castellon and Olajide Williams

CLINICAL FEATURES AND DIAGNOSIS

Cerebral venous thrombosis (CVT) is a rare disorder representing 0.5–1% of all strokes and affecting mainly young adults and children. The estimated annual incidence is 5 per million in adults and 7 per million in children and neonates. CVT is three times more frequent in women and complicates approximately 12 per 100,000 deliveries. The clinical presentation is highly variable depending on the location of the thrombosis within the cerebral venous sinuses. The most common symptoms are headaches (92%), focal deficits (45%), seizures (37%), and mental status changes (25%). The diagnosis of CVT should be considered in all young and middle-aged patients presenting with headache or stroke symptoms without the usual risk factors. The diagnosis of CVT is usually made with clinical suspicion and imaging confirmation. Brain MRI with magnetic resonance venography (MRV) is the gold standard for diagnosis of CVT. Computed tomography (CT), either with or without contrast, is not recommended, as it can be normal in up to 30% of patients. CT venography is as accurate as MRV and is a good alternative for patients that cannot undergo MRV. Once the diagnosis has been made, all patients should be screened for risk factors associated with CVT such as malignancy hypercoagulable state, especially thrombophilia, since approximately a third of patients will have it, either as a genetic or acquired disorder.

TREATMENT

Once the diagnosis of CVT has been made treatment should be started immediately. The goals of treatment are preventing thrombus progression, improving neurological deficits and managing complications. Table 10.1 summarizes treatment options.

Anticoagulation

Anticoagulation may be beneficial for the treatment of CVT regardless of the presence of pretreatment intracerebral hemorrhage (ICH); however, available data are inconclusive. A meta-analysis of two small randomized trials involving 79 patients showed a 13% absolute risk reduction in death or dependency at 3 months in the anticoagulation arm that did not reach statistical significance. No new ICH or increase in size was seen when comparing anticoagulation (UFH or LMWH) versus placebo. If anticoagulation

Table 10.1 Treatment of Cerebral Venous Thrombosis

Heparin	1000 to 2000 units/h
	aPTT 1.5–2.0 × control
Low Molecular Weight	Enoxaparin 1.5 mg/kg/day or 1 mg/kg q12h
Heparin	Dalteparin sodium 200 units/kg/day or 100 units/kg q12h
Thrombolysis	Urokinase bolus 100,000 to 600,000 IU followed by 100,000
	U/h infusion for 24h
	rtPA bolus 1 to 5 mg followed by 1 to 2 mg/h infusion × 24 h
Endovascular	AngioJet
treatment	Penumbra system
	Merci retrieval device
Intracranial	Acetazolamide 500 to 1000 mg daily
hypertension	Mannitol 1 g/kg as a 20% solution IV bolus
	Head of bed 30°
	Hyperventilation
Seizures	AED prophylaxis might be indicated for patients with
	supratentorial lesions for 15 days

rtPA, recombinant tissue plasminogen activator.

From Ferro JM, Canhao P. Acute treatment of cerebral venous and dural sinus thrombosis. Curr Treat Opt Neurol 2008;10:126–137.

is considered, patients should be treated with intravenous unfractionated heparin (UFH) with a goal of 2 times the baseline PTT or weight based low-molecular-weight heparin (LMWH). The European Federation of Neurological Societies (EFNS) and American Heart Association (AHA) guidelines acknowledge that LMWH has fewer hemorrhagic complications, thrombotic events, and deaths than UFH when used to treat patients with extracranial thrombosis. Regarding long-term oral anticoagulation with warfarin after the acute phase, the duration of treatment is unknown, and a paucity of data exists. Most recommendations are derived from prior experience treating venous thromboembolism and are driven by underlying risk factors and the likelihood of CVT recurrence (Table 10.2). There is no evidence that direct thrombin inhibitors (dabigatran) or factor Xa inhibitors (apixiban, rivaroxaban) are indicated for the treatment of CVT.

Antiplatelet Therapy

There are limited data on the use of antiplatelet therapy for CVT. There are no randomized data in support of antiplatelet therapy for CVT, and only anecdotal reports of use of aspirin for CVT exist.

Thrombolysis

There are no randomized trials on the benefit of thrombolysis in patients with CVT. In one systematic review in which most patients were severely ill (78% in coma), the most commonly used agent was urokinase (75%) followed by recombinant tissue plasminogen activator (22%) and streptokinase (2%). Although good functional outcomes were

Table 10.2 Risk Factors for CVST and Suggested Treatment Duration

Risk Factor for CVST	Suggested Treatment Duration
Malignancy	Indefinite or until malignancy resolves, LMWH for initial 3–6 months
Transient thrombophilic state*	3 months
Mild thrombophilia†	3–6 months
Severe thrombophilia‡	6–12 months
Oral contraceptives	3 months
Pregnancy/puerperium	LMWH for remainder of pregnancy + at least 6 weeks post-partum, total 6 months

* Dehydration, drugs, infection, trauma, surgical precipitants.

† Heterozygous prothrombin gene mutation, heterozygous factor V Leiden, high levels of factor VIII.

‡ Homozygous prothrombin gene mutation, homozygous factor V Leiden, protein C/protein S/ antithrombin III deficiency, combined thrombophilias, antiphospholipid syndrome.

From Caprio F, Bernstein RA. Duration of anticoagulation after cerebral venous sinus thrombosis. Neurocrit Care 2012;16:335–342.

reported, major complications were intracranial and extracranial hemorrhage, 17% and 21%, respectively, and death was observed in 5% of the cases. The International Study on Cerebral Vein and Dural Sinus Thrombosis (ISCVT) reports poor outcomes (death or dependency) in 38.5% of patients treated with thrombolysis at 6 months. Overall, to date, there is no concrete evidence of the safety and efficacy of thrombolytic therapy in CVT.

Endovascular Therapy

There are no randomized trials on the benefit of endovascular therapy in patients with CVT. However, anecdotal reports have shown that the use of mechanical clot retrieval devices may increase the chances of recanalization and good outcomes, although these outcomes may be overrepresented due to publication bias. Different devices have been used for endovascular therapy: AngioJet (MEDRAD, Inc., Warrendale, PA), Merci retrieval device (Concentric Medical, Mountain View, CA), and Penumbra System (Penumbra, Inc., Alameda, CA).

Intracranial Hypertension

Approximately 40% of patients with CVT will present with signs and symptoms of increased intracranial pressure, and 50% will have brain edema. Most patients will improve once the venous occlusion starts to resolve. Patients with diffuse brain edema should be treated like any other patient with elevated intracranial pressure: elevation of the head of bed to 30°, hyperventilation with a target $Paco_2$ of 30–35 mm Hg, and osmotic diuretics (i.e., mannitol 1 g/kg as 20% solution IV bolus or hypertonic saline). In patients with chronic elevated intracranial pressure, no midline shift and threatened vision, intravenous acetazolamide 500–1000 mg per day can be tried; other options include serial lumbar punctures and shunts. In patients with severe intracranial hypertension refractory to medical therapy with signs of impending herniation, hemicraniectomy should be considered, although there are no randomized trials proving the benefit of this procedure in patients with "malignant CVT."

Seizures

Approximately 40–45% of patients with CVT will experience symptomatic seizures and up to 13% can develop status epilepticus. Patients that present with seizures or develop seizures during treatment should be treated with antiepileptic drugs (AEDs). In patients that present with seizures, treatment with AEDs for 1 year may be reasonable as late seizures can occur up to 1 year after CVT. Prophylactic treatment with AED is controversial and lacks strong supporting evidence. However, some centers consider prophylactic AEDs for patients at high risk for seizures such as those with focal signs, lesions anterior to the central sulcus, and parenchymal lesions. The length of prophylaxis is variable; in most reports, AEDs were prescribed for approximately 15 days.

SUMMARY

a. Cerebral venous thrombosis is a rare cause of stroke. CVT should be considered in patients without traditional stroke risk factors with unusual territory infarcts.

b. Clinical presentation is highly variable. Symptoms can be grouped in 4 categories: isolated intracranial hypertension, focal syndrome, cavernous sinus syndrome, and sub-acute encephalopathy.

c. Anticoagulation with unfractionated heparin or low molecular weight heparin followed by long-term anticoagulation may be considered in patients with CVT although data is not conclusive.

d. Thrombolysis and mechanical thrombectomy may be considered in patients with progressive thrombosis despite anticoagulation, although data lacking.

e. Anticoagulation duration depends on the underlying etiology and usually ranges from 3 to 6 months to lifetime.

f. Hemicraniectomy may be considered as a life-saving measure in patients with impending herniation who failed to respond to medical therapy.

g. Seizures complicate up to 40% of patients with CVT. Prophylactic use of antiepileptic drugs is controversial, although use in patients who are at high risk for seizures, particularly those with supratentorial lesions, may be considered.

SUGGESTED READING

Bousser MG, Ferro JM. Cerebral venous thrombosis: an update. Lancet Neurol 2007;6:162–170.

Caprio F, Bernstein RA. Duration of anticoagulation after cerebral venous sinus thrombosis. Neurocrit Care 2012;16:335–342.

Einhaupl K, et al.; European Federation of Neurological Sciences. EFNS guideline on the treatment of cerebral venous and sinus thrombosis in adult patients. Eur J Neurol 2010;17:1229–1235.

Ferro JM, Canhao P. Acute treatment of cerebral venous and dural sinus thrombosis. Curr Treat Opt Neurol 2008;10:126–137.

Ferro JM, Canhao P, Bousser MG, et al. Early seizures in cerebral vein and dural sinus thrombosis: risk factors and role of antiepileptics. Stroke 2008;39:1152–1158.

Ferro JM, Canhao P, Stam J, et al. Prognosis of cerebral vein and dural sinus thrombosis: results of the International Study on Cerebral Vein and Dural Sinus Thrombosis (ISCVT). Stroke 2004;35:664–670.

Ferro JM, Crassard I, Coutinho JM, et al. Second International Study on Cerebral Vein and Dural Sinus Thrombosis. Decompressive surgery in cerebrovenous thrombosis: a multicenter registry and a systematic review of individual patient data. Stroke 2011;42:2825–2831

Piazza G. Cerebral venous thrombosis. Circulation 2012;125:1704–1709.

Saposnik G, Barinagarrementeria F, Brown RD, et al; American Heart Association Stroke Council on Prevention. Diagnosis and management of cerebral venous thrombosis: a statement for healthcare professionals from the American Heart Association/American Stroke Association. Stroke 2011;42:1158–1192.

Stam J. Thrombosis of the cerebral veins and sinuses. N Engl J Med 2005;352:1791–1798.

SECTION THREE

EPILEPSY AND SYNCOPE

11 Seizures and Epilepsy in Adults and Children

Rafael Toledano and Antonio Gil-Nagel

INTRODUCTION

Epileptic *seizures* are the clinical expression of excessive activation of neuronal populations or networks, with a capacity for recruitment and propagation to other neurons. Epileptic seizures are stereotyped within a particular patient and are usually self-limited. They originate from an imbalance between neuronal excitation and inhibition. *Epilepsy* is a disorder of the central nervous system (CNS), manifesting as repetitive spontaneous seizures or a single seizure in a patient with an enduring neurological disorder, which has a potential to provoke additional seizures. Most patients with recurrent seizures and some with a single seizure require chronic treatment with antiepileptic drugs (AEDs).

DIFFERENTIAL DIAGNOSIS

Diagnosis of epilepsy is based on analysis of semiology described by witnesses. However, it is not always easy to differentiate seizures from other nonepileptic paroxysmal events, even with direct observation. When diagnosis is uncertain, capturing the episodes with prolonged video-electroencephalographic (EEG) monitoring must be attempted.

Nonepileptic Conditions That Mimic Seizures

Syncope

Loss of consciousness and postural tone in syncope can be associated with convulsion-like movements, eye–head version, and symmetric or asymmetric tonic posturing, mimicking epileptic seizures. The most striking difference is the lack of confusion or amnesia after recovery of consciousness. However, lack of a postictal phase is also possible in focal seizures.

Migraine

Certain features might confound seizures and migraine. Seizures are often preceded or followed by headache, migraines and seizures may be present in the same patient, and aura in occipital migraine may mimic occipital seizures (Table 11.1).

Table 11.1 Differential Diagnosis between Migraine and Occipital Lobe Seizures

	Migraine	Epilepsy
Aura duration	Minutes to 1 h	Seconds to a few minutes
Visual aura	Flickering, uncolored zigzags, spreading peripherally, might leave scotoma	Bright, multicolored curved or rounded shapes, might arise in one hemifield and move Complex hallucinations
Headache	Usually present, unilateral, pulsating, worse on exertion, moderate or severe intensity, often with photophobia, phonophobia	Variable features, ipsilateral to seizure focus, often mild
Other semiology	Allodynia, tingling/numbness of hand that may slowly progress to ipsilateral face	Confusion, other symptoms indicating rapid propagation to different brain areas

Psychogenic Nonepileptic Seizures

Psychogenic nonepileptic seizures (PNES) are episodes of altered consciousness, movement, sensation, or experience mimicking epileptic seizures but related to a psychological process and not associated with abnormal bioelectrical activity in the brain. Several clinical features can help in the identification of PNES (Table 11.2). However, video-EEG monitoring is recommended to prove a nonepileptic origin and differentiate it from epileptic seizures, which often are also present in the same patient.

Panic Attacks

Panic attacks are periods of intense fear or apprehension, with abrupt onset and varying duration (minutes to hours). Differential diagnosis needs to be done with ictal fear and ictal panic in patients with focal epilepsy, mostly involving temporal and parietal lobes (Table 11.3).

Transient Global Amnesia

Transient global amnesia (TGA) is defined by a sudden onset of an anterograde and retrograde amnesia that lasts up to 24 hours. In TGA, there is no impairment of other cognitive functions, clouding of consciousness, or loss of personal identity. TGA should be differentiated from transient epileptic amnesia (TEA), an impairment of memory commonly seen in patients with complex partial seizures (Table 11.4).

Paroxysmal Dyskinesia

Paroxysmal dyskinesia is a movement disorder featured by brisk episodes of hyperkinetic movements such as dystonia, ballism, chorea, or a mixture of them. Movements can occur spontaneously or triggered by different stimuli. Differential diagnosis with hypermotor seizures arising from the frontal lobe and insula of the temporal pole can be challenging, since ictal EEGs are usually masked by movement artifact.

Table 11.2 Differential Diagnosis between Epileptic Seizures and PNES

Semiology	Epileptic Seizure	PNES
Ictal course		
Stereotyped nature	Yes	No
Duration	Short (<2 minutes)	Longer duration (>2 minutes)
Occurrence during sleep	Common in focal seizures	May appear patient is sleeping
Course pattern	Brisk and progressive	Waxing and waning
Motor manifestations		
Asynchronous movements	Uncommon	Common
Discontinuity	Uncommon	Common
Pelvic thrusting	Very rare (frontal seizures)	Common
Eyes	Eyes open during episode	Closed
Bites	Lateral tongue or cheek	None or tip of the tongue
Resistance to exploration	No	Yes
Emotional and autonomic manifestations		
Pupillary response	Altered	Normal
Heart rate	Elevated	Normal
Crying	Uncommon	Common
Cyanosis	Common during convulsion	No
Postictal period		
Breathing	Altered	Normal
Confusion	Common	Uncommon
Postictal fatigue	Common	No
Memory of the event	Impaired	Preserved

Table 11.3 Differential Diagnosis between Seizures and Panic Attacks

	Seizures	Panic Attacks
Duration	Short episodes of seconds to 1 min	Longer episodes of several minutes
Triggers	None	Common
History of psychiatric disorders	Less common	Common
Hyperventilation during the episode	Infrequent	Frequent
Amnesia	Frequent	Rare
EEG	Epileptiform activity but not always	Normal

Table 11.4 Differential Diagnosis between TGA and TEA

	TEA	TGA
Frequency	Multiple per year	One in the same year
Duration of episode	Minutes	Several hours
Additional signs	Automatisms, confusion, focal deficits. Other seizures types are frequent. Persistent memory difficulties after the episode	No alteration of other cognitive functions. Repetition of the same questions. Perplexity
Other features	Response to AEDs Epileptiform activity on EEG Abnormal MRI (hippocampal atrophy)	Workup is usually normal MRI can show transient focal hyperintense lesions in the hippocampus

Postconcussion Tonic Movements

This syndrome, also known as "impact seizures," is characterized by episodes of tonic stiffening and clonic movements associated with loss of consciousness with onset immediately following head trauma that can be mild.

Paroxysmal Extreme Pain Disorder

Paroxysmal extreme pain disorder (PEPD; also known as familial rectal pain) is a sodium channelopathy that affects neonates and infants. Bursts of extreme pain circumscribed to the rectal area, eyes, or mouth are triggered by local stimuli such as defecation, cold, eating, and bathing. Pain is commonly associated with tonic stiffening and variable autonomous changes.

Hyperekplexia

This is an inherited disorder characterized by excessive startle reflexes, causing falls in relation to unexpected tactile and auditory stimuli. Neonates might present with tonic stiffening caused by auditory and tactile startle. Its differential diagnosis with startle seizures and epilepsy is usually based on accompanying epileptic signs after the fall, as well as brain magnetic resonance imaging (MRI) and EEG findings, usually showing epileptogenic abnormalities on the frontal lobes or mesial frontoparietal regions.

Brainstem Stroke

Involuntary convulsive-like movements may be the presentation semiology in patients with brainstem strokes. These movements vary in nature, frequency, and trigger, including fasciculation-like, shivering, jerky, tonic-clonic, and intermittent shaking movements. It is important to recognize this type of motor phenomenon since it may be a diagnostic clue for early diagnosis and treatment of brainstem strokes, especially in patients with thrombosis of the basilar artery.

Seizures and Stroke

Inhibitory motor seizures, also known as focal akinetic seizures, originate in the peri-central area (negative motor areas) and typically manifest with ictal limb paralysis. In patients with focal brain lesions, postictal limb paralysis (Todd paralysis) is also commonly found after a first phase of focal clonic movements. Aphasia may also be the isolated manifestation on seizures that involve the dominant perisylvian region, the temporal pole and the basal temporal language area.

Seizures and Movement Disorders

The differential diagnosis between epilepsy and movement disorders is extensive, and there are some diseases in which epilepsy and movement disorders coexist. For instance, progressive myoclonic epilepsies typically show different types of movements disorders and seizures. In glucose transporter type 1 deficiency syndrome (GLUT1), patients may develop absences and dystonia. Myoclonus can have an epileptic origin and is commonly seen in different types of epilepsies that normally manifest with other types of seizures. Tremor-like jerks are seen in patients with epilepsia partialis continua. Autosomal dominant nocturnal frontal lobe epilepsy (ADNFLE) is characterized by clusters of nocturnal motor seizures that vary from simple arousals from sleep to hyperkinetic seizures with tonic or dystonic features, similar to paroxysmal hypnogenic dyskinesia. Bilateral akinetic seizures arise from the presupplementary motor area located at the mesial aspect of the frontal lobe, and their distinctive feature is the inhibition of bilateral movements giving the appearance of motor freezing. Faciobrachial dystonic seizures are the hallmark of LGI1 antibody limbic encephalitis, a type of seizure that might imitate acute dystonia and precede the onset of a forthcoming subacute confusional/amnesic state. In most cases, the clinical characteristics and typical semiology identified during prolonged video-EEG monitoring can lead to their diagnosis. Other neurophysiological tests (recording of tremor, back-averaging, evoked potentials) can be of help in some cases.

Seizures and Parasomnias

Parasomnias or Non-REM (NREM) behaviour disorder are unpleasant or undesirable behavioral or experiential phenomena that occur predominantly or exclusively during sleep. Within this group of diseases, it might be difficult to make the differential diagnosis between nocturnal frontal lobe seizures and parasomnias with prominent motor behaviors (Table 11.5).

PHARMACOLOGICAL TREATMENT

When Should Treatment Be Started?

The recommendation to initiate treatment after a seizure is based on the risk of seizure recurrence, the severity of the episode, potential side effects of antiepileptic drugs (AEDs), working/social consequences of seizure recurrence, and preferences of the patient.

Table 11.5 Differential Diagnosis between NREM Arousal Disorders and Nocturnal Frontal Lobe Epilepsy (NFLE)

	NREM arousal disorders	NFLE
Age at onset	<10 y	Childhood-adolescence
Family history	60%–90%	<40%
Frequency of episodes	1–3 per month	Many episodes per month, clustering is common
Episode duration	Seconds to 30 min	<2 min
Evolution	Tends to disappear by adolescence	Continuous over years although stable with increasing age
Trigger factors	Alcohol, fever, stress	Not common
Sleep stage at onset	NREM III–IV, usually after 90 min of sleep	NREM II, usually within the first 90 min–2 h of sleep
Semiology	Variable complexity; not highly stereotyped; usually not recall	Highly stereotyped on video monitoring; hyperkinetic movement; there might be recall of the event
EEG	Normal (arousal)	Epileptiform in 50% of patients

Around 50% of patients with a first unprovoked seizure who are not treated will never have a second seizure. The risk of recurrence is about 44% in the first 6 months after the first seizure and thereafter falls to 17% in the second year. If two or more seizures had occurred, the risk of further events increases to 80%. The risk is higher in patients with structural brain disease, abnormal neurological exploration, mental retardation, epileptiform activity on the EEG, and, in particular, epilepsy syndromes. AED therapy prevents or reduces the risk of seizure recurrence during its use but does not modify long-term evolution of the disease.

Overall treatment is indicated in the following scenarios:

1. After two seizures, if their severity is relevant for the patient and the interval between them is short (1 to 2 years).
2. After one seizure when the risk of recurrence is high, such as when there is a brain tumor or cortical dysplasia, or a recognizable syndrome associated with a high rate of recurrence (e.g., juvenile myoclonic epilepsy or nocturnal frontal lobe epilepsy), and when the consequences of recurrence are not tolerable.

Selection of AEDs is based principally in the evidence of efficacy in different seizure types and epileptic syndromes, adverse event profile, drug interactions, patient characteristics, and existing comorbidities (Tables 11.6 through 11.13).

Failure of Initial Treatment

Antiepileptic treatment can result in seizure freedom for 60% to 70% of patients. In those who seizure freedom is not reached, subsequent steps in treatment will be led by the cause of the failure:

Table 11.6 Mechanism of Action and Pharmacokinetic Properties of AEDs

AED	Primary Mode(s) of Action	Oral Bioavailability (%) Protein binding (% bound)	Clearance route Elimination Half-life (h)	Active Metabolites Clinically Significant Target Serum Concentration (mcgr/mL)
Carbamazepine (CBZ)	Blocks fast-inactivated state of Na+ channel	75–80 70–80	>95% Hepatic 8–24	CBZ-epoxide 4–12
Clobazam (CLB)	Activates GABAA receptor	90–100 87–90	>95% Hepatic 10–30	N-Demethylclobazam
Clonazepam (CLN)	Activates GABAA receptor	80–90 80–90	>95% Hepatic 7–56	
Eslicarbazepine acetate (ESL)	Blocks fast and possibly slow-inactivate state of Na+ channel	90 40	60% Hepatic 40% Renal 13–20	
Ethosuximide (ETH)	Blocks low-voltage–activated Ca2+ channel	90–95 0	65% Hepatic 20–60	40–100
Felbamate (FBM)	Various actions on multiple targets	95–100 22–36	50% Hepatic 50% Renal 13–23	
Gabapentine (GBP)	Blocks high-voltage–activated Ca2+ channel	60 0	100% Renal 6–9	
Lacosamide (LCM)	Blocks slow-inactivated state of Na+ channel	95–100 <15	60% Hepatic 40% Renal 13	

(continued)

Table 11.6 Continued

AED	Primary Mode(s) of Action	Oral Bioavailability (%) Protein binding (% bound)	Clearance route Elimination Half-life (h)	Active Metabolites Clinically Significant Target Serum Concentration (mcgr/mL)
Lamotrigine (LTG)	Blocks fast-inactivated state of Na^+ channel/other mechanisms	95–100 55	90% Hepatic 22–36	2.5–15
Levetiracetam (LEV)	Modulates synaptic vesicle protein 2A	95–100 <10	66% Renal 7–9	
Oxcarbazepine (OXC)	Blocks fast-inactivated state of Na^+ channel	95–100 40 (active metabolite)	45% Hepatic 45% Renal 8–10 (active metabolite)	Monohydroxylated active metabolite of OXC
Perampanel (PER)	AMPA glutamate receptor antagonist	90–100 95	Hepatic and renal 105	Multiple
Phenobarbital (PB)	Activates $GABA_A$ receptor	95–100 48–54	75% Hepatic 25% Renal 72–144	10–40
Phenytoin (PHT)	Blocks fast-inactivated state of Na^+ channel	85–90 90–93	>95% Hepatic 9–40	10–20
Pregabalin (PGB)	Blocks high-voltage–activated Ca^{2+} channel	90–100 0	100% Renal 6	
Primidone (PRM)	Activates $GABA_A$ receptor	90–100 20–30	50% Hepatic 50% Renal 4–12	Phenobarbital 5–10

Retigabine (RTG)	Opens Kv7 K⁺ channel	60	<80	60% Hepatic, 20–30% Renal	6–10	
Rufinamide (RFM)	Sodium channel blockade (fast inactivation) others	85	34	>95% Hepatic	6–10	
Tiagabine (TGB)	Blocks synaptic GABA reuptake	95–100	96	>90% Hepatic	5–9	
Topiramate (TPM)	Various actions on multiple targets	80	9–17	30–50% Hepatic, 50–70% renal	20–24	
Valproic acid (VPA)	Various actions on multiple targets	100	88–92	>95% Hepatic	7–17	50–100
Vigabatrin (VGB)	Inhibits GABA transaminase activity	60–80	0	100% Renal	5–7	0.8–36
Zonisamide (ZNS)	Various actions on multiple targets	95–100	40–60	>90% Hepatic	50–68	10–40

Enzyme-inducing antiepileptic drugs (EIAEDs): PHT, PHB, CBZ, PRM.

AMPA, α-amino-3-hydroxy-5-methyl-4-isoxazolepropionic acid; GABA, γ-aminobutyric acid.

Table 11.7 Usual Dosage and Frequency of Administration of Currently Available AEDs

AED	Initial Dosage	Titration Rate	Maintenance Dose
Carbamazepine	A: 100–200 mg/d C: 4 mg/kg/d	Increase to target dose over 1–4 wk	A: 400–1600 mg (2–3 doses) C: 20–30 mg/kg/d (2–3 doses)
Clobazam	A: 5–15 mg/d C: 0.25–1 mg/kg/d	Increase to target dose over 1–3 wk	A: 10–40 mg (1–3 doses) C: 0.5–1 mg/kg/d (1–3 doses)
Clonazepam	A: 0.25 mg/d C: 0.95 mg/kg/d	Increase to target dose over 1–3 wk	A: 0.5–4 mg (1–3 doses) C: 0.1–0.2 mg/kg/d (1–3 doses)
Eslicarbazepine acetate	A: 400 mg/d	Increase to target dose over 1–2 wk	A: 400–1200 mg (1 dose)
Ethosuximide	A: 250 mg/d C: 10 mg/kg/d	Increase to target dose over 1–4 wk	A: 500–2000 mg (2–3 doses) C: 20–30 mg/kg/d (1–3 doses)
Felbamate	A: 600 mg/d C: 15 mg/kg/d	Increase to target dose over 2–3 wk	A: 1600–3600 mg (3–4 doses) C: 30–45 mg/kg/d (2 doses)
Gabapentin	A: 300–900 mg/d C: 5–10 mg/kg/d	Increase to target dose over 1–2 wk	A: 900–3600 mg (3 doses) C: 20–100 mg/kg/d (2–3 doses)
Lacosamide	A: 100 mg/d C: 1 mg/kg/d	Increase to target dose over 1–4 wk	A: 200–400 mg (2–3 doses) C: 2–10 mg/kg/d
Lamotrigine	Monotherapy A: 25 mg/d C: 0.5 mg/kg/d With valproate A: 25 mg on alternate days C: 0.15 mg/kg/d With EIAEDs A: 25–50 mg/d C: 0.5 mg/kg/d	Monotherapy (A) 25 mg 1st–2nd wk 50 mg 3rd–4th wk 50 mg/d every 1–2 wk With valproate (A) 25 mg on alternate days 1st–2nd wk 25 mg 3rd–4th wk 25–50 mg/d every 1–2 wk With EIAEDs (A) 25–50 mg 1st–2nd wk	Monotherapy A: 100–400 mg (2 doses) C: 2–10 mg/kg/d (2 doses) With valproate A: 100–250 mg (2 doses) C: 1–5 mg/kg/d (2 doses) With EIAEDs A: 200–500 mg (2 doses) C: 5–15 mg/kg/d (2 doses)

50–100 mg 3rd–4th wk
50–100 mg/d every 1–2 wk

Drug	Starting dose	Titration	Target/maintenance dose
Levetiracetam	A: 250–500 mg/d C: 5 mg/kg/d	Increase to target dose over 1–2 wk	A: 1000–3000 mg (2–3 doses) C: 20–60 mg/kg/d (2–3 doses)
Oxcarbazepine	A: 300–600 mg/d C: 5–10 mg/kg/d	Increase to target dose over 1–3 wk	A: 600–2400 mg (2–3 doses) C: 30–50 mg/kg/d (2–3 doses)
Perampanel	A: 2–4 mg C: 2 mg	Increase by 2 mg/wk, to target dose	A: 4–12 mg (1 dose) C: 2–8 mg (1 dose)
Phenobarbital	A: 50–100 mg/d C: 3 mg/kg/d	Increase to target dose over 2 wk	A: 50–200 mg (1–2 doses) C: 3–5 mg/kg/d (1–2 doses)
Phenytoin	A: 50–100 mg/d C: 5 mg/kg/d	Increase to target dose over 1–2 wk	A: 100–400 mg (2–3 doses) C: 5–10 mg/kg/d (2–3 doses)
Pregabaline	A: 75–150 mg/d	Increase to target dose over 2–4 wk	A: 150–600 mg (2–3 doses)
Primidone	A: 62.5–125 mg/d C: 10 mg/kg/d	Increase to target dose over 3–4 wk	A: 500–1500 mg (2–3 doses) C: 20 mg/kg/d (2–3 doses)
Retigabine	A: 100–300 mg/d	Increase to target dose over 3–4 wk	A: 600–1200 mg (3 doses)
Rufinamide	A: 200–400 mg/d C: 5 mg/kg/d	Increase to target dose over 1–2 wk	A: 400–3200 mg (2 doses) C: 45 mg/kg/d (2 doses) Maximum dose of 1000 mg <30 kg Maximum dose of 600 mg <30 kg with VPA
Tiagabine	A: 2.5–5 mg/d C: 0–25 mg/kg/d	Increase to target dose over 1–3 wk	A: 15–50 mg (2–3 doses) C: 0.5–2 mg/kg/d (2 doses)
Topiramate	A: 25–50 mg/d C: 0.5–1 mg/kg/d	Increase to target dose over 2–4 wk	A: 100–400 mg (2 doses) C: 2–10 mg/kg/d (2 doses)
Valproic acid	A: 200–500 mg/d C: 10 mg/kg/d	Increase to target dose over 1–4 wk	A: 400–2500 mg (2–3 doses) C: 15–40 mg/kg/d (2–3 doses)
Vigabatrin	A: 250–500 mg/d C: 50 mg/kg/d	Increase to target dose over 1–2 wk	A: 1000–3000 mg (2–3 doses) C: 100–150 mg/kg/d (2 doses)
Zonisamide	A: 50 mg/d C: 2 mg/kg/d	Increase to target dose over 2–4 wk	A: 100–500 mg (1–3 doses) C: 4–12 mg/kg/d (2 doses)

Table 11.8 Efficacy Spectrum of the Main Antiepileptic Drugs in Different Seizure Types

Effective against Focal Seizures and Some Generalized Seizure Types	Primarily Effective Against Focal Seizures, with or without Secondary Generalization
Benzodiazepines	Carbamazepine
Broad spectrum	*May worsen absence and myoclonic seizures*
Ethosuximide	Eslicarbazepine acetate
Effective against absence seizures.	
Ineffective against focal and GTC seizures.	
Felbamate	Oxcarbazepine
Effective against focal seizures and drop attacks associated with Lennox-Gastaut syndrome	*May worsen absence and myoclonic seizures*
Lamotrigine	Gabapentin
Broad spectrum, also effective against drop attacks associated with Lennox-Gastaut syndrome	*May worsen myoclonic seizures*
May worsen myoclonic seizures	
Levetiracetam	Lacosamide
Broad spectrum	
Phenobarbital	Perampanel
Ineffective against absence seizures	
Primidone	Phenytoin
Ineffective against absence seizures	*May worsen absence and myoclonic seizures*
Topiramate	Pregabalin
Broad spectrum, also effective against drop attacks associated with Lennox-Gastaut syndrome	*May worsen myoclonic seizures*
Zonisamide	Retigabine
Broad spectrum	
Rufinamide	Tiagabine
Focal seizures and Drop attacks associated with Lennox-Gastaut syndrome	*May worsen absence and myoclonic seizures*
Valproic acid	Vigabatrin
Broad spectrum	*May worsen absence and myoclonic seizures*

1. Reassessing of initial diagnosis and compliance.
2. Increasing the dose of AED if there was an initial response and no side effects.
3. Switching to another monotherapy if the cause of the failure is toxicity.
4. In case of lack of response proceed to either substitution of the initial AEDs or therapy with two drugs. The later might be recommended if there was a partial response to the first AED (Figure 11.1).
   1. It might be necessary to reduce the dose of the first AED to improve tolerability.

Table 11.9 Selection of AEDs Taking into Account Comorbidities

Comorbidity	AEDs that Can Aggravate Condition	AEDs that Can Improve Condition
Acne	Phenytoin, lamotrigine	
Alopecia	Valproic acid	
Anorexia	Topiramate, zonisamide	Vigabatrin, valproic acid, gabapentin, pregabalin
Anxiety		Benzodiazepines, gabapentin, pregabalin
Cardiac (arrhythmias)	Carbamazepine, lacosamide, retigabine, rufinamide	
Diabetes	Valproic acid	
Hepatic insufficiency	Benzodiazepines, EIAEDs, lamotrigine, valproic acid	AEDs without hepatic metabolism are preferable
HIV	EIAEDs	
Hyponatremia	Carbamazepine, oxcarbazepine, eslicarbazepine acetate	
Insomnia	Lamotrigine	
Migraine		Lamotrigine, topiramate, valproic acid, zonisamide
Mood disorders	Levetiracetam, phenobarbital, topiramate, vigabatrin, zonisamide *(depression and psychotic episodes)*	Carbamazepine, lamotrigine, valproic acid *(mood stabilizers)* Topiramate *(impulsivity)*
Neuropathic pain		Carbamazepine, gabapentin, lamotrigine, oxcarbazepine, pregabalin, topiramate, zonisamide?
Obesity	Gabapentin, pregabalin, valproic acid, vigabatrin	Topiramate, zonisamide
Osteoporosis	EIAEDs, valproic acid	
Parkinsonism	Valproic acid	
Renal calculi		Topiramate, zonisamide *(especially if combined with ketogenic diet)*
Renal insufficiency	AEDs with renal elimination require dose adjustment Levetiracetam, gabapentine, pregabalin	
Restless leg syndrome		Benzodiazepines, pregabalin
Tumors	EIAEDs *(interaction with chemotherapy)*	Valproic acid *(might improve survival in brain tumors)*
Tremor	Valproic acid *(especially if combined with lamotrigine)*	Primidone, pregabalin, topiramate, zonisamide

EIAEDs: Enzyme-inducing antiepileptic drugs.

Table 11.10 Dose-Related Side Effects Associated with Individual AEDs

Arrhythmias	CBZ, PHT, LCM, and RTG
Hyponatremia and water intoxication	CBZ and OXC
Metabolic acidosis, paresthesias, oligohidrosis	ZNS and TPM
Macrocitosis and anemia in relation to folate deficiency	CBZ, PHT, and PB
Tremor	VPA
Leukopenia	CBZ and PHT
Thrombocytopenia and abnormal platelet function	VPA
Insomnia	LTG and PB
Urinary retention	RTG

CBZ, carbamazepine; CLB, clobazam; LCM, lacosamide; LTG, lamotrigine; OXC, oxcarbazepine; PB, phenobarbital; PHT, phenytoin; RTG, retigabine; TPM, topiramate; VPA, valproic acid; ZNS, zonisamide.

2. Polytherapy might be indicated from the beginning in patients with epileptic syndromes that are usually associated with high rates of refractoriness

Refractory Epilepsy

Drug-resistant epilepsy, which affects approximately 30% of patients, is considered in case of failure to achieve complete seizure control after adequate trial of two appropriate and well-tolerated AEDs, given alone or in combination. In this case, patients should be evaluated to establish the diagnosis of epilepsy, the type of epilepsy, and the possibility of epilepsy surgery. Chances of reaching remission diminish accordingly to the number of drugs taken; however, further AED changes may improve seizure frequency or severity.

Treatment in Special Conditions

Elderly

Focal epilepsies are the most common in the elderly patient; seizures are usually milder and more difficult to identify; and response to AEDs is higher than in other age groups. Because cerebrovascular disease is the most common cause of epilepsy in the elderly, patients presenting with seizures at this age should have a cardiovascular workout. Age-related physiological changes, namely hypoalbuminemia, reduction of hepatic and renal drug clearance, and CNS changes contribute to increase toxicity to AEDs. Sedation and cognitive difficulties are among the most common and preventable adverse events. Cognitive adverse events are more pronounced with barbiturates, benzodiazepines, topiramate, and other drugs given at high dose (levetiracetam, carbamacepine, and valproid acid). Lower daily doses and slower titration schedules decrease the risk of CNS-related side effects.

Pediatric Age

Most of the principles followed when treating adult patients apply to children. The epileptic syndrome will guide the choice of the AED and monotherapy will prevail over polytherapy when possible. Despite these common criteria, as the pharmacokinetics

Table 11.11 Acute Idiosyncratic Side Effects Associated with Individual AEDs

Cutaneous reactions	*High risk:* PHT, LTG, CBZ *Moderate risk:* ZNS, PB, CLB, OXC, TGB *Low risk:* LEV, GBP, VPA, FBM, TPM, VGB, PRM, LCM, RTG From minor cutaneous reactions to Stevens-Johnson syndrome or toxic epidermal necrolysis. More common if there are antecedents of similar reactions with other drugs.
Hepatotoxicity	VPA, FBM Age younger than 2 y, polytherapy with enzyme-inducing AEDs, inborn errors of metabolism, previous hepatic disease, and mental retardation have been identified as risk factors. Routine biochemical monitoring is not efficient for screening idiosyncratic hepatic reactions. Unfortunately, there is no correlation with serum levels of this drug.
Hematological toxicity	FBM: Aplastic anemia (around 127 cases per 1 million users) CBZ: Aplastic anemia (5–20 cases per 1 million users) CBZ and PHT: agranulocitosis
Psychiatric adverse events	PB, benzodiazepines, and LEV: Irritability, hyperactivity, and anxiety. TPM, TGB, VGB, LEV, PHT: Increased rates of psychotic and depressive episodes. Psychiatric adverse events are not exclusive of any particular AED and should be taken into account in any patient who develops these symptoms independently of the AED that he/she might be taking. Rapid-dose escalation, previous personal or family psychiatric history, and refractory epilepsy have all been found to increase the risk of affective and psychotic symptoms in patients taking AEDs
Paradoxical aggravation of seizures	PHT, CBZ, and OXC: Absences, myoclonic, atonic, tonic seizures PHB: Absences VGB, TGB, GBP, and PGB: Absences and myoclonus CBZ, PHB, and LTG: Benign focal epilepsy of childhood Benzodiazepines: Tonic status in LGS CBZ, LTG: Epileptic encephalopathy with continuous spike-and-wave during sleep/Landau-Kleffner syndrome CBZ, PHT: Progressive myoclonic epilepsies Exacerbation of seizures as an expression of a "paradoxical reaction" occurs when an AED increases the frequency of seizures, changes the pattern, and/or provokes new seizure types in individuals with seizure disorders expected to be responsive to the therapeutic effect of the AED. AEDs associated with the greatest risk of worsening seizures are those with a single mechanism of action, either GABAergic enhancement or blockade of Na^+ channels. Broad-spectrum AEDs, particularly VPA, appear to have a low potential for seizure aggravation.
Other idiosyncratic reactions	VPA: pancreatitis TPM: Acute myopia and secondary angle closure glaucoma RTG: blue discoloration of skin and retina

CBZ, carbamazepine; CLB, clobazam; FBM, felbamate; GBP, gabapentine; LCM, lacosamide; LEV, levetiracetam; LTG, lamotrigine; OXC, oxcarbazepine; PB, phenobarbital; PHT, phenytoin; PRM, primidone; RTG, retigabine; TGB, tiagabine; TPM, topiramate; VGB, vigabatrin; VPA, valproic acid; ZNS, zonisamide.

Table 11.12 Most Common Chronic Adverse Events

Changes in body weight	*Weight gain:* PGB, GBP, CBZ, VGB, and principally with VPA Clinical variables such as gender, age, dose, and pretreatment body weight have failed to identify those patients at a higher risk for weight gain. When managing VPA-induced weight gain, dietary restriction and regular exercise appear not to be sufficient, and changing VPA to a weight-neutral AED is the preferable option when it is possible *Weigh loss:* FBM, ZNS, and most commonly with TPM The degree of TPM-associated weight loss correlates both with pretreatment weight and with the dose employed.
Bone health	PHT, PHB, CBZ, and VPA have been associated with a higher risk of fractures, osteoporosis, and rickets. Although controversial, periodic bone health screening (biochemical markers such as serum calcium, phosphate, PTH, and 25-OHD as well as follow-up bone densitometry) and supplementary treatment with biphosphonates, calcium, and/or high doses of vitamin D should be considered from the beginning when using AEDs that induce cytochrome P450.
Sexual and reproduction function	PHT, CBZ, barbiturates, and VPA: men on these AEDs suffer most commonly from higher rates of sexual dysfunction caused by disturbances of reproductive endocrine function. Women on VPA are at a higher risk for menstrual disorders, hyperandrogenism, and possibly for polycystic ovary syndrome.
Visual impairment	VGB: Bilateral peripheral reduction of visual fields with sparing of visual acuity; patients generally do not report visual deterioration. In patients on this AED regular visual peripheral screening is mandatory.
Other chronic adverse events	ZNS, TPM: kidney stones PHT, CBZ, GBP: dystonia and paroxysmal movement disorders VPA: parkinsonism PHT: cerebellar atrophy, gingival hyperplasia PHB: connective disorders such us frozen shoulder, Dupuytren's contractures, palmar nodules, and joint pain

CBZ, carbamazepine; CLB, clobazam; FBM, felbamate; GBP, gabapentine; LCM, lcaosamide; LEV, levetiracetam; LTG, lamotrigine; OXC, oxcarbazepine; PB, phenobarbital; PHT, phenytoin; PRM, primidone; RTG, retigabine; TGB, tiagabine; TPM, topiramate; VGB, vigabatrin; VPA, valproic acid; ZNS, zonisamide.

of AEDs change with age, one will have to adjust doses over time; the absorption and metabolism of many AEDs are usually faster in infants and young children, thus requiring higher doses per unit of weight.

Table 11.13 Interactions between AEDs

Current AED	Effect of the Added AED over the First Drug	Clinical Implications
Carbamazepine	⇓ EIAEDs, ↓OXC, ↓FBM, ↓ ZNS, ⇑VPA	1. Lower serum concentrations of CBZ with EIAEDs. There can be at the same time a increase of CBZ-10, 11-epoxide, an active metabolite responsible of toxicity with normal/low concentration of CBZ 2. Inhibition of CBZ-10, 11-epoxide metabolism by VPA, with higher risk of toxicity by this metabolite with normal values of CBZ
Clobazam	⇓ EIAEDs ⇑ Stiripentol	1. Lower serum concentration of CBZ 2. EIAEDs increase N-desmethyl-CLB, an active metabolite and can produce toxicity with low/normal concentration of CLB 3. Stiripentol increases serum concentration of CBZ, increasing the risk of toxicity
Clonazepam	⇓EIAEDs	Lower serum concentration of CZP
Eslicarbazepine acetate	↓EIAEDs	Not significant interactions
Ethosuximide	⇓EIAEDs, ↓↑ VPA	Lower serum concentration of ESM with EIAEDs
Felbamate	⇓EI, ↑ VPA, ↑GBP	Lower serum concentration of FBM with EIAEDs
Gabapentine	—	Not significant interactions
Lacosamide	↓EIAEDs	Not significant interactions
Lamotrigine	⇓EIAEDs, ↓ OXC, ⇑VPA	1. Lower serum concentration of LTG with EIAEDs 2. VPA inhibits metabolism of LTG increasing the risk of toxicity by LTG
Levetiracetam	↓EIAEDs	Not significant interactions
Oxcarbazepine	↓EIAEDs	Not significant interactions
Perampanel	↓EIAEDs	Lower serum concentration of PER
Phenobarbital	⇑VPA, ⇑FBM, ↑OXC, ↑stiripentol, ↑PHT	Higher serum concentration of PB when added VPA or FBM, increasing the risk of toxicity by PB
Phenytoin	↑ RFM, ↑↓ EIAEDs, ↑OXC, ↑TPM, ⇑FBM, ↓VGB, ↓VPA	1. Interactions difficult to predict with other EIAEDs 2. VPA displaces protein binding of PHT increasing the serum free fraction with a higher risk of toxicity by PHT with "total" serum concentration within the limits
Pregabalin	↓EIAEDs	Not significant interactions

Table 11.13 Continued

Current AED	Effect of the Added AED over the First Drug	Clinical Implications
Primidone	⇓EIAEDs	Lower serum concentration of PRM with a increase of it metabolite PB, therefore there is higher risk of toxicity by PB
Retigabine	↓EIAEDs	Not significant interactions
Rufinamide	↓EIAEDs, ⇑VPA	Increase of serum concentration of RFM when associated with VPA (specially in children <30 kg of weight)
Tiagabine	⇓EIAEDs	Lower serum concentration of TGB
Topiramate	⇓EIAEDs, ↓VPA	Lower serum concentration of TPM.
Valproate	⇓EIAEDs, ↓ETM, ↓TPM, ⇑FBM, ↑stiripentol	Lower serum concentration of VPA
Vigabatrin	—	Not significant interactions
Zonisamide	⇓EIAEDs	Lower serum concentration of ZNS

EIAED, enzyme-inducing antiepileptic drug; CBZ, carbamazepine; CLB, clobazam; FBM, felbamate; GBP, gabapentine; LCM, lcaosamide; LEV, levetiracetam; LTG, lamotrigine; OXC, oxcarbazepine; PB, phenobarbital; PHT, phenytoin; PRM, primidone; RTG, retigabine; TGB, tiagabine; TPM, topiramate; VGB, vigabatrin; VPA, valproic acid; ZNS, zonisamide.

⇓⇑: Clinically significant decrease/increase of the serum concentration of the first AED when a second AED is added.

↓↑: Not clinically significant decrease/increase of the serum concentration of the first AED when a second AED is added.

Women

Pregnancy

The mayor points in the treatment of women of child-bearing potential are based in general principles and AED use and selection.

a. General principles
   - Plan pregnancy in advance and discuss risk of unwanted pregnancy in all women of childbearing potential.
   - Supplementation with folic acid of higher 3 mg/d to reduce the risk of major birth defects.
   - Monitor serum AED levels at the beginning of pregnancy and during it to establish the individual therapeutic range that might guide dose adjustment in case there are breakthrough seizures or toxicity.
   - In women on Enzyme-inducing AEDs, vitamin K 20 mg/wk after the 34th week of pregnancy might reduce the risk of hemorrhage in both the mother and the neonate.

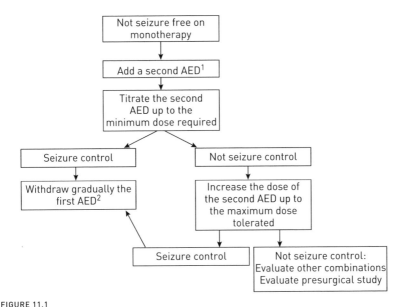

FIGURE 11.1

Treatment algorithm in patients in whom there is failure of initial treatment.

1. It might be necessary to reduce the dose of the first AED to improve tolerability.

2. Polytherapy might be indicated from the beginning in patients with epileptic syndromes that are usually associated with high rates of refractoriness.

b. AED selection and use during pregnancy
  - Simplify to monotherapy antiepileptic treatment if epilepsy has been controlled easily over the years and there are no risk factors of recurrence.
  - Use AEDs at their minimal effective dose, based on prescription information or on the patient's past history when available.
  - Low dose of lamotrigine (<300 mg/d) and low dose of carbamazepine (<400 mg/d) are the safest AEDs with an overall risk comparable to that of women not taking AEDs (risk of 2% and 3.4%, respectively).
  - Valproic acid is associated with the highest risk of teratogenicity when used in polytherapy or with doses higher than 700 mg/d (5.6% for a dose <700 mg, 10.4% for 700 to <1500 mg, and 24.2% for >1500 mg). Children of women who took valproic acid during pregnancy had also lower intelligence quotients.
  - Based on some studies, topiramate is associated with a high risk while levetiracetam might be associated with a low risk of congenital malformations.

Breastfeeding

AEDs pass into breast milk in levels that are inversely proportional to the serum protein binding. However, breastfeeding in women with epilepsy is not contraindicated as the benefits of it are much higher that the possible effects of AEDs on the newborn. The most common side effects in the newborn are sedation and irritability, especially with barbiturates and benzodiazepines. Night breastfeeding should be avoided if lack of sleep is a trigger for seizures.

Contraception

EIAEDs, oxcarbamazepine, eslicarbazepine acetate, and topiramate (>400 mg/d) reduce the efficacy of oral contraceptives. Women taking these AEDs together with oral contraceptives should use formulations containing at least 50 mcg of ethinyl estradiol and/or barrier methods. If injections of depot medroxyprogesterone acetate are used, they should be administered at shorter intervals (10 weeks instead of the usual 12 weeks).

Polycystic Ovary Syndrome

The endocrine disorder polycystic ovary syndrome (PCOS), characterized by ovulatory dysfunction and hyperandrogenism, has a higher prevalence in women with epilepsy. The risk of developing PCOS is higher in patients on valproic acid and is usually reversible on withdrawal of this AED.

When to Withdraw Antiepileptic Treatment

Withdrawal of AEDs needs to be individualized based on the epileptic syndrome, the characteristics of the patient, and the repercussion of recurrence on the patient. In general, discontinuation of treatment is considered after 2 to 5 years of seizure freedom. Overall, the probability of remaining seizure free after AED withdrawal at 2 years is around 61% to 91% for children and 35% to 57% for adults. The risk of recurrence is increased in patients with symptomatic epilepsies, focal seizures, and certain epileptic syndromes such as juvenile myoclonic epilepsies. Once the decision of AED discontinuation is taken, if the patient is on monotherapy the general recommendation is to gradually withdraw the AED over a period of 2 to 3 months (longer than 6 months when discontinuing barbiturates and benzodiazepines). When the patient is on polytherapy, withdrawal will take longer and must be sequential: the first AED to be removed will be the AED associated with more side-effects and/or the AED that is lest efficacious. In a second step the last AED introduced that controlled seizure will be eliminated. Recurrence of seizures should be managed by restoring the last AED which controlled seizures, however there is group of patients in whom reinstitution of the same treatment will not control seizure as well as before.

STATUS EPILEPTICUS

Definition

Status epilepticus (SE) is defined as a seizure that persists for a sufficient length of time, or repeated frequently enough, that recovery between attacks does not occur; it is usually defined as 30 or more minutes of ongoing or recurrent seizures without recovery to baseline state. However, a lower limit of 5 minutes has been set for practical reasons, to initiate treatment before CNS damage has occurred, and because most of generalized tonic-clonic seizures usually subside before, while the risk of continuous seizures increases substantially beyond this 5-minute cutoff. Refractory SE (RSE) refers to SE that persists despite adequate administration of benzodiazepines and at least one AED. SE is the second most frequent neurological emergency, with an annual incidence of

Table 11.14 Classification of Status Epilepticus (SE)

*With motor symptoms**	*Nonconvulsive SE (NCSE)†*	*Boundary syndromes‡*
– Convulsive SE (tonic-clonic seizures) – Myoclonic SE – Focal motor (including epilepsia partialis continua) – Hyperkinetic SE	Degree of unresponsiveness: 1. NCSE with coma 2. NCSE without coma – Generalized: • Typical absence status • Atypical absence status myoclonic absence status – Focal: • Aura continua • With vegetative symptoms • With sensory symptoms • With visual symptoms • With olfactory symptoms • With gustatory symptoms • With emotional symptoms • Aphasic SE • SE with dyscognitive symptoms	– Epileptic encephalopathy – Acute forms of coma with status-like EEG pattern – Epileptic behavioral disturbance and psychosis – Drug-induced or metabolic confusional state with epileptiform EEG changes

*The type of seizure defines the type of SE.

†NCSE has been defined as "an enduring epileptic condition with reduced or altered consciousness, behavioral and vegetative abnormalities, or merely subjective symptoms without major convulsive movements."

‡Boundary syndromes are conditions in which it is not clear to what extent the symptoms are explained by the continuous epileptiform activity. In this group of patients it might be difficult to distinguish whether impairment of alertness is solely caused by the current disease of precipitated by NCSE.

10 to 40 per 100.000 population. SE is associated with a high morbidity and mortality. Around 15% of patients with epilepsy have had an episode of SE during their disease, and it is the first clinical manifestation in 12% of epilepsy patients.

Types

SE is clinically classified based on the presence/absence of motor symptoms as well as the preservation/impairment of consciousness. According to these criteria, three main categories have been proposed (see Table 11.14).

Prognosis

The prognosis depends on the type of SE, etiology, duration, level of consciousness at presentation, and age of onset. Mortality is up to 20% in SE lasting longer than 1 hour. Mortality rates for RSE have been estimated to be between 16% and 39%; mortality after RSE is about three times higher than that for non-RSE. The likelihood of a return to baseline clinical conditions after convulsive RSE is as low as 20%. The risk of epilepsy after an incident symptomatic SE event, especially if refractory, is three times higher than that after a first symptomatic seizure. On the other extreme, SE caused by sudden AED withdrawal is less devastating and not necessarily associated with neuropsychological damage. Prognosis in nonconvulsive *status epilepticus* (NCSE) is less clear and mainly associated with the cause of it.

Management

Treatment of SE should be tailored according to the type of status and the cause. There is general consensus that NCSE without coma such as absence SE and other forms of focal NCSE may be managed less aggressively than tonic-clonic SE. Most of these patients will respond to a loading dose of AEDs. In patients with previous history of idiopathic generalized epilepsy (IGE), intravenous valproate and benzodiazepines are the preferred drugs. In patients with focal NCSE, phenytoin and levetiracetam can also be selected. On the other hand, convulsive SE should be considered as a life-threatening condition, requiring a more rapid and aggressive management; all common measures for intensive care treatment need to be implemented at the beginning of the status. At the same time, an extensive workup is mandatory to identify the cause of the SE and to rule out medical conditions that might require specific treatment (e.g., electrolyte alterations, hypoglycemia, ketoacidosis, CNS infections, brain tumor, stroke). In convulsive SE, there is a general agreement of a stage-approach management:

Stage 1: Stage of early status (5 to 10 minutes). Choose among the following benzodiazepines:
  a) Lorazepam: intravenous bolus 0.1 mg/kg *pediatric dose*; 0.007 mg/kg (usually 4 mg) *adult dose*
  b) Diazepam: intravenous bolus 0.25 to 0.5 mg/kg *pediatric dose*; 10 to 20 mg *adult dose*
  c) Clonazepam: intravenous bolus 200 to 500 mcg *pediatric dose*; 1 to 2 mg *adult dose*
  d) Midazolam: intramuscular 5 mg *pediatric dose* (or 0.3 mg/kg to a maximum of 10 mg); 10 mg *adult dose*
     – Buccal/intranasal midazolam (0.5 mg/kg) or rectal diazepam (0.5 mg/kg) might be specially indicated in patients with frequent clusters of seizures and prolonged seizures that could evolve to SE.

Stage 2: Stage of established status (10 to 30 minutes). Choose among:
  a) Phenytoin: intravenous infusion 15 to 20 mg/kg *adult dose*; 20 mg/kg *pediatric dose*; maximum rate of 50 mg/min
  b) Fosphenytoin: intravenous infusion 15 to 20 mg phenytoin equivalents/kg *adult dose*; maximum rate of 100 phenytoin equivalents/min
  c) Valproic acid: intravenous infusion 15 to 30 mg/kg *adult dose*; 20 to 40 mg/kg *pediatric dose*; rate of 10 mg/kg/min
  d) Phenobarbital: intravenous infusion 10 to 20 mg/kg *adult dose*; 15 to 20 mg/kg *pediatric dose* maximum rate of 100 mg/min
  e) Levetiracetam (the evidence for use in SE is limited): intravenous infusion 20 to 30 mg/kg *adult dose*; maximum rate of 500 mg/min

- Phenytoin/phosphenytoin and phenobarbital are associated with a higher risk of cardiorespiratory depression compared with valproic acid and levetiracetam.
- Lacosamide is just being studied as an alternative to the conventional treatment although there are still limited data.

Stage 3: Stage of refractory status (30 to 60 min). Choose among:

a) Midazolam: 0.1 to 0.3 mg/kg at 4 mg/min bolus followed by infusion of 0.05 to 0.4 mg/kg/h
b) Propofol: 3 to 5 mg/kg intravenous bolus followed by an infusion of 5 to 10 mg/kg/h
c) Thiopental: 100 to 250 mg bolus over 20 seconds, then further 50-mg boluses every 2 to 3 minutes until seizures are controlled. Then an infusion of 3 to 5 mg/kg/h
d) Pentobarbital: 10 to 20 mg/kg bolus at 25 mg/min followed by an infusion of 1 to 3 mg/kg/h

- In this stage, all patients need cardiorespiratory assistance.
- Titrate the dose of anesthetics to maintain a burst suppression pattern on the EEG.
- It necessary, various anesthetics can be combined (for instance: midazolam and propofol).
- Other AEDs should be added in association with any of the anesthetics (this drugs can be loaded intravenously or orally).
- Midazolam and propofol have a shorter half-life compared with barbiturates, allowing for a rapid clinical assessment after drug reduction or discontinuation.
- Propofol can induce propofol infusion syndrome, a fatal cardiocirculatory collapse with lactic acidosis, hypertriglyceridemia, and rhabdomyolysis. This syndrome is mostly described in young children and patients with suspected mitochondrial disorders, some recommend avoiding prolonged infusion (>48 hours) in this age group.
- Anesthesia should be reversed after 24 to 48 hours of a maintained burst-suppression pattern on EEG monitoring. If seizures continue, a new cycle of anesthetic should be started and the cycle prolonged over time.

Stage 4: Super-refractory SE (SSE)

SSE refers to an SE that continues 24 hours or longer after the onset of anesthesia, including those cases in which the SE recurs on the reduction or withdrawal of anesthesia. In this setting, higher doses of current anesthetics might be considered, along as other unusual anesthetics such as ketamine and inhaled anesthetics. Second-line treatment at this stage should be individualized as clear guidance has not been established; hypothermia, magnesium infusion, pyridoxine infusion 100 mg intravenous (indicated in children with SE and no cause determined), ketogenic diet, and emergency neurosurgery (in patients with focal lesions such as brain tumors and cortical dysplasia) should be considered in cases where other conventional therapies have failed.

Epilepsy Surgery

Up to a third of patients with epilepsy are refractory to medical therapy. Epilepsy surgery is an effective therapeutic option in a selected subset of these patients, leading to seizure control in around 60% to 70% of cases. In addition, when effective, epilepsy surgery improves quality of life and reduces the risk of death related to epilepsy. Epilepsy surgery should be considered at some point in every patient with refractory focal epilepsy, when two appropriately chosen AEDs have failed to control seizures. When considering a patient for surgery, both the patient and the treating physician should take into account the severity and frequency of seizures, the natural history of the underlying epilepsy syndrome, and whether there are other alternatives less aggressive. Surgery should not be delayed in patients with a surgically remediable epilepsy syndromes (SRES) when seizures are frequent and associated with high risk of morbidity (such as falls, accidents, or Sudden Dead in Epilepsy), produce cognitive deterioration and/or impairment of daily life activities.

Surgically Remediable Epilepsy Syndromes

These epilepsy syndromes are featured by frequent and disturbing seizures with low chances of controlling with AEDs. The shared characteristics of SRES are:

- The epileptogenic zone has been correctly identified after the presurgical evaluation with video-EEG monitoring, brain MRI, neuropsychological evaluation, and additional tests as needed.
- The evolution of the disease is predictable and it is not likely that there will be a long-lasting response after forthcoming medical changes.
- Surgery itself is very likely to help the patient without assuming a high risk of a permanent severe neurological deficit.

Recent data show that chances of complete seizure control without surgery after the failure of two AEDs is less than 16% and that after failure of six AEDs is almost zero. Because of this, once SRES is identified and refractoriness to AEDs has been ascertained, surgery should not be delayed beyond a reasonable time.

The main SRES are those associated with structural abnormality in brain MRI, such as hippocampal sclerosis, some types of malformations of cortical development (e.g., Taylor II cortical dysplasia), brain tumors (e.g., low-grade gliomas, dysembrioplastic neuroepithelial tumors, and ganglioglioma), and cavernous angioma. In these cases, the probability of seizure control after surgery is 70% to 80%. In focal epilepsy associated with normal brain MRI or extensive pathology (e.g., type I cortical dysplasia, diffuse malformations of cortical development, or perinatal hypoxia), the probabilities of complete seizure control may fall to 50%. In hemispheric syndromes (e.g., Sturge-Weber syndrome, hemimegalencephaly, extensive porencephalic lesions, and Rasmussen´s syndrome), hemispherectomy, when possible, is the treatment of choice and can bring complete seizure control in up to 50% to 60% of patients. One-third to one-fourth of patients evaluated for surgery will be identified as surgical candidates. The extension of the evaluation will be tailored according to the epilepsy syndrome we are facing:

Stage I

1. Video-EEG monitoring
   - Diagnosis of the epilepsy syndrome
   - Analysis of the severity of epilepsy
   - Identification of the epileptogenic zone through analysis of seizure semiology and EEG findings
2. Neuroimaging
   a. MRI
      - Identification of a lesion responsible of the seizures
      - Functional evaluation of language and sensorimotor function
   b. Positron emission tomography/single-photon emission computed tomography/ magnetoencephalography
      - Indicated when MRI does not show any lesion or the lesion is not definitive
3. Neuropsychological evaluation
   - Identification of the epileptogenic zone
   - Evaluation of the surgical risk
   - Evaluation of psychiatric comorbidity
   - Baseline for comparison after surgery

Stage II

1. Evaluation with intracranial electrodes (stereo-EEG, subdural electrodes, or combination of both). Indicated when:
   - MRI does not show any epileptogenic lesion or the findings are not definitive
   - Incongruence among the results obtained through stage I
   - Mapping of eloquent brain areas that may be close to the epileptogenic zone

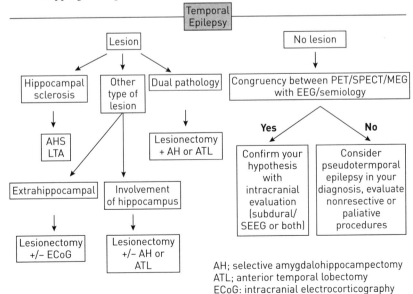

AH; selective amygdalohippocampectomy
ATL; anterior temporal lobectomy
ECoG: intracranial electrocorticography

FIGURE 11.2
Algorithm for evaluation of surgery in temporal lobe epilepsy.

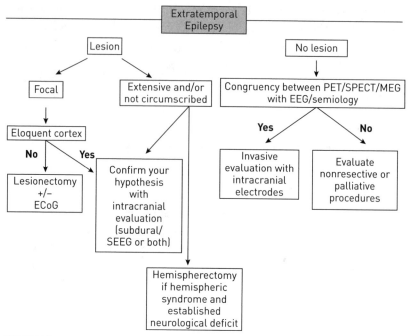

FIGURE 11.3

Algorithm for evaluation of surgery in extratemporal epilepsy.

2. Wada test. Indicated to evaluate the risk of memory decline when:
   - Surgery is planned to be done on the dominant temporal lobe
   - When there is suspicion of bitemporal pathology
   - Normal hippocampus on MRI
   - Normal memory on neuropsychological evaluation

Figures 11.2 and 11.3 summarize the evaluation of surgery in focal epilepsies according to the data showed by the presurgical evaluation.

Surgical Procedures

See Table 11.15.

OTHER NONPHARMACOLOGICAL TREATMENTS

Ketogenic Diet

The ketogenic diet (KD) is a high-fat, low-carbohydrate, and normal-protein diet used for the treatment of medically refractory epilepsy as an adjunctive therapy with AEDs. The KD includes 80% fat, 15% protein, and 5% carbohydrate; the ratio of fat to carbohydrate plus protein ranges from 2:1 to 4:1. Most of the fat in the classic, most commonly used KD is provided as long-chain triglycerides, although there are different variants that improve tolerability while maintaining ketosis. KD is effective in both focal and generalized refractory epilepsies. It is generally used in children and adults with developmental disabilities, with very frequent seizures, who are resistant to AEDs

Table 11.15 Surgical Procedures

Type of Surgery	Description	Indication
Lesionectomy and focal cortical resection	Resection of the epileptogenic lesion and the neocortex surrounding the lesion	Cavernomas Glial tumors (ganglioglioma and DNET) Low grade astrocitomas
Selective amygdalohippocampectomy	Resection of the amygdala and hippocampus	Hippocampal sclerosis Better outcomes in term of memory preservation compared with anterior temporal lobectomy
Anterior temporal lobectomy	Resection of temporal medial structures (hippocampus and amygdala) and neocortex	Hippocampal sclerosis and temporal lesions that involve the hippocampus With the standard procedure, the anterior 3–3.5 cm of temporal lobe measured along the middle temporal gyrus is resected
Lobectomy	Anatomic resection of a brain lobe	Large lesions or non circumscribed lesions such as porencephalic cysts, traumatic lesions, and malformations of cortical development
Corpus callosotomy	Bihemispheric disconnection through a longitudinal incision of the corpus callosum. The aim of this procedure is to interrupt the spreading pathways of seizures rather than to eliminate the epileptogenic zone.	Patients with Lennox-Gastaut syndrome and other generalized symptomatic epilepsies Indicated as a palliative procedure to treat tonic-clonic and atonic seizures (drops attacks) It can be limited to the anterior third portion of the corpus callosum or complete in patients with severe cognitive impairment
Hemispherectomy	Disconnection of the hemisphere responsible of the epilepsy. There are different techniques according to the extension of the resection.	Hemispheric syndromes: Hemimegalencephaly, Sturge-Weber syndrome, Rasmussen's syndrome, extensive cortical dysplasias, and porencephalic lesions This procedure might be indicated in patients that at the time of the surgery have already a established neurological deficit
Multiple subpial transactions	The intent of the procedure is to interrupt laterally spreading fibers and spare vertical axons. This limits seizure spread and preserves descending cortical function. Commonly is combined with limited cortical resections.	Controversial indications, usually in patients with focal epilepsies that arise in eloquent cortex areas that therefore are not amenable to total resection

and are not surgical candidates. In addition, it is the treatment of choice for pyruvate dehydrogenase deficiency and glucose transporter type 1 deficiency syndrome.

Electrical Stimulation for Epilepsy

Vagus nerve stimulation (VNS) is an open-loop device approved for the adjunctive treatment of refractory partial seizures in adults and adolescents older than 12 years. The generator is surgically placed subcutaneously on the left chest wall and connected to the left vagus nerve in the neck through a bipolar lead. Pulse sequences are programmed by means of radiofrequency signals with a programming wand and a computer. Most adverse effects occur during the stimulation period of each sequence, are usually well tolerated, and tend to disappear over time; they include hoarseness or voice alteration, throat pain, coughing, dyspnea, and paresthesia. The device is indicated as a palliative treatment for patients with focal refractory epilepsy, although there are also reports indicating efficacy in patients with generalized epilepsy. Studies show a mean seizure reduction of 30% within the first 3 months and greater than 50% seizure reduction after 1 to 2 years.

Bilateral stimulation of the anterior nuclei of the thalamus (deep brain stimulation) is approved in Europe but not in the United States for the treatment of refractory focal epilepsy. In clinical trials, treated patients had a median decrease in seizures of 40.4% after 3 months of therapy compared with 14.5% in the control group and a 56% median reduction in seizure frequency after 2 years, while 54% of patients had a 50% reduction in seizure frequency.

By means of a closed-loop with a seizure detection algorithm, responsive neurostimulation (RNS) can detect seizure onset directly from the cortex and then electrically stimulate the seizure focus to abort propagation. From clinical trials, it appears that efficacy is comparable to that of the other devices.

At the present time, VNS, DBS, and RNS are considered a last choice for patients with severe refractory epilepsy who are not candidates for surgical resection and have been resistant to most available AEDs. VNS has been used in thousands of patients and is less invasive and therefore is usually considered first. It is not clear whether patients should be treated with VNS before attempting DBS. RNS might be more convenient when we know where seizures start; patients has been studied with the use of intracranial electrodes, and surgical resection is found to be associated with a high risk of neurological deficit.

Stereotactic Radiosurgery

Stereotactic radiosurgery using the Leksell Gamma Knife is an option for the treatment of mesial temporal epilepsy, hypothalamic hamartoma, and other epileptogenic lesions that are well defined on brain MRI and have a volume of less than 7.5 cm². Results from different studies show that radiosurgery can be as effective as conventional surgical procedures; however, long-lasting control of the seizures usually takes from 1 to 2 years after the treatment.

de Tisi J, Bell GS, Peacock JL, et al. The long-term outcome of adult epilepsy surgery, patterns of seizure remission, and relapse: A cohort study. Lancet 2011;378:1388–1395.

Derry CP, Duncan JS, Berkovic SF. Paroxysmal motor disorders of sleep: The clinical spectrum and differentiation from epilepsy. Epilepsia 2006;47:1775–1791.

Devinsky O, Gazzola D, LaFrance WC Jr. Differentiating between nonepileptic and epileptic seizures. Nat Rev Neurol 2011;7:210–220.

Engel J Jr, Wiebe S, French J, et al. Practice parameter: Temporal lobe and localized neocortical resections for epilepsy: Report of the Quality Standards Subcommittee of the American Academy of Neurology, in association with the American Epilepsy Society and the American Association of Neurological Surgeons. Neurology 2003;60;538–547.

French JA, Kanner AM, Bautista J, et al. Efficacy and tolerability of the new antiepileptic drugs I: treatment of new onset epilepsy: Report of the Therapeutics and Technology Assessment Subcommittee and Quality Standards Subcommittee of the American Academy of Neurology and the American Epilepsy Society. Neurology 2004;62:1252–1260.

French JA, Kanner AM, Bautista J, et al. Efficacy and tolerability of the new antiepileptic drugs II: treatment of refractory epilepsy: Report of the Therapeutics and Technology Assessment Subcommittee and Quality Standards Subcommittee of the American Academy of Neurology and the American Epilepsy Society. Neurology 2004;27:62:1261–1273.

Glauser T, Ben-Menachem E, Bourgeois B, et al. ILAE treatment guidelines: Evidence-based analysis of antiepileptic drug efficacy and effectiveness as initial monotherapy for epileptic seizures and syndromes. Epilepsia 2006;47:1094–1120.

Kwan P, Arzimanoglou A, Berg AT, et al. Definition of drug resistant epilepsy: Consensus proposal by the ad hoc Task Force of the ILAE Commission on Therapeutic Strategies. Epilepsia 2010;51:1069–1077.

Neal EG, Chaffe H, Schwartz RH, et al. The ketogenic diet for the treatment of childhood epilepsy: A randomised controlled trial. Lancet Neurol 2008;7:500–506.

Novy J, Logroscino G, Rossetti AO. Refractory status epilepticus: A prospective observational study Epilepsia 2010;51:251–256.

Perucca E, Tomson T. The pharmacologic treatment of epilepsy in adults. Lancet Neurol 2011;10:446–456.

Raspall-Chaure M, Neville BG, Scott RC. The medical management of the epilepsies in children: conceptual and practical considerations. Lancet Neurol 2008;7:57–69.

Schiller Y, Najjar Y. Quantifying the response to antiepileptic drugs. Effect of past treatment history. Neurology 2008;70:54–65.

Shorvon S, Baulac M, Cross H, et al. The drug treatment of status epilepticus in Europe: Consensus document from a workshop at the first London Colloquium on Status Epilepticus. Epilepsia 2008;49:1277–1285.

Tomson T, Battino D, Bonizzoni E, et al; EURAP Study Group. Dose-dependent risk of malformations with antiepileptic drugs: An analysis of data from the EURAP Epilepsy and Pregnancy Registry. Lancet Neurol 2011;10:609–617.

Trinka E, Höfler J, Zerbs A. Causes of status epilepticus. Epilepsia 2012;53:127–138.

12 Syncope

Luisa Sambati and Pietro Cortelli

INTRODUCTION

Transient loss of consciousness (TLoC) is defined as a self-limited loss of consciousness with a rapid onset, a short duration, and a spontaneous and complete recovery. This definition includes functional TLoC (i.e., epilepsy, concussion, metabolic disturbances or intoxications) and mimics (i.e., narcolepsy or psychogenic) of TLoC.

Syncope can be defined as self-limited TLoC caused by cerebral hypoperfusion, with or without a brief warning (e.g., lightheadedness, nausea, sweating, weakness, visual disturbances), usually associated with rapid and complete recovery. A decrease in systolic blood pressure (BP) to 60 mm Hg or lower is associated with syncope, and a sudden cessation of cerebral blood flow for as short as 6 to 8 seconds has been shown to be sufficient to cause complete LoC.

Syncope is a prevalent disorder, accounting for 1% to 3% of emergency department visits and as many as 6% of hospital admissions each year in the United States. As many as 50% of the population may experience a syncopal event during their lifetime, and at least 20% experience it recurrently.

The initial evaluation, consisting of careful history assessment, physical examination, including orthostatic BP measurements and electrocardiogram (ECG), help to categorize syncope into reflex, orthostatic, and cardiac (Figure 12.1, Table 12.1).

Additional examinations should be performed when the diagnosis is not clear or when cardiac syncope is suspected: (1) immediate ECG monitoring should be carried out if there is suspicion of arrhythmic syncope and echocardiogram when data are suggestive of structural heart disease or previous known heart disease; and (2) in patients over 40 years, carotid sinus massage could be useful to exclude carotid sinus hypersensitivity and orthostatic challenge (lying-to-standing orthostatic test and/or head-up tilt testing) is useful to reveal syncope related to the standing position or to a reflex mechanism.

REFLEX SYNCOPE

Reflex syncope is the most common form of syncope and includes vasovagal syncope (VVS), syncope caused by carotid sinus hypersensitivity (CSH), and situational syncope (i.e., syncope occurring during micturition, defecation, swallowing, coughing, etc.) (Figure 12.2). VVS is a common and distressing problem, and up to 0.9% of primary care visits are for VVS. There is an early peak incidence around 15 years for young women and a later significant rise in visits for both sexes over the age of 65 years, with a familial occurrence.

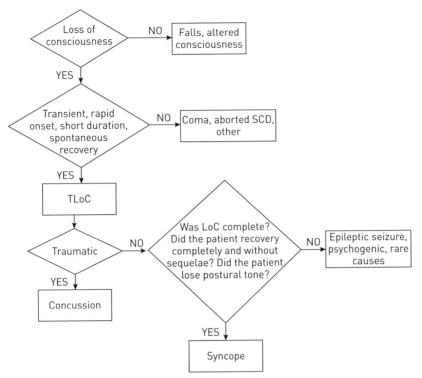

FIGURE 12.1

Diagnostic algorithm of syncope. TLoC, transient loss of consciousness; SCD, sudden cardiac death.

VVS can be diagnosed if the patient experiences the symptoms in the presence of hypotension and/or bradycardia after more than 3 minutes' stability of these parameters from tilt-up.

Orthostatic VVS occurs when cardiac output decreases by around 50%. Unconsciousness ensues when mean cerebral BP falls to around 40 mm Hg. It is due to both vasodilatation and cardioinhibition. Syncope in which bradycardia is thought to be a more important contributory factor than low BP is termed cardioinhibitory VVS. By contrast, if BP drops but the heart rate shows little or no decrease, the reflex is termed *vasodepressive VVS*.

Acute therapy for VVS consists if lying down. Falling usually helps to restore consciousness in syncope by increasing venous return and cardiac output, leading to a rise in BP. Further, drinking 500 mL of cold water should help to resolve the acute phase.

Preventive therapy for VVS starts with lifestyle measures. The patient should be educated to recognize prodromal symptoms and to avoid or attenuate the triggering event. Further, he should be reassured regarding the benign nature of the condition, with a low short-term risk (schooling and psychological trauma, employment, and driving problems).

Salt and fluid-volume adjustments, alcohol, and hot and crowded environment avoidance; physical maneuvers including isometric muscle tensing such as leg crossing or hand grip; and arm tensing and tilt training are usually useful to prevent syncope.

Pharmacological therapy could be used to reduce anxiety, which precipitate events: midodrine could be used as pill-in-the-pocket strategy, and paroxetine could be used in depressed patients.

Table 12.1 Short-term, High-risk Criteria that Require Prompt Hospitalization or Intensive Evaluation

Family history	Sudden death, especially in relatives <30 y
	Cardiac diseases
Age at onset	Young patients tolerate increased heart rates better than do older patients
	Syncope can be one of the symptoms of hereditary channelopathies
Comorbidities	Severe anemia
	Electrolyte disturbances
	History of severe structural cardiac diseases
	History of coronary artery diseases
	Heart failure, low left ventricular ejection fraction, or previous myocardial infarction
Clinical features	Sudden occurrence, without warning or palpitations, during physical exercise
	While lying down and with facial cyanosis, preceded by chest pain or palpitation
	Syncope at night is frequent in prolonged QT and Brugada syndromes; in children, consider: loud noise, fright, extreme emotional stress
ECG features	Bifascicular block (left bundle branch block [BBB] or right BBB with left anterior or posterior hemiblock or QRS >120 ms
	Ssinus bradycardia (<40 bpm) or sinoatrial block
	Preexcited QRS
	Prolonged or short QT interval
	ST elevation in ECG leads V1–3 (Brugada pattern)
	Pattern suggesting arrhythmogenic right ventricular cardiomyopathy
	Q waves suggesting myocardial infarction
Structural cardiovascular disease	Acute myocardial ischemia or infarction
	Acute aortic dissection, pulmonary embolism, congestive heart failure
	Hemodynamically important aortic or mitral valvular stenosis
	Severe pulmonary hypertension
Ongoing treatment	β-Blockers
	Ca^{2+} blockers
	Antiarrythmic
	Psychotropic
	Antibiotics

The family physician in charge of the follow-up should avoid prescribing hypotensive drugs, such as α-blockers and diuretics (Figure 12.3).

Carotid sinus hypersensitivity (CSH) is a disease of older people with a prevalence between 25% and 48% in patients referred to hospital for unexplained syncope. Massage of carotid sinus (CSM) during tilt table testing is diagnostic: if massage results in a short asystole of at least 3 seconds and/or a BP drop of more than 50 mm Hg but no syncope, then the response is considered to be hypersensitive. If CSM results

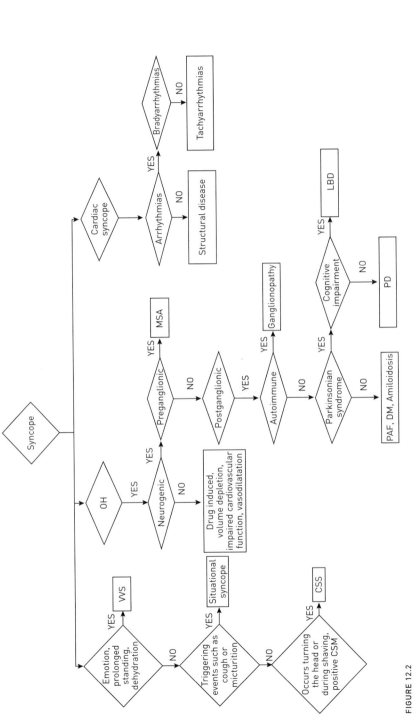

FIGURE 12.2
Diagnostic algorithm of causes of syncope.

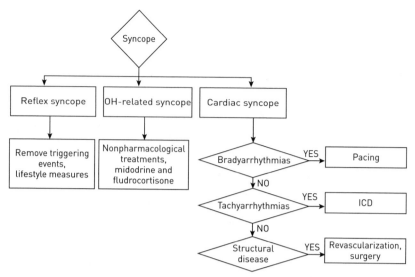

FIGURE 12.3

Algorithm of syncope treatment.

in syncope, due to a longer period of asystole and lower BP, the response is named *induced carotid sinus syncope*. Carotid sinus syndrome (CSS) causing syncope can be spontaneous, in less than 1% of cases, or induced, usually by external pressure. Cardiac pacing appears to be beneficial in patients with cardioinhibitory CSH (i.e., when bradycardia has been documented) with a clear history of syncope in association with head turning or carotid sinus pressure when symptoms are reproduced during CSM.

SYNCOPE DUE TO ORTHOSTATIC HYPOTENSION

Orthostatic hypotension (OH) is defined as a fall in systolic BP of 20 mm Hg or more and a drop in diastolic BP of 10 mm Hg or more, within 3 minutes of standing up. OH can be caused by neurodegenerative postganglionic disease (pure autonomic failure [PAF], Parkinson disease plus autonomic failure, or Lewy body dementia); neurodegenerative preganglionic disease (i.e., multiple system atrophy); autoimmune autonomic ganglionopathy due to ganglionic acetylcholine receptor autoantibodies; secondary autonomic failure (diabetes mellitus, amyloid, hereditary sensory, and autonomic neuropathies [HSAN IB and IV] and inflammatory neuropathies, peripheral neuropathies accompanying porphyria, vitamin B12 deficiency, and HIV infection); drug-induced autonomic failure; volume depletion (low intravascular volume: blood or plasma loss, fluid or electrolyte loss); impaired cardiac function because of structural heart disease; and vasodilatation because of drugs, alcohol, and heat (Figure 12.2).

Treatment of OH causing syncope (Figure 12.3) starts with nonpharmacological measures. First, drugs that potentially induce syncope should be reduced or removed. Hot environment, carbohydrate-rich meals, alcohol, and prolonged recumbence during daytime should be avoided. Intake of at least 8 g of NaCl daily and water repletion (2–2.5 L) should be recommended. The patient should be educated to move to head-up position slowly, particularly in the morning when BP may be lowered by nocturnal polyuria; to sit on the edge of the bed for some minutes after recumbence and to activate calf muscle while supine and to do physical counter maneuvers (leg crossing with tension of the thigh, buttock, and calf muscle—party position—bending over forward, squatting) at the onset of presyncopal symptoms. Sleeping with an elevation of the bed's head-end (20–30 cm) could be useful to prevent supine hypertension, polyuria, and early morning OH. Rapid cool water ingestion is reported to be effective in combating orthostatic intolerance and postprandial hypotension. Abdominal binders or compression stockings may help to treat gravitational venous pooling in older patients. Constant physical exercise, such as isotonic exercise and swimming, could be useful to ameliorate the venous return and the orthostatic tolerance. Pharmacological treatment is often required if lifestyle measures are not effective.

Midodrine is recommended with a level of evidence "A" for monotherapy or combined therapy. The prodrug is activated to desglymidodrine, the active α-adrenoreceptor agonist, which is rapidly absorbed from the gastrointestinal tract. The peak plasma concentration of midodrine occurs in 20 to 40 minutes, and the half-life time is 30 minutes. The half-life time of desglymidodrine is 4 hours. Patient sensitivity to this agent varies and the dose should be titrated from 2.5 mg to 10 mg three times a day. The peak effect of this agent occurs 1 hour after ingestion. It increases the receptor number and affinity and reduces baroreceptor modulation. The effectiveness of indirect agonists is at least in part due to the release of norepinephrine from the postganglionic neuron. The pressor effect of midodrine is a consequence of both arterial and venous constriction. Potential side effects of this agent include pilomotor reactions, pruritus, paresthesia, supine hypertension, gastrointestinal complaints, and urinary retention and chills. Midodrine does not cross the blood–brain barrier and does not have the central sympathomimetic side effects. It has been demonstrated that midodrine reduces exercise-induced OH in PAF, increasing BP via vasoconstriction. The last dose should be administered 4 hours before bedtime because supine hypertension is a common adverse effect; it should be administered with caution in patients with hepatic dysfunction and not administered in a patient with severe heart disease, acute renal failure, urinary retention, pheochromocytoma, or thyrotoxicosis.

9-α-Fluorohydrocortisone (fludrocortisone acetate 0.1–0.2 mg/d), recommended as level of evidence "C," is a synthetic mineralocorticoid, has a long duration of action, and is well tolerated by most patients. It increases renal sodium reabsorption, expands plasma volume, and enhances the sensitivity of blood vessels to circulating catecholamines and norepinephrine release from sympathetic neurons, through the sensitization of α-adrenoreceptors, and increases vascular fluid content. Treatment is initiated with a 0.1-mg tablet and can be increased up to 1 mg. Higher doses can result in fluid overload and congestive heart failure, severe supine hypertension, and hypokalemia. Treatment may unfortunately be limited by supine hypertension due to an increase in the peripheral vascular resistance. Other side effects include ankle edema, especially in patients with low serum albumin, hypokalemia, and rarely congestive heart failure. Headache may occur. Potassium supplementation is usually required, particularly when higher doses are used.

Octreotide 25 to 50 mcg subcutaneous inhibits release of gastrointestinal peptides with vasodilatory properties. It is recommended with level of evidence "C," an hour before a meal to reduced postprandial but also postural and exertion-induced hypotension, without increasing nocturnal hypertension.

Erythropoietin corrects the normochromic normocytic anemia that frequently accompanies autonomic failure. It is administered subcutaneously or intravenously at doses between 25 and 75 U/kg three times a week until a hematocrit value that approaches normal is attained. Lower maintenance doses (approximately 25 U/kg three times a week) may then be used. Iron supplementation is usually required, particularly during the period when the hematocrit is increasing.

The synthetic vasopressin analogue desmopressin acetate (DDAVP) acts on the V2 receptors in the collecting ducts of the renal tubules and has no V1 receptor vasoconstricting potential. DDAVP, which can be taken as a nasal spray (10–40 mcg) or orally (100–800 mcg), prevents nocturia and weight loss and reduces the morning postural fall in BP in patients with autonomic failure. Fluid and electrolyte status should be carefully monitored during therapy to avoid hyponatremia.

CARDIAC SYNCOPE

Syncope secondary to cardiovascular disease is the second most common cause of TLoC. Cardiac arrhythmias and structural heart problems are major risk factors for sudden cardiac death (SCD) and overall high mortality rates. Cardiac syncope doubled the risk of death with a 6-month mortality rate greater than 10% (Soteriades et al. 2002) (Figure 12.2).

Considering the high short-term risk related to cardiac syncope, the diagnostic algorithm in a patient presenting syncope should be oriented to exclude cardiac causes.

Arrhythmias are the most frequent cause of cardiac syncope; the electrical disorder can be primitive or associated with structural heart abnormalities or be induced by a reversible cause, such as drug toxicity, electrolyte disturbances, or implanted device malfunction .

Both tachyarrhythmia (supraventricular or ventricular tachycardias) and bradyarrhythmia (a sustained low ventricular rate <30 bpm for 15–20 seconds or a prolonged pause in heart rhythm of more than 5 seconds) can cause syncope; prognosis and treatment are quite different and depend on the kind of arrhythmias and the clinical contest.

The higher risk of mortality is related to ventricular tachyarrhythmia due to ischemic heart disease or cardiomyopathies but also to some genetic disorder like channelopathies that can induce life-threatening arrhythmias in patients with a normal heart; there could be an high risk for SCD, particularly in young people.

Pacemakers are indicated for use in the treatment of symptomatic bradyarrhythmias, and they control or replace the heart's intrinsic electrical activity. Patients may require intermittent or permanent pacing (Figure 12.3).

Pacing systems are electrical devices that consist of a small battery-powered generator and one or more pacing leads that are in contact with the inner wall of the right atrium and/or the right ventricle. The pacemaker senses whether an intrinsic depolarization has occurred. On the contrary, the pacemaker generates an electrical impulse, which is delivered to the heart muscle via the pacemaker leads to initiate contraction.

Heart block should be treated with permanent pacing in the case of chronic symptomatic atrioventricular block, asymptomatic second- and third-degree heart block, and symptomatic first-degree heart block. Patients with bundle branch block and syncope progress to complete heart block with a 5% to 11 % incidence per year; in these patients, pacemaker implantation, following a negative electrophysiological study to exclude concurrent tachyarrhythmias, is recommended.

Sinus node dysfunction (including bradycardia/tachycardia syndrome) is the second most common indication for permanent pacing. Pacemakers may be categorized as single- or dual-chamber devices, depending on whether leads are applied to one or two heart chambers.

The choice between a dual-chamber or single-chamber pacemaker depends on the individual patient, their underlying heart disease, and atrioventricular (AV) node–His–Purkinje function.

Patients with pure sinus node dysfunction benefit from the use of a dual-chamber pacemaker, due to a small but progressive need for ventricular pacing, in relation to the possible development of heart block. Treatment of heart block or AV nodal dysfunction requires a dual-chamber pacemaker to avoid a significant 25% to 30% incidence of pacemaker syndrome (i.e., a suboptimal AV synchrony or AV dyssynchrony, regardless of the pacing mode, after the pacemaker implantation, that can cause syncope).

Patients with chronic AF with a slow ventricular response need a single-chamber ventricular pacemaker.

In supraventricular tachyarrhythmias (paroxysmal AV nodal reciprocating tachycardia, AV reciprocating tachycardia, or typical atrial flutter), catheter ablation is the first-choice treatment. In patients with syncope associated with atrial fibrillation or atypical left atrial flutter, the decision should be individualized (drugs or ablation).

In patients with syncope due to ventricular tachycardia (VT) without heart disease or with mild left ventricular dysfunction, catheter ablation or drug therapy should be considered.

Life-threatening ventricular tachyarrhythmias such as VT and ventricular fibrillation (VF) can be treated with an implantable cardioverter-defibrillator (ICD). An ICD is an electrical device similar to a pacemaker that monitors heart rhythms. If it senses VF or very fast VT, it delivers shocks capable to restore normal rhythm; it has also pacemaker function.

ICD is indicated in patients with syncope and depressed ventricular function and in patients with VT and VF without correctable cause. In these patients, ICD usually does not prevent syncopal recurrences, but it is indicated to reduce the risk of SCD. Torsade de pointes is usually an acquired ventricular tachyarrhythmia due to drugs that prolong the QT interval; the immediate suspension of suspected drug and eventually temporary pacing provide the therapy.

ICD is indicated in patients with arrhythmogenic right ventricular cardiomyopathy/dysplasia, particularly if the patient is young with extensive right ventricular dysfunction, left ventricular involvement, polymorphic ventricular tachycardia, late potentials, epsilon waves, or family history of SCD.

In patients with inherited cardiac ion channel abnormalities (long QT syndromes, Brugada syndrome, short QT syndrome, catecholaminergic polymorphic ventricular tachycardia), ICD should be carefully considered if ventricular tachyarrhythmia cannot be excluded as the cause of syncope and when pharmacological treatment (i.e., β-blockers for type 1 long QT syndrome) failed.

Structural cardiovascular disease can cause syncope when the circulatory demand outweighs the impaired ability of the heart to increase its output. Syncope associated with myocardial ischemia should be treated with pharmacological therapy or revascularization (Figure 12.3).

In ischemic and nonischemic cardiomyopathies, if revascularization may not ameliorate the risk of malignant ventricular arrhythmia, patients should be treated with ICD.

In hypertrophic cardiomyopathy (with or without left ventricular outflow tract obstruction), ICD therapy is effective as specific treatment of ventricular arrhythmia; surgical myectomy is also capable of reducing syncope in the obstructive form of hypertrophic cardiomyopathy. In cardiovascular congenital abnormalities, severe aortic stenosis, acute aortic dissection, and left atrial myxoma, syncope is related to mechanical obstruction of cardiac output. These conditions require surgical treatment. Syncope due to pericardial tamponade may require immediate surgical treatment including emergency intervention.

Syncope occurs frequently in patients with pulmonary hypertension and contributes to morbidity and mortality. Many patients reveal a vasoconstrictive component in their lung vessels that is potentially reversible therapeutically. Accurate noninvasive diagnostic methods and an understanding of the mechanisms causing pulmonary hypertension are necessary, as is appropriate therapy based on these results.

CONCLUSION

Syncope is a TLoC caused by cerebral hypoperfusion; if not treated properly, it can be a dramatic, life-threatening event. Differentiation between different causes and determination of the underlying etiology should be achieved with a careful, standardized initial evaluation. Risk stratification should be undertaken as soon as possible to decide which patients require in-hospital management and which are suitable for outpatient care. Reflex syncope is a common medical problem, and VVS is the most frequent form. Although the prognosis of the disorder is excellent, it may impose substantial changes in lifestyle and cause profound psychological distress. Thus, management of this disorder is an important issue. In other conditions such as syncope due to OH, most patients can be treated successfully with a combination of fludrocortisone and a sympathomimetic agent. The existing treatments for this condition lack efficacy for those patients with more than minor symptoms, since lifestyle measures are the greatest advances in treatment. In some patients, drugs alone are largely ineffective and not without adverse effects. Important treatment challenges include developing a safe, once-daily medication that offers a real reduction in syncope recurrence. In cardiac syncope, the higher risk is SCD that should be prevented with drug and implanted therapy. Further studies should evaluate the effectiveness of these therapies for outcomes of mortality, stroke, heart failure, atrial fibrillation, and pacemaker syndrome. The principal goals of treatment for patient with syncope are prevention of symptom recurrence, improvement of quality of life, prolongation of survival, and limitation of physical injuries. The importance and priority of these goals depend on the cause of the syncope.

Further understanding of the mechanism of syncope in different diseases could help to devise a patient-tailored symptomatic or etiological therapy to prevent syncope recurrence and related risks.

SUGGESTED READING

Corcoran SJ, Davis LM, Cardiac implantable electronic device therapy for bradyarrhythmias and tachyarrhythmias. Heart Lung Circ 2012;21:328–337.

Lahrmann H, Cortelli P, Hilz M, et al. EFNS guidelines on the diagnosis and management of orthostatic hypotension. Eur J Neurol 2006;13:930–936.

Soteriades ES, Evans JC, Larson MG, et al. Incidence and prognosis of syncope. N Engl J Med 2002;347:878–885.

Sutton R, Benditt D, Brignole M, Moya A. Syncope: Diagnosis and management according to the 2009 guidelines of the European Society of Cardiology. Pol Arch Med Wewn 2010;120:42–47.

Sutton R, Brignole M, Benditt DG. Key challenges in the current management of syncope. Nat Rev Cardiol 2012;9:590–598. doi:10.1038/nrcardio.2012.102. Epub 2012 Jul 17.

Task Force for the Diagnosis and Management of Syncope; European Society of Cardiology (ESC); European Heart Rhythm Association (EHRA); Heart Failure Association (HFA); Heart Rhythm Society (HRS), Moya A, Sutton R, Ammirati F, et al. Guidelines for the diagnosis and management of syncope (version 2009). Eur Heart J 2009;30:2631–2671. Epub 2009 Aug 27.

van Dijk JG, Thijs RD, Benditt DG, Wieling W. A guide to disorders causing transient loss of consciousness: Focus on syncope. Nat Rev Neurol 2009;5:438–448. Epub 2009 Jul 14.

SECTION FOUR
SLEEP DISORDERS

13 Insomnia

Juan A. Pareja and Teresa Montojo

INTRODUCTION TO SLEEP DISORDERS

Sleep-wake cycles are regulated by a complex interaction between homeostatic and chronobiological processes as well as environment factors. Homeostatic regulation results from sustained wakefulness that builds a pressure to fall asleep. Chronobiological regulation synchronizes the wake-sleep period with the day-night cycle of the earth through the action of a pacemaker (the suprachiasmatic nucleus of the hypothalamus) trained primarily by the intensity of light received through the retinohypothalamic pathway. Melatonin is released from the pineal gland at night and has the abilities to synchronize circadian rhythms and to promote sleep. The three states of being—wake, NREM sleep (N1, N2, and N3 stages), and REM sleep—oscillate through the 24-hour geophysical period in a predictable and orderly way: sleep and wakefulness with a circadian rhythm and the different stages of sleep with an ultradian rhythm.

Most sleep disorders cause daytime sleepiness and/or insomnia at night and, in a lesser proportion, abnormal movements or behaviors. The medical history and polysomnogram (PSG) often suffice for diagnosis. The PSG allows identification and documentation of each of the stages of sleep and circumstances, normal or pathological, that occur in real time and disrupt the quality or continuity of sleep. Sometimes it is necessary to complete the study with a multiple sleep latency test (MSLT) to determine a patient's propensity to fall asleep. It allows a quantitative and qualitative estimation of daytime hypersomnia.

INSOMNIA

Insomnia is defined by a persistent difficulty with sleep initiation, duration, consolidation, or quality that occurs despite enough time and opportunity for sleep and results in some form of daytime impairment. Child insomnia usually manifests as a resistance to go to bed or to sleep independently (without parents or caregivers). Insomnia should be differentiated from "short sleepers" who need only a few hours of sleep to feel rested and fully awake during the day.

The underlying mechanisms of insomnia include a constitutional vulnerability (weak homeostatic pressure and/or a persistent state of hiperarousal) that leads the patients to develop insomnia spontaneously or when copying with precipitating factors (life stressors, medical, psychiatric, and sleep disorders). In addition, behavioral and maladaptive responses (e.g., attributing excessive importance to sleep, preoccupation of the consequences of insomnia, exaggerated expectations on the function of sleep) may perpetuate insomnia beyond the duration of precipitating stressors. A positive family history is frequently encountered, but involved genes are largely unknown. However, a genetic factor is relevant in fatal family insomnia.

Insomnia is the most common of all sleep disorders (10%–20% of adults). Although insomnia is found in all age groups, it increases with age, being more common in females and in the elderly. Insomnia can be acute (lasting up to 4 weeks) or chronic (persisting longer than 1 month). Etiologically, it may be divided into primary or secondary cases (Table 13.1); the vast majority of insomnia cases are secondary.

The diagnosis of insomnia relies on the clinical history that can be complemented by a sleep diary. PSG is generally not indicated in patients with insomnia, except to rule out a comorbid sleep disorder or if insomnia is severe and unresponsive to conventional therapy.

TREATMENT OF INSOMNIA

Hypnotics

Benzodiazepine hypnotics are the most useful agents, providing the patients with a shortened sleep latency and an increased sleep time (Table 13.2). They are nonselective agonists of the $GABA_A$ receptor, with hypnotic, anxiolytic, and anticonvulsive actions. Adverse effects include daytime sedation, cognitive impairment, and rebound insomnia and abstinence syndrome on withdrawal. They may also worsen respiratory

Table 13.1 Major Categories of Insomnia

	Primary
Idiopathic	Long-standing insomnia, with no significant remission periods, with onset in infancy or early childhood. A family history is frequently encountered
Psychophysiological	Conditioned insomnia due to learned associations between the bed and bedroom with arousal. The disorder is often acute (related to a particular stressful event), but can perpetuate (chronic psychophysiological insomnia).
Paradoxical	Complain of severe insomnia without evidence of daytime impairment and with a large discrepancy between subjective estimation of sleep latency and total amount of sleep and objective findings by PSG or actigraphy.
	Secondary
Inadequate sleep hygiene	Insomnia caused by sleep-wake irregular routines, lifestyle, and activities that interfere with sleep
Adjustment	Insomnia related to an identifiable stressor, usually short term
Psyquiatric disorders	Depression, anxiety, schizophrenia, alcohol and drug abuse. Abstinence from CNS depressant drugs (rebound insomnia)
Medical disorders	Medical illnesses producing night symptoms such as pain, dyspnea, cough, esophageal reflux, nocturia, etc., as well as medical treatments (steroids, α-adrenergic agents, etc.) that disturb sleep
Neurological disorders	Sleep-related headaches, neurodegenerative disorders, restless legs syndrome, traumatic brain injury, posttraumatic syndrome, fatal familial insomnia

Table 13.2 Pharmacologic Treatment with Hypnotics

Drug	Half-life (h)	Dose (mg)
Benzodiazepine Hypnotics		
Short acting		
Midazolam	1–4	7.5
Triazolam	2–5	0.125–0.25
Lorazepam	10–20	1–2
Lormetazepam	12–20	1–2
Intermediate acting		
Temazepam	8–15	7.5–30
Estazolam	10–24	0.5–2
Clonazepam	18–40	0.5–4
Flurazepam	24–100	15–30
Nonbenzodiazepine Hypnotics		
Short acting		
Zaleplon	1	5–20
Zolpidem	3	5–10
Intermediate acting		
Zopiclone	5–7	7.5
Eszopiclone	5–7	1–3

function in patients with sleep apnea and chronic pulmonary diseases. At high doses, they can induce tolerance and dependence.

Nonbenzodiazepine hypnotics are selective agonists of the $GABA_A$ receptor, lacking relevant anxiolytic and anticonvulsive properties and thus minimizing all the adverse effects attributed to benzodiazepine hypnotics (Table 13.2).

Short-acting hypnotics are indicated for sleep-onset insomnia, while intermediate-acting drugs can be used for sleep maintenance insomnia with or without sleep-onset insomnia.

Antidepressants

Sedative antidepressants are mostly indicated to treat insomnia coexisting with mood disorders. These drugs have less risk of dependency and abuse. Antidepressants stabilize sleep architecture, diminish sleep latency and frequency of awakenings, and increase sleep efficiency and total sleep time. Commonly used antidepressants, with doses given at bedtime, include trazodone (50–300 mg), amitriptyline (10–25 mg), and mirtazapine (15–30 mg).

Melatonin and Melatonin Receptor Agonists

Melatonin (3–9 mg at night) is a nonmedicinal substance that may be indicated in elderly patients with insomnia, who presumably have low melatonin levels. Agomelatin (25–50 mg at night) is a melatonergic agonist and serotonergic antagonist, with antidepressive, anxiolytic, and hypnotic properties, indicated in insomnia comorbid with depression. Ramelteon (8 mg at night) is a powerful melatonergic agonist useful in sleep-onset insomnia.

Neuromodulators, Neuroleptics, and Antihistamines

Gabapentin (300–600 mg at night) and pregabalin (50–100 mg at night) are indicated in insomnia in the context of restless legs syndrome (see Chapter 15) or chronic pain. Quetiapine (25–200 mg at night) is useful to treat insomnia comorbid with dementia and with bipolar or psychotic disorders. Antihistamines (e.g., dyphenhydramine 25–50 mg at night) are over-the-counter medications that may be helpful for mild, short-term insomnia, but the patients should be advised that antihistamines quickly induce tolerance and cognitive impairment.

Behavioral Treatment

Behavioral and psychological therapies are intended to diminish the influence of perpetuating or exacerbating factors in insomnia, unrealistic expectations of the quality and quantity of sleep, excessive focus on limited sleep, distorted interpretations of insomnia, and worry about the consequences of poor sleep. This therapy is indicated in chronic insomnia.

> *Sleep hygiene*: trains the insomniacs to avoid habits that promote wakefulness and stimulates behaviors that facilitate somnolence (Table 13.3)
> *Relaxation therapy*: the goal is to reduce both physic and phsychic tension by the means of several techniques such as abdominal breathing, yoga, biofeedback, hypnosis, etc.
> *Stimulus control*: the technique tries to reassociate/strengthen the relationship between night, bedroom, bed, and sleep, by means of a set of behavioral instructions (Table 13.4).
> *Sleep restriction*: uses the homeostatic control of sleep by shortening the sleep time to increase sleep pressure and promote drowsiness at night. In practice, time in bed is reduced to the patient's stimated nocturnal sleep time but no less than 5 hours. This is increased by 15 minutes every week if sleep efficiency (time asleep/time in bed) is 90% or greater.
> *Cognitive therapy*: tries to modify maladaptive attitudes in regard to insomnia, such as attributing excessive importance to sleep, preoccupation of the consequences of insomnia, and exaggerated expectations on the function of sleep.

CIRCADIAN RHYTHM SLEEP DISORDERS

Circadian rhythm sleep disorders occur when there is an asynchrony between the timing of sleep and the 24-hour social and geophysical day-night cycle. As a result,

Table 13.3 Sleep Hygiene

Avoid all stimulants (e.g., caffeine, nicotine) several hours before bedtime.

Do not drink alcohol around bedtime.

Finish eating at least 3–4 h before bedtime.

Keep the bedroom environment quiet, dark, and comfortable. Sleep on a comfortable mattress and pillows.

Exercise regularly particularly in the late afternoon or early evening. Avoid vigorous physical activity close to bedtime.

Avoid naps.

Table 13.4 Stimulus Control

1. Go to bed only when sleepy.
2. Use the bed only for sleep and sex.
3. If unable to sleep for 15 minutes, get out of bed and go to another room and do something relaxing. Return to bed only when sleepy.
4. Repeat step 3 as often as necessary.
5. Get up at the same time every morning.
6. Do not nap during the day.

the patient cannot sleep when desired, though when sleep is at the preferred time, it is normal. Insomnia and/or hypersomnia is the main complaint. Light exposure and melatonin administration can be used to shift the timing of the circadian clock. The response to melatonin is the opposite of the response to light. Melatonin given in the evening and bright light exposure in the morning will phase-advance the circadian clock, while melatonin in the morning and bright light in the evening will phase-delay the circadian clock.

Advanced Sleep Phase Syndrome

The intrinsic period of the circadian human pacemaker is shortened, causing a characteristic pattern of early sleep onset and early morning awakening. The disorder mostly often affects the elderly. The patients complain of waking up too early in the morning and of evening hypersomnia. Treatment can be based on the administration of melatonin in the morning and/or bright light during the early evening.

Delayed Sleep Phase Syndrome

The intrinsic period of the circadian human pacemaker is lengthened, causing a characteristic pattern of delayed sleep onset and wake-up time. This condition is typical of the youth. Treatment may include melatonin given in the evening and early morning exposure to bright light.

Irregular Sleep-Wake Pattern

This consists of the chaotic periods of sleep and wakefulness distributed during the day and night. This pattern is common in adult patients suffering from neurodegenerative diseases and in intellectually retarded children. Treatment is mostly based on strict sleep hygiene (Table 13.3). Exposure to bright light in the morning and melatonin given in the evening may help.

Free-Running Disorder (Non–24 Hours Sleep-Wake Disorder or Hypernychthemeral Disorder)

This disorder is characterized by a progressive delay in the circadian clock and the sleep-wake cycle that results in insomnia and hypersomnia depending on when sleep is attempted in relation to the phase of the circadian clock. The disorder is most commonly seen in blind individuals but has also been reported after brain injury and in normal persons. Recommended treatment includes sleep hygiene (Table 13.3) and melatonin 1 to 2 hours before the desired bedtime.

Shift Work Sleep Disorder

Shift work changes can cause insomnia or excessive sleepiness temporarily. To facilitate the adaptation to changes in working schedules, light intensity should be increased during working hours, whereas a strict darkness by wearing sunglasses is recommended from leaving work to sleep onset. Melatonin 1 to 3 mg before bedtime may help.

Rapid Time Zone Change Syndrome (Jet Lag)

Transoceanic travel (by plane) produces a transient offset in the sleep-wake cycle caused by the mismatch between the geophysical clock from the point of departure and at arrival. In other words, the internal biological clock is exposed to other geophysical cycle to one must adapt. During the desynchronization period, subjects experience daytime hypersomnia, insomnia, irritability, and cognitive disturbances. Treatment on eastward flights is based on avoiding morning light and exposure to afternoon light. On westward flights, it is advisable to stay awake while it is light outside. Melatonin 2 to 5 mg before bedtime on arrival during 4 consecutive nights may be helpful.

SUGGESTED READING

American Academy of Sleep Medicine. The International Classification of Sleep Disorders. Second Edition. Diagnostic and Coding Manual. Westchester, IL: American Academy of Sleep Medicine; 2005.

Jennum P, Santamaría J, Bassetti C, et al. Sleep disorders in neurologic disease. In R Hughes, M Brainin, and NE Gilhus, editors. European handbook of neurological management. Ames, IA: Blackwell; 2006.

Smith MT, Perlis ML, Park A, et al. Comparative meta-analysis of phramacotherapy and behavior therapy in persistent insomnia. Am J Psychiatry 2002;159: 5–11.

Spielman AJ, Nunes J, Glovinsky PB. Insomnia. In MS Aldrich, guest editor. Neurologic Clinics: Sleep Disorders I. Philadelphia, PA: WB Saunders; 1996:513–544.

14 Parasomnias

Juan A. Pareja

INTRODUCTION

Parasomnias are unexpected or undesirable phenomena that occur at the beginning of sleep, during sleep, or at waking up. Parasomnias present clinically with behavioral, emotional, perceptual, sensory, oneiric, or vegetative signs and symptoms. Parasomnias should be differentiated from nocturnal seizures and psychiatric disorders (see Chapter 11).

DISORDERS OF AROUSAL

Normal sleep is frequently interrupted by intermittent brief arousals that usually produce either a transition to a lighter stage of sleep or—less frequently—a full awakening. In abnormal arousals known as partial arousals, the person seems to be trapped in a mixed state, unable to resume sleep and to awake in full. In this pathophysiological context, activation of the skeletal motor and/or autonomic nervous system emerges, and the subject displays behavior but is unaware of it. Disorders of arousal are associated with NREM sleep.

Sleepwalking and Sleep Terrors

Sleepwalking (SW) and sleep terrors (ST) typically emerge, and spontaneously remit, during childhood but may persist beyond adolescence, into adulthood, or may reappear in adulthood after a variable latency. SW and ST are constitutional disorders with relevant genetic factors.

SW is characterized by complex automatic behavior ranging from suddenly sitting up in bed with a glassy stare to automatic ambulation. During episodes, meaningful or any type of communication with a sleepwalker is often useless. There may be quite calm behavior but also vigorous, problematic, or even aggressive and violent behavior that can result in injury.

ST is characterized by abrupt onset of loud, inconsolable screaming with impressive autonomic manifestations such as tachycardia, elevated blood pressure, tachypnea, mydriasis, and profuse sweating. Patients usually sit up in bed staring with fear and engage in frenzied activity.

Episodes of SW-ST usually start in the first third of the night, mostly arising during arousals from slow-wave sleep (N3 stage). Interictally, polysomnography (PSG) is normal but may show hyperabrupt arousals without behavior arising from slow-wave sleep. Although there is often amnesia of the parasomnia, adults can remember a vivid dream with scenes of imminent danger that invites to escape. However, in children, oneiric memory hardly ever exists.

Overall, many circumstances that increase slow-wave sleep or produce arousals may ultimate trigger the SW-ST episodes, such as obstructive sleep apnea, periodic limb movements, nocturnal seizures, febrile illness, alcohol use, sleep deprivation, pregnancy, menstruation, and psychotropic medications—especially lithium carbonate and anticholinergic agents. Psychopathology does not seem to play a decisive role in the development and persistence of SW-ST, although life events and stress may act as precipitating mechanisms in predisposed persons.

Confusional Arousals (Sleep Drunkenness)

Confusional arousals is a milder variant of SW-ST and represents a disturbance of cognition and attention despite the motor behavior of wakefulness, resulting in complex behavior without conscious awareness. Confusional arousals can be precipitated by sleep deprivation, alcohol intake, sedatives, or obstructive sleep apnea and typically induce the patient to wander confused and disoriented.

Treatment of Arousal Disorders

Simple reassurance, sleep hygiene, and maintaining a safe bedroom environment are sufficient in the majority of cases. However, in arousal disorders associated with either vigorous behavior or injury or with extremely frequent episodes, pharmacological treatment is indicated. In such instances, benzodiazepines, in particular clonazepam (0.5–4 mg at bedtime), provide extraordinary benefit in controlling such nocturnal behaviors. Alprazolam, diazepam, imipramine, paroxetine, carbamazepine, and melatonin can also be effective.

PARASOMNIAS USUALLY ASSOCIATED WITH RAPID EYE MOVEMENT SLEEP

Rapid eye movement (REM) sleep behavior disorder (RBD) is clinically characterized by the presence of complex behavior often resulting in injury, which represents attempted enactment of violent dreams. It usually affects men over age 50, but it can also affect women and it can begin at any age, even in childhood.

In RBD, the protective muscle atonia that usually features REM sleep is partially lost. The PSG can display elevated muscle tone and/or excessive phasic submental and/or limb EMG twitching during REM sleep.

Nocturnal behavior are usually brief but complex and vigorous, often causing injury to the patient as well as to the bed partner. On awakening from an episode, there is usually rapid return to alertness and the patient may report a vivid, violent dream that correlates with the displayed behavior.

Although this disorder is usually chronic, there are acute forms, often caused by medications (tricyclic antidepressants, venlafaxine, fluoxetine, selegiline, monoamine oxidase inhibitors) or deprivation (alcohol, barbiturates, meprobamate). The acute form is usually of short duration.

The chronic form is idiopathic between 25% and 60% of cases. Many patients have the onset of the disorder linked with the onset of a neurological disorder, usually a degenerative disease, generally a synucleinopathy such as Parkinson's disease, multisystem atrophy, and dementia with Lewy bodies. RBD may precede the onset of the comorbid neurological illness by more than 10 years. RBD can also be another manifestation of narcolepsy.

Clonazepam is the treatment of choice. Doses between 0.5 and 4 mg, administered at bedtime, are very effective for controlling both the dreams and the behavioral disturbances. Clonazepam can suppress excessive muscle phasic activity but fails to reverse excessive tonic activity. Other, less effective treatments include melatonin (3–9 mg at bedtime) and antidepressants (intended to reduce REM sleep time).

Recurrent isolated sleep paralysis is characterized by periods of flaccid paralysis of all but the respiratory and extraocular muscles, occurring during the waking stage immediately preceding (hypnagogic) or succeeding (hypnopompic) sleep. The experience lasts from seconds to minutes and is frequently frightening. The familial and sporadic or "isolated" cases occur in otherwise normal subjects. Antidepressants given at bedtime are effective preventive drugs.

Sleep-related hallucinations include hallucinations experiences at sleep onset (hypnagogic hallucinations), as well as complex visual hallucinations on waking during the night. Although hypnagogic hallucinations may be associated with narcolepsy (see Chapter 16), in isolation they are benign. Antidepressants given at bedtime are effective preventive drugs.

Nightmare disorder is a vivid and frightening dream, often provoking a feeling of dread, oppression on the chest, or the conviction of paralysis, occurring during REM sleep and leading to awakening with intense fear, anxiety, and feeling of impending harm. Both alertness and recall of the dream are full immediately on awakening. It can be conceived as the combination of hallucinations and sleep paralysis.

OTHER PARASOMNIAS

Sleep-related eating disorder (SRED) is characterized by recurrent episodes of involuntary eating and drinking during sleep. The patients partially awake and sleepwalk to the kitchen where they may cook and eat. This condition can emerge from any stage of sleep and represents a dissociation of consciousness and eating behavior often associated with sleepwalking but can also be associated with periodic limb movements disorder, restless legs syndrome, obstructive sleep apnea, and other disturbances. Medications such as triazolam, anticholinergics, lithium carbonate, and zolpidem have been reported as precipitating of SRED.

One-third of these patients can suffer injury resulting from his or her confused and impulsive behavior when cooking (burns or collisions with the furniture of the kitchen) or eating hot, high-caloric foodstuffs or inappropriate substances.

SRED must be differentiated from nocturnal eating syndrome (NES), a condition in which the subject is fully awake during episodes of compulsive nocturnal eating (Table 14.1). The patients typically need to eat between dinner and sleep onset and on awakenings, being unable to start or resume sleep without eating or drinking. There may be some overlap between SRED and NES.

The differential diagnosis of SRED should include other conditions that can cause recurrent eating during both wakefulness and sleep: hypoglycaemia, peptic ulcer disease, reflux esophagitis, Kleine-Levin syndrome, Kluver-Bucy syndrome, and nocturnal extension of daytime anorexia nervosa, bulimia nervosa, and binge eating disorder.

Table 14.1 Abnormal Nighttime Eating

Sleep-Related Eating Disorder	Nocturnal Eating Syndrome
Eating on awake from sleep	May eat before going to bed
Partial arousal from sleep	Full arousal from sleep
Amnesia for the event	Full recall for the event
Intake of inappropriate food	Intake of normal foods
Temerary cooking	Normal cooking
No daytime food cravings	Food cravings in the evening
Comorbid sleep disorders*	Absence of comorbid sleep disorders

*Sleepwalking, obstructive sleep apnea, restless legs syndrome, periodic leg movements of sleep.

The effective treatment of comorbid disorders tends to control SRED. Idiopathic cases may respond to topiramate (100–150 mg/d) or a combination of L-dopa and clonazepam or opioids. NES is better treated with standard doses of fluoxetine, sertraline, or paroxetine.

Sleep-related expiratory groaning (catathrenia) is characterized by inspirations followed by prolonged expirations during which the patient makes a monotonous vocalization that closely resembles groaning. Some cases respond to continuous positive airway pressure.

Sleep-related dissociative disorders are psychogenic dissociative events that occur during wakefulness after arousal from sleep. Most patients with this disorder also manifest dissociative behaviors during the day. It is important to differentiate this entity from disorders of arousal. Management of these conditions by experienced specialists is strongly recommended.

Exploding head syndrome is characterized by an impression of a usually painless explosion in the head or a sudden loud noise that occurs as the patient is falling asleep or waking during the night. It is considered a sensory analogue of sleep starts. If the number of attacks is important, treatment with clomipramine or nifedipine may be of help.

Sleep enuresis consists of the involuntary voiding of urine after an age (about 5 years) at which the child can generally maintain bladder control throughout the night. Treatment involves the use of behavioral techniques and the administration of imipramine or desimipramine, or intranasal desmopressin.

SUGGESTED READING

American Academy of Sleep Medicine. The International Classification of Sleep Disorders. Second edition. Diagnostic and Coding Manual. Westchester, IL: American Academy of Sleep Medicine; 2005.

Jennum P, Santamaría J, Bassetti C, et al. Sleep disorders in neurologic disease. In R Hughes, M Brainin, and NE Gilhus, editors. European handbook of neurological management. Ames, IA: Blackwell; 2006.

Mahowald MW, Ettinger MG. Things that go bump in the night—the parasomnias revisited. J Clin Neurophysiol 1990;7:119–143.

Schenck CH, Hurwitz TD, Mahowald MW. REM sleep behavior disorder: An update on a series of 96 consecutive cases and a review of the literature. J Sleep Res 1993;2:224–231.

15 Sleep-Related Movement Disorders

Juan A. Pareja

INTRODUCTION

Sleep-related movement disorders are characterized by simple or stereotypic movements with sufficient frequency or intensity to disturb sleep and produce daytime hypersomnia or tiredness.

RESTLESS LEGS SYNDROME AND PERIODIC LEG MOVEMENTS IN SLEEP

Restless legs syndrome (RLS) is a sensorimotor disorder consisting of an urge to move attributed to the need to get rid of an in crescendo discomfort located mainly in the legs. The unpleasant sensation (described as tingling, creeping, burning, crawling, or throbbing) is transitorily relieved on movement but soon recurs, thus producing a cycle of abnormal sensation–movement. Symptoms of RLS appear in quiescent periods, with a circadian preponderance at night and the symptoms interfering with sleep onset. Taking altogether, these are key features for the diagnosis.

RLS is frequently associated with periodic leg movement in sleep (PLMS). PLMS is characterized by the presence of periodic contractions of the dorsiflexors of the foot occurring every 15 to 40 seconds. Associated flexion of the knee and hip may also occur. PLMS may cause intermittent arousals resulting in sleep fragmentation. Accordingly, fatigue and daytime sleepiness are the main complaints of these patients.

RLS is very common, affecting 5% to 10% of European adults. Almost 50% of patients have a family history of the syndrome. The majority of cases are primary, but there are secondary cases to iron deficiency, chronic renal disease, pregnancy, and peripheral neuropathies. Certain drugs such as antihistamines, neuroleptics, and most antidepressants can precipitate or exacerbate the syndrome.

Iron deficiency in the central nervous system (which has a negative influence in the dopaminergic neurotransmission), a dopaminergic alteration, and a constitutional factor seem to be the decisive factors for declaration of the syndrome. In fact, patients improve with dopaminergic agonists or after replenishing of iron deposits and get worse with dopamine antagonists (neuroleptics).

Treatment with dopamine (L-dopa) or dopaminergic agonists is very effective (Table 15.1). Treatment can be taken at night when symptoms appear or predominant. With time, the symptoms may expand through the day, with the patients needing daytime treatment. Possible limitations to dopaminergic therapy are rebound and

Table 15.1 Treatment of Restless Legs Syndrome

Dopaminergic	Usual Doses (mg/d)
L-Dopa	50–200
Ropirinol	1.5–4.6
Extended-release ropirinol	2–4
Pramipexol	0.18–1
Extended-release pramipexol	0.26–2.1
Rotigotine (transdermal patch)	1–4
Neuromodulators	
Gabapentin	300–3600
Pregabaline	25–300
Clonazepam	0.5–2
Opioids	
Codeine	30–180
Propoxyphene	100–600
Tramadol	50–300
Oxycodone	5–20
Hydrocodone	5–30
Methadone	5–20

augmentation. Rebound is related to short-lasting medications (such as L-dopa) that lead to the reappearance of symptoms as drug levels decline. Treatment of rebound includes use of dopaminergic drugs with prolonged effect or administration of the drug three times per day. Augmentation produces advance and exacerbation of symptoms, even extension to the arms. Augmentation is a relatively frequent iatrogenic effect of long-term dopaminergic therapy, especially with L-dopa. Management of augmentation includes a change of L-dopa for a dopaminergic agonist, stopping dopaminergic therapy and changing to neuromodulators, and the use of dopaminergic drugs with slow release or continuous delivery (via skin patch). There seems to be a better prognosis with continuous dopaminergic stimulation that likely provides stability of the symptoms and prevents augmentation.

Other effective treatments include some neuromodulators and opiates (Table 15.1). Even with normal serum iron levels, ferrotherapy is recommended to achieve ferritin serum levels greater than 45 mcg/mL.

SLEEP-RELATED RHYTHMIC MOVEMENT DISORDER

Sleep-related rhythmic movement disorder (SRRMD) is characterized by stereotypic and repetitive movements of the head, neck, trunk, or extremities that occur during drowsiness or sleep. This motor activity occurs unpredictably, often several nights a week. It usually occurs in the N2 sleep period, although it can occur at any sleep stage.

SRRMD disorders include head banging (jactatio capitis nocturna), leg banging, headrolling, bodyrolling, and body rocking. SRRMD occurs most frequently in infants, but adult persistence is not uncommon. The etiology is unknown and family incidence can be seen in some cases. The majority of affected children have no associated significant behavioral or emotional problems.

SRRMD is usually benign and often remits spontaneously. There is no effective treatment, although some cases have responded to imipramine and hypnosis.

BRUXISM

Bruxism is characterized by unconscious intermittent tight jaw closure, with rhythmic grinding of the teeth during all stages of sleep, mostly stage N2. This condition may result in damage to the teeth, to the periodontal structures, and to the temporomandibular joints.

Although it can occur at any age, the disorder predominates in children, and a genetic tendency has been observed. Bruxism may represent a manifestation of different alterations such as orofacial dyskinesia, mandibular dystonia, and tremor.

There is no convincingly effective treatment. Injections of botulinum toxin in the masticatory muscles may be indicated in diskinetic bruxism. Other treatments with psychotherapy, hypnosis, tryciclic antidepressants, muscle relaxants, or anti-inflammatory drugs have shown little or no efficacy. A variety of dental devices and intraoral splints are available to protect the teeth.

SLEEP-RELATED LEG CRAMP

Leg cramps are characterized by sudden painful spasms of leg muscles that wake the patient from sleep. The involved muscles are felt hard or tight on palpation, indicating a strong muscle contraction. Most cases are idiopathic. Immediate relief can be obtained by stretching the affected muscle. Quinine sulfate, magnesium, gabapentin, or verapamil may prevent nocturnal cramps.

SUGGESTED READING

Allen R, Earley C. Restless legs syndrome: A review of clinical and pathophysiologic features. J Clin Neurophysiol 2001;18:128–147.

American Academy of Sleep Medicine. The International Classification of Sleep Disorders. Second edition. Diagnostic and Coding Manual. Westchester, IL: American Academy of Sleep Medicine; 2005.

Jennum P, Santamaría J, Bassetti C, et al. Sleep disorders in neurologic disease. In R Hughes, M Brainin, and NE Gilhus, editors. European handbook of neurological management. Ames, IA: Blackwell; 2006.

Silber MH. Sleep-related movement disorders. Continuum (Minneap Minn) 2013;19 (1 Sleep Disorders):170–184.

16 Hypersomnia

Juan A. Pareja

INTRODUCTION

Sleepiness is normal after prolonged wakefulness or when approaching a normal sleep period. *Excessive sleepiness, hypersomnia,* or *daytime sleepiness* is defined as the propensity to enter sleep at an inappropriate time or setting. The patients are unable to stay awake and alert during the major part of the day, resulting in unintended lapses into drowsiness or sleep. The severity of hypersomnia ranges from occurring in boring monotonous situations to bouts of irresistible sleep or sleep attacks. Overall, hypersomnia can be produced by disorders that produce sleep fragmentation or can be centrally driven (Table 16.1). Sleepiness can be documented by using the Multiple Sleep Latency Test (MSLT) or estimated subjectively by using the Epworth Sleepiness Scale (Table 16.2).

SLEEP-RELATED BREATHING DISORDERS

Sleep-related breathing disorders encompass a variety of disordered breathing problems that appear exclusively in sleep or are exacerbated by sleep. Although lung diseases can disrupt sleep, the majority of respiratory disturbances during sleep occur in patients with healthy lungs.

Central Sleep Apnea/Hypopnea Syndrome

Central sleep apnea/hypopnea syndrome is characterized by the presence of central apneas and/or hypopneas (Table 16.3) recurring with intermittent or periodic patterns during sleep. According to the underlying level of ventilation, the syndrome may be classified in normocapnic and hypercapnic. Moreover, the syndrome can be idiopathic or secondary to brainstem structural lesions/dysfunctions or medical conditions. Treatment must be directed to the correction of the origin of the syndrome.

Normocapnic Central Sleep Apnea/Hypopnea Syndrome

Idiopathic Central Sleep Apnea Syndrome Central apneas may occur in patients with an exaggerated ventilatory response to the levels of $Paco_2$. These patients tend to have waking low levels of $Paco_2$ (less than 40 mm Hg) and thus are close to the apnea threshold, which is reached with a minimum increase in ventilation. The main complaints are daytime hypersomnia, disrupted sleep, insomnia, and night asphyctic episodes. The polysomnogram (PSG) shows more than five central apneas per hour of sleep.

Table 16.1 Major Categories of Hypersomnia

157

Hypersomnia

Sleep-related breathing disorders (SRBD)
  Central Sleep Apnea syndrome
  Obstructive Sleep Apnea syndrome
Hypersomnia of central origin
  Narcolepsy
  Idiopathic hypersomnia
  Recurrent hypersomnia
    Kleine-Levin syndrome
    Menstrual-related hypersomnia
Hypersomnia due to medical condition
  Parkinson´s disease
  Posttraumatic hypersomnia
  Central nervous system (CNS) lesions
  Genetic disorders associated with primary CNS hypersomnia
    Fragile X syndrome
    Niemann-Pick type C disease
    Moebius syndrome
    Norrie´s syndrome
  Genetic disorders associated with primary CNS hypersomnia and SRBD
    Prader-Willi syndrome
    Myotonic dystrophy
  Endocrine disorders
  Metabolic and toxic conditions
Sleep deprivation
Depression (pseudohypersomnia)

Cheyne-Stokes Breathing Syndrome The syndrome is characterized by the presence of repeated ventilatory cycles with periods of apnea or hypopnea alternating with periods of hyperpnea. The PSG may document gradually growing amplitude breathing excursions, followed by respiratory excursions of gradually descending amplitude, culminating in an apnea or hypopnea of central type. This disorder is usually due to heart failure, kidney failure, or stroke. The patients hyperventilate during wakefulness and sleep, either via stimulation of vagal receptors in congestive lungs or via chemoreceptors hypersensitivity.

Hypercapnic Central Sleep Apnea/Hypopnea Syndrome

This syndrome is associated with high waking $Paco_2$ levels due to daytime hypoventilation in the context of diminished chemoreceptor responsiveness or impaired respiratory muscles (neuromuscular diseases).

Sleep-Related Hypoventilation/Hypoxemic Syndrome

Sleep-related hypoventilation/hypoxemic syndrome is defined as hypoventilation during sleep related to decreased alveolar ventilation that results in hypercapnia and hypoxemia.

Table 16.2 Epworth Sleepiness Scale

How likely are you to doze off or fall asleep in the following situations, in contrast to feeling just tired?. This refers to your usual way of life in recent times. Even if you have not done some of these things recently, try to work out how they would have affected you. Use the following scale to choose *the most appropriate number* for each situation:

    0 = would *never* doze

    1 = *slight* chance of dozing

    2 = *moderate* chance of dozing

    3 = *high* chance of dozing

Situation	Chance of Dozing
Sitting and reading	....
Watching TV	....
Sitting, inactive in a public place (e.g., theatre or a meeting)	....
As a passenger in a car for an hour without a break	....
Lying down to rest in the afternoon when circumstances permit	....
Sitting and talking to someone	....
Sitting quietly after a lunch without alcohol	....
In a car, while stopped for a few minutes in traffic	....
Global score	....

The numbers for the eight situations are added together to give a global score between 0 and 24. The mean normal score is <6.

From Johns MW. A new method for measuring daytime sleepiness: The Epworth Sleepiness Scale. Sleep 1991;14:540–545.

- **Idiopathic**: Alveolar hypoventilation with normal properties of the lungs.
  Congenital central alveolar hypoventilation syndrome. It is characterized by the onset of hypoventilation in infancy, owing to failure of automatic central control of breathing.
  Idiopathic sleep-related nonobstructive alveolar hypoventilation. The symptoms start in adolescence or early adulthood. The underlying mechanisms are a reduced responsiveness to hypercapnia or hypoxia during wakefulness and sleep owing to a dysfunction/lesion of the medullary chemoreceptors controlling ventilation.
- **Secondary**: Alveolar hypoventilation is due to medical disorders, typically chronic pulmonary diseases, morbid obesity, anatomical disorders of the chest wall, and neuromuscular diseases.

Table 16.3 Definitions of Respiratory Events During Sleep

Apnea Complete cessation of ventilation for a duration >10 sec

Hypopnea Reduction of >50% from baseline in the amplitude of air flow signal lasting ≥10 sec. A clear amplitude reduction that does not reach the above criterion but is accompanied by microarousal or oxygen desaturation of oxyhemoglobin of ≥3%

Central apnea Cessation of air flow and thoracoabdominal respiratory effort for >10 sec

Obstructive apnea Cessation of air flow in the presence of respiratory effort with duration of >10 sec, which can be accompanied by greater than 4% oxygen desaturation and/or microarousals

Mixed apnea Apnea that starts as central and continues as obstructive, >10 sec in length, which can be accompanied by a desaturation >4% or microarousals

Treatment with nasal intermittent positive pressure ventilation, bilevel positive airway pressure BiPAP), variable positive airway pressure, and noninvasive volumetric ventilation is useful for central apnea syndrome, Cheyne-Stokes breathing syndrome, and alveolar hypoventilation. Invasive ventilation may be required in patients with severe—life threatening—hypoventilation. Nonspecific treatment of central apneas includes acetazolamide, oxygen, or theophyline, but the evidence for its therapeutic use is poor.

Obstructive Sleep Apnea/Hypopnea Syndrome

Obstructive sleep apnea/hypopnea syndrome (OSA) is characterized by the occurrence of multiple episodes of complete (apnea) or partial (hypopnea) upper airway obstructions during sleep (Table 16.3). Respiratory pauses cause intermittent arousals and oxygen desaturations.

Snoring and excessive daytime sleepiness are the chief complaints of these patients. They may also report insomnia with recurrent awakenings from sleep, chocking and gasping during sleep, unrefreshing sleep, early morning headaches, and daytime fatigue with impaired concentration. The prevalence of OSA is 2% to 4%, with predominance in males, usually older than 40 years. This disorder is due to a hypotonia of muscles of the upper airway, which collapse during sleep and hinder the inflow of air. Collapsibility of upper airway muscles and narrow airway passage (craniofacial abnormalities) are mostly constitutional. Acquired factors such as obesity; cardiac, pulmonary, neurological (cerebrovascular, neuromuscular disorders), and endocrine (acromegaly, hypothyroidism) diseases; alcohol; and sedative drugs may all contribute to the final outcome of these patients.

Nasal continuous positive airway pressure (CPAP) is the treatment of choice for OSA. Either fixed-pressure CPAP or auto-adjusted pressure CPAP reverses all the symptoms of OSA. BiPAP may be indicated in OSA patients with neuromuscular disorders. Oral appliance may be useful in patients who do not tolerate CPAP. Surgery of the upper airway should be restricted to selected patients.

HYPERSOMNIA OF CENTRAL ORIGIN

Hypersomnia of central origin include a group of disorders in which daytime sleepiness is the cardinal symptom and cannot be attributed to a disturbed nocturnal sleep or chronobiological disorder.

Narcolepsy

Narcolepsy is a neurological condition characterized by excessive daytime sleepiness with or without cataplexy, often associated with the occurrence of manifestations of rapid eye movement (REM) sleep (hypnagogic hallucinations, sleep paralysis) during waking periods. Other possible symptoms include automatic behavior, insomnia, diplopia, and blurred vision.

The symptoms typically start between 15 and 25 years of age and affect both sexes with similar incidence. Only 20% to 30% of narcoleptics will display a full range of symptoms. Hypersomnia is always present, whereas REM sleep symptoms may appear decades later. In about 15% of narcoleptics, cataplexy is absent. This has prompted a nosological distinction between narcolepsy with cataplexy and narcolepsy without cataplexy.

Narcolepsy is a primary disorder. There is a genetic predisposition as *DQB1-0602* haplotype is present in 95% of patients with narcolepsy with cataplexy and in 41% of patients with narcolepsy without cataplexy. Loss of hypocretin-1–secreting neurons in the hypothalamus (presumably on a degenerative or autoimmune basis) plays a major pathogenic role in the majority of patients with narcolepsy. Depletion of hypocretin-ergic neurons determines a decrease or almost total absence of hypocretine-1 in the cerebrospinal fluid (CSF) in 90% of patients with narcolepsy with cataplexy and in 10% to 20% of patients with narcolepsy without cataplexy.

Most patients recognize a precipitating factor (generally related to sleep-wake schedule changes) in the onset of symptoms. Traumatic brain injury and febrile states have also been reported as possibly triggers. Symptomatic narcolepsy is extremely rare. In virtually all such cases, a structural lesion in the diencephalon or hypothalamus has been documented.

A diagnosis of narcolepsy relies on the presence of typical symptoms and confirmation by either PSG followed by an MSLT or CSF hypocretin-1 levels of 110 pg/mL or less. Sleepiness not attributable to other causes and a convincing history of cataplexy strongly suggest the diagnosis. Definite diagnosis requires an MSLT showing a mean sleep latency of 8 or fewer minutes and the presence of REM periods in at least two naps. MSLT should be performed after a PSG. Typical findings in PSG include short sleep latency, sleep-onset REM, sleep fragmentation, and periods of ambiguous sleep (REM sleep without atonia or fast transitions from non-REM and REM sleep).

The treatment of narcolepsy includes regular sleep-wake schedules and one or several short naps that may provide transitory increased alertness. Otherwise, treatment is aimed at counteracting the symptoms (Table 16.4). Hypersomnia is treated with stimulants taken in the morning or in the morning and noon to avoid insomnia. Extended-release stimulants are taken once in the morning. Sodium oxybate is administered at night, with its very short half-life requiring patients to take the first dose at bedtime and to wake up at night for a middle-of-the night second dose. Antidepressants (counteracting REM-related symptoms) can be taken at night or twice (morning/night). It should be mentioned that sodium oxybate is effective for all the symptoms of narcolepsy. Association of sodium oxybate and modafinil is very useful.

Owing to the fact that reduction of hypocretins is the primary defect in narcolepsy future potential therapies may include hypocretin agonists. Immunomodulation aimed at reducing a putative immunological reaction against hypocretinergic neurons has not been validated yet.

Idiopathic Hypersomnia

Idiopathic hypersomnia (IH) is characterized by excessive daytime somnolence despite having a normal (6–10 hours) nocturnal sleep time (IH without long sleep duration) or a prolonged (>10 hours) nocturnal sleep time (IH with long sleep duration). Otherwise, sleep architecture is normal.

Regardless of the duration of night sleep, the patients have an important disability to get out of bed in the morning even with confusion upon waking (sleep inertia). Unlike narcolepsy, unintended naps in IH are longer and typically unrefreshing.

Table 16.4 Treatment of Narcoleptic Symptoms

Treatment	Common Daily Dose	Maximum Daily Dose
Hypersomnia		
Modafinil	100 mg	400 mg
Sodium oxibate	4.5 g	9 g
Methylphenidate	30 mg	100 mg
Extended release methylphenidate (Concerta)	18 mg	54 mg
Dextroamphetamine	15 mg	100 mg
Extended release dextroamphetamine (Dexedrine spansuls)	10 mg	60 mg
Methamphetamine	15 mg	80 mg
Mazindol	1 mg	8 mg
Cataplexy, Sleep Paralysis, Hypnagogic Hallucinations		
Sodium oxybate	4.5 g	9 g
Imipramine	25 mg	200 mg
Clomipramine	10 mg	200 mg
Protryptiline	5 mg	30 mg
Fluoxetine	20 mg	80 mg
Venlafaxine	37.5 mg	300 mg
Insomnia		
Sodium oxybate	4.5 g	9 g
Short-acting benzodiazepines	See Chapter 13, Table 13.2	

The diagnosis relies on the clinical features and requires both a normal PSG and a MSLT showing a mean sleep latency less than 8 minutes (often <5 minutes), with one or fewer REM sleep periods. IH could be confused with monosymptomatic narcolepsy (presenting only with hypersomnia). Absence of ancillary symptoms of narcolepsy (cataplexy, hypnagogic hallucinations, and sleep paralysis) differentiates IH from narcolepsy. In addition, IH has neither HLA correlation nor CSF hypocretin deficiency.

The management of hypersomnia in IH is similar to that of narcolepsy, with modafinil and other stimulants at similar doses (Table 16.4).

Recurrent Hypersomnia

Recurrent hypersomnia presents with periods of daytime sleepiness alternating with phases of normality.

Kleine-Levin Syndrome

It usually affects teenager boys and consists of symptomatic periods lasting days or weeks, in which the patients present with marked somnolence and a variable combination of abnormal behavior, hyperphagia, and hypersexuality. These periods can turn every few months and may resolve spontaneously after a variable period of recurrence. Hypersomnia can be treated with modafinil. It has been claimed that treatment with lithium carbonate may reduce the frequency and duration of symptomatic periods.

Menstrual-Related Hypersomnia

Hypersomnia periods recur with catamenial periodicity. Symptoms are restricted to the menstrual days and seem to be dependent on a hormonal dysfunction since anovulatory treatment leads to prolonged remission of the syndrome.

SUGGESTED READING

American Academy of Sleep Medicine. *The International Classification of Sleep Disorders. Second edition. Diagnostic and Coding Manual.* Westchester, IL: American Academy of Sleep Medicine; 2005.

Arnulf I, Zeitzer JM, File J, Farber N, Mignot E. Kleine-Levin syndrome: A systematic review of 186 cases in the literature. Brain 2005;128:2763–2776.

Carskadon MA, Dement WC, Mitler MM, et al. Guideliness for the Multiple Sleep Latency Test (MSLT): A standard measure of sleepiness. Sleep 1986;9:519–524.

Jennum P, Santamaría J, Bassetti C, et al. Sleep disorders in neurologic disease. In R Hughes, M Brainin, and NE Gilhus, editors. European handbook of neurological management. Ames, IA: Blackwell; 2006.

Johns MW. A new method for measuring daytime sleepiness: The Epworth Sleepiness Scale. Sleep 1991;14:540–545.

SECTION FIVE
NEUROMUSCULAR DISEASES

17 Motor Neuron Disease (Amyotrophic Lateral Sclerosis)

Ole-Bjørn Tysnes

INTRODUCTION

Amyotrophic lateral sclerosis (ALS) occurs at an annual incidence of approximately 2:100,000. It has been reported an increase in incidence over the past decades, but most of this is probably related to increasing age of the populations studied. The overall picture is that the incidence is rather stable with some higher numbers for more northern countries. It occurs with slightly higher incidence in men than in women, and the mean age of onset is approximately 60 years. ALS is rare at ages younger than 40, but it can occur as early as in the teenage years. Most reports are consistent with decreasing incidence in very old age.

CLINICAL CHARACTERISTICS

The onset of ALS is usually a focal motor symptom. It can be from bulbar or spinal motor neurons. Spinal onset is more frequent (60%) than bulbar onset. Bulbar onset becomes more frequent at higher age. Combination of a paresis with atrophy and fasciculations is the typical spinal onset. The paresis will increase and spread and the neurophysiological examination will reveal generalized affection of the anterior horn motor neuron. In bulbar cases, the typical onset symptom is dysarthria. Swallowing difficulties occur later in the disease. On examination, atrophy of the tongue is evident and fasciculations in the tongue can be identified. In some cases, upper motor neuron involvement is predominant. Atrophy may then be absent or difficult to identify. Cases with spinal onset ALS then present with predominant spastic pareses, and in bulbar cases, tongue atrophy is absent, but tongue movements are severely affected (pseudobulbar palsy). Cases with predominant upper motor neuron involvement can be difficult to diagnose, especially early in the disease course. Normal EMG is often observed in cases with pseudobulbar onset. Some cases of ALS have very early insufficient respiratory function. This symptom may be present before the ALS diagnosis has been made; most often, this occurs in cases with bulbar onset ALS.

During the past 10 years, it has become evident that neuropsychological frontal symptoms are relatively frequent in ALS. Today, the disease therefore cannot in general be considered a pure motor disease. In some cases, there is an obvious overlap between frontotemporal dementia and ALS. While frontotemporal dementia occurs rarely in

ALS (5%), more subtle frontal symptoms may occur in approximately 50% of all ALS cases. The knowledge of frontal symptoms in ALS must have an impact on decisions taken in the management of ALS patients, especially in the late course of the disease.

ETIOLOGY

ALS in more than 90% of cases is considered a sporadic disease (SALS). Most inherited cases (FALS) have an autosomal dominant presentation. Thus, in general clinical work, FALS cases are relatively easy to identify, and most patients will already be aware that ALS exists in their family. For 20 years, the *SOD* mutation was the known major cause of FALS (20%), but recently a C9orf72 expansion (hexanucleotide) has been identified in more than 30% of cases of FALS and, in some series, up to 10% of SALS cases. This challenges our view on SALS. We do not know if apparent sporadic cases with the C9orf72 expansion have an increased risk for ALS in their offspring. Today, genetic testing is not recommended in daily ALS work. Some centers perform testing in familial cases. The identification of specific mutations can be of importance in genetic counseling and may give information on the probable evolution of symptom severity.

We still have little knowledge on the etiology of true cases of SALS. Several hypotheses on intoxication or physical exercise have been proposed after publications on ALS clustering, but knowledge of the SALS etiology remains sparse.

MEDICAL TREATMENT

ALS is still without effective medical treatment. Riluzole was introduced almost 20 years ago and is the only approved medical treatment (standard dosage is 50 mg twice daily). From the trials, it was demonstrated that riluzole increased survival by approximately 3 months, but it seems that the drug can have a more pronounced effect in some cases, especially when given early in the disease course. This challenges the way we work when diagnosing ALS. There is a pressure to decide on the ALS diagnosis to be able to start medical treatment. This increases the risk of treating patients who do not have a final diagnosis of ALS. Side effects of riluzole treatment may be serious but are usually mild (nausea, especially during the initial days of treatment). Serious side effects are liver toxicity and bone marrow depletion. These potential side effects must always be ruled out by repeated serological testing after the onset of treatment. If riluzole is well tolerated over a month or two after treatment initiation, the risk of serious side effects can be considered low.

MANAGEMENT

In addition to the breakthrough in genetic causes of ALS, the most important changes during the past decades have been in the management of these patients. In earlier years, ALS patients were offered little to be able to continue a respectful life after an ALS diagnosis. Most patients were left with their families and they were admitted to hospitals or palliative units in the late course of the disease. Today, most ALS patients have the possibility to live in their home until they die. The treatment of respiratory insufficiency has had a significant impact on survival time from diagnosis even when

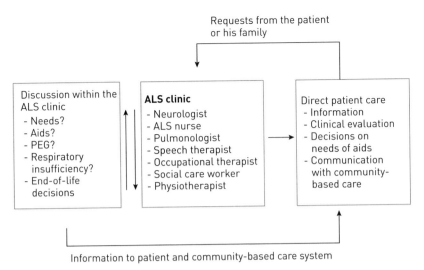

FIGURE 17.1
Organization of the ALS clinic.

excluding patients on permanent ventilation support. Management of ALS patients is currently often organized in ALS clinics (Figure 17.1).

Communication

Communication problems occur early in ALS with bulbar onset but are also frequent in later stages of spinal onset ALS. Speech therapists or occupational therapists will be consulted. The effect of traditional speech therapy is usually sparse because the disease progresses rapidly and even single-syllable words can be difficult to understand. Most cases with bulbar onset and anarthria will use pen and paper to communicate. Some will also use electronic aids like Lightwriter or i-Pad. Mobile phones or i-Pad also allow for electronic communication via SMS or e-mail. Electronic aids can also be used in the later stages of the disease when it becomes impossible to use pen and paper. The ALS patients should therefore be encouraged early to use electronic communication aids. If or when paralysis of the hands occurs, computer-based systems must be established such that the ALS patient can use head or eye movements to control the computer. Actions must be taken early enough for the patient to be able to learn how to use the communication aid before the disease has progressed too far. The use of eye-movement markers in advanced ALS is useful for the communication of "new thoughts." The method is rather laborious for the untrained physician, but trained carers of ALS patients may use the device or even communicate directly by watching the patient's eye movements without any devise, at an impressive speed.

Nutrition

Most cases with ALS come sooner or later to a situation of malnutrition. This usually occurs earlier in cases with bulbar onset. The patient's weight should be registered regularly. The time the patient requires for a meal can give an idea of the onset of nutrition problems. Physicians and carers should encourage patients to accept percutaneous endoscopic gastrotomy (PEG) before the disease is too advanced. Respiratory problems represent a risk factor when establishing the PEG. For patients, it is difficult to "give up" eating. They must be informed that they still can eat even if they have the PEG. The PEG is to protect against malnutrition, and it will often improve the general condition of the patient. The risk when establishing the PEG is low in most cases. Procedure-related complications like subcutaneous emphysema occur but are very rare. The only serious complications I have seen are when the PEG is established in patients with severe respiratory failure. The patients may then experience increased dyspnea, which is not reversible, and that may lead to earlier end-stage respiratory failure.

Sialorrhea

Drooling or sialorrhea occurs together with increasing dysarthria and dysphagia. It is embarrassing for the patient, can cause some skin problems, and affects the use of noninvasive ventilation devises. Atropinergic drugs like scopolamine have an effect on the drooling but may not be tolerated due to mental side effects like fatigue or decreased cognitive function. During the past years, the use of botulinum toxin injections in the parotid glands has been established, eventually in the submandibular glands. Some centers prefer one-fraction irradiation of the salivary glands, which has a more prolonged effect than botulinum toxin injections. At our center, we use salivary gland radiation. It is my experience that a second treatment is rarely required, as patients who receive this treatment are in a terminal phase of the disease.

Physical Problems

It is the nature of ALS that the patients have increasing and changing physical problems with the development of the disease. The engagement of community-based physiotherapists and occupational therapists is obliged. Aids must be available when required, and the complexity and availability of such aids vary considerably. Aids to prologue the functioning of the hands or to walk comfortably are usually easy to acquire. A manual wheelchair is in the same category. Electrical wheelchairs to use indoor or outdoor, with or without integrated communication systems, require more planning and may need economy decisions in the social care system. The need for transportation systems is obvious. In some cases with slow progression, it is recommended that the patient can have a car to move outdoors. It is more usual to give support to a car that the spouse can drive and that is suitable for the transportation of even electric wheelchairs.

A frequent question is whether ALS patients should do physical exercise to prevent the development of increasing paresis. In general, it is not recommended for ALS patients to perform hard exercise and it has not been demonstrated that such training prolongs physical functions or survival.

Home Situation

Almost all ALS patients prefer to stay at home as long as possible, and it is a major task for the ALS team to facilitate this. Physicians must introduce the problem to the patient early and to the spouse. The idea to move to a more appropriate apartment or to make changes in the actual place of living must mature. Decision making is difficult and involves both the patient and the spouse. The speed of ALS symptom development, personal relation to the place they live, and thoughts on the future of both patient and spouse are important factors, in addition to technical issues regarding the current place of living. An occupational therapist should always be part of the patient's care group and must give indications early on what is possible to organize in the patient's place of living. Patients and spouses hesitate to discuss these kinds of questions. Physicians must engage in the couple's problems with such questions. Information on prognosis and how nursing can be organized will influence the decision making of the couple. The possibility to live outside an institution will often influence the ALS patient's decisions when it comes to ventilation support.

Work Toward the Social Care System

All patients with ALS will require aids that involve the social care system. At the time of the diagnosis, the patient can take care of himself but he can have problems continuing at work if desired, transportation can be needed, and the ALS diagnosis can influence the work of the spouse. Later, there may be a need for a personal assistant to allow the patient to get out of the house or to take part in a social life. It can be questions of what arrangements exist that makes it possible for the couple to spend time together without the spouse doing all nursing himself. A social care worker should be part of the ALS team to inform the patient and the spouse of their rights and what possibilities may exist.

Respiration

Respiratory failure is the final outcome in all ALS patients. During the past decade, it has become increasingly frequent to use noninvasive ventilation support (NINV). It has been demonstrated that such treatment reduces symptoms related to nighttime hypoxia such as headache and fatigue, and the longer survival in ALS is attributed to more extensive use of NINV. Respiratory support must be considered actual treatment in all ALS patients. NINV can be used without ethical concerns as the treatment always will be self-limiting. Patients can always decide to continue treatment or to stop treatment. A great advantage using NINV is that patients with early respiration symptoms can survive long enough to have experience with the helpless feeling of being more and more paralyzed. This makes it clearer for the patient to make decisions on a more permanent ventilation support. The treating physician must early decide if the patient's cognitive status is such that he can understand the impact of permanent ventilation support through tracheostomy. As many as 50% of ALS patients develop frontal symptoms during the disease. They have reduced understanding of what impacts their decision of a permanent ventilation solution can have on the spouse and other members of the family. This is especially important if children still live at home. Patients may have the idea that spouse or children may help to keep the ventilation support going. In such cases, the physician must inform the patient directly about the impact on the family of a permanent ventilation-support situation and about the difficulties with family members having such kind of responsible duties at home. In principle, all care must be given by professional carers. The patient must be able to understand that that his house will take the form of a small "hospital unit" and that his family also will have to live there. Family members of ALS patients very rarely object to patient's decision making on respiratory issues. Neurologists and pulmonologist in the ALS team have a duty to take an active part in the discussion and the decision making when it comes to permanent ventilation support. Only patients who are able to understand the full consequences of permanent ventilation through tracheostomy should be offered such a possibility.

Ethical Issues

Treating ALS patients takes physicians into several problems where ethical questions are apparent. Today the information of the diagnosis must be given as early as possible. After the consultation with the neurologist, the patent will have enough information of find the diagnosis on the Internet on his own. Although diagnostic uncertainty may exist, it is better to inform about the diagnosis and the uncertainty than leaving it to the patient to search for the diagnosis. Some patients want all kinds of information early;

ALS treatment and management

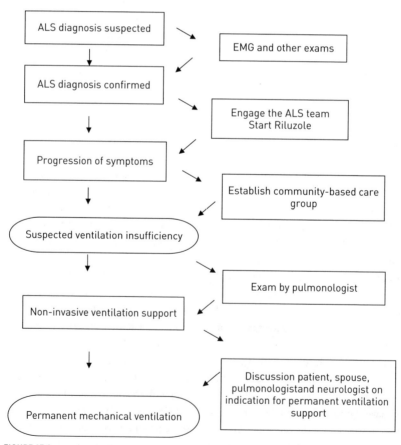

FIGURE 17.2

ALS treatment and management.

others hesitate to learn anything. The physician must balance the information having in mind an idea of what kind of information the patient requires. Both offering and stopping ventilation support represent ethical problems. The situation of both the patient and spouse must be considered when permanent ventilation support is discussed. Is the patient sufficiently informed about all the consequences of permanent ventilation? How will such a decision affect the family? How can the patient be sure that he will come out of the ventilation support when he wants? Can he be sure that he can communicate clearly enough such that carers and family understand his wishes? Can he be sure that there is anyone to take him off the ventilation support? Reidun Førde, professor in medical ethics at the University of Oslo, finds it from an ethical point of view similar to let an ALS patient on respiratory support continue to live against his will, as to stop the ventilation with his will. It cannot be considered euthanasia.

CONCLUSIONS

Diagnosing and treating ALS patients offer great challenges, especially regarding the information and management throughout the disease (Figure 17.2). Great advantages come to the patients through better management with new technological possibilities. Innovations in communication, nutrition, treatment of drooling, organization of the patient's home, and better noninvasive and invasive ventilation systems have made this possible. In the near future, we will understand how or if we can use genetic information in the treatment and management of ALS patients.

SUGGESTED READING

Andersen PM et al. EFNS Task Force on Diagnosis and Management of Amyotrophic Lateral Sclerosis: Eur J Neurol 2012;19:360–375.
EFNS guidelines on the clinical management of amyotrophic lateral sclerosis (ALS)—revised report of an EFNS task force.

18 Acute and Chronic Neuropathies

Christian A. Vedeler

GUILLAIN-BARRÉ SYNDROME

Clinical Findings

In about two-thirds of the cases, Guillain-Barré syndrome (GBS) is a postinfectious disease most often following an upper respiratory or a gastrointestinal infection. After approximately 1 to 2 weeks, patients develop a symmetric weakness that can affect both proximal and distal muscles. Cranial nerve involvement is common and paresthesias are also frequent with reduced distal sensation affecting all modalities. Tendon reflexes are usually reduced or lost within the first week of the disease. Autonomic affection is common and can give rise to temporary bladder and gastrointestinal retention, variations in sweating and blood pressure, and, of special concern, cardiac arrhythmia, which may be associated with bradycardia and asystole.

GBS has three phases; a progressive phase lasting a maximum of 4 weeks; a plateau phase, which may last for several months; and a recovery phase, which may last for more than 1 year.

The cerebrospinal fluid (CSF) may be normal within the first week but thereafter usually shows an "albuminocytological dissociation," meaning there is an increased total protein concentration and normal amount of leukocytes. Electrodiagnostic testing confirms a segmental demyelinating polyneuropathy with slowed nerve conduction velocities with conduction blocks, abnormal temporal dispersion, and prolonged distal and proximal (F-wave) latencies. These findings are usually most prominent in the second week of the disease.

GBS consists of three variants: *Acute inflammatory demyelinating polyneuropathy (AIDP)* is the most common variant and has clinical features as described earlier. *Miller Fisher syndrome (MFS)* is a mild form of GBS with ophthalmoplegia, areflexia, and sensory ataxia with normal muscle strength. If the muscle strength is affected, it is defined as AIDP. GQ1b antibodies are associated with MFS. *Acute motor axonal neuropathy (AMAN)* or *acute motor and sensory axonal neuropathy (AMSAN)* is usually preceded by a gastrointestinal infection with *Campylobacter jejuni* and is associated with GM1 IgG antibodies. Electrodiagnostic testing shows primary axonal affection.

Treatment and Prognosis

GBS patients should be admitted to hospital in the acute phase of the disease because of the risk that they become rapidly tetraparetic with respiratory distress and develop cardiac arrhythmia. Such severely affected patients should be treated in an intensive care unit. Subcutaneous heparin should be given if the patient has severe weakness, and skin care is essential to prevent decubitus ulceration. Active physiotherapy should be avoided in the acute phase as this may worsen the autonomic instability. Pain can be severe in the acute phase of GBS and is treated as other causes of neuropathic pain with anticonvulsants or antidepressants.

If the patient is moderately affected [a GBS disability scale of ≥3 (i.e., inability to walk unaided)], treatment with intravenous immunoglobulin (IVIg) should be started (Figure 18.1). The normal dose is 2 g/kg and is usually given in divided doses of 0.4 g/kg every day for 5 days. Plasma exchange is equally effective but is less used because IVIg is more easily administrated and has fewer complications. Such immune modulatory treatments should be started within the first 2 weeks of disease onset. If there are contraindications for IVIg treatment, such as IgA deficiency, plasma exchange should be performed. Such treatment consists of 5 exchanges in 1 to 2 weeks with a total exchange of 5 plasma volumes.

So far, it is not known if IVIg or plasma exchange is effective in MFS or mild GBS with GBS disability scale of ≤2. If GBS patients relapse, they will usually benefit from another round of treatment, IVIg, or plasma exchange. If they deteriorate despite such treatment, they will still probably benefit with another course of IVIg or plasma exchange. If the patient is severely affected with no signs of improvement 2 to 3 weeks after the first treatment has been completed, another course of IVIg or plasma exchange may also be tried. However, there is no proved effect of retreatment of such patients. Corticosteroids have not been shown to be effective in GBS.

The prognosis of GBS is usually good; a mortality rate of 3% to 5% has nevertheless been been reported, usually due to respiratory or cardiac failure complications that should be avoidable if severely affected patients are treated in intensive care. About 20% to 30% of patients have permanent sequelae despite rehabilitation. These are most commonly permanent distal weakness and sensory disturbance. Residual disability correlates with increasing age, severe weakness, and axonal loss. Some patients also experience temporary fatigue during the recovery phase.

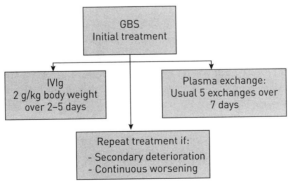

FIGURE 18.1
Algorithm for treatment of Guillain-Barre syndrome (GBS).

CHRONIC INFLAMMATORY DEMYELINATING POLYNEUROPATHY

Clinical Findings

Chronic inflammatory demyelinating polyneuropathy (CIDP) is usually a slowly progressive disease over more than 8 weeks. In up to 5% of cases, it can start acutely (within 4 weeks) and resemble acute inflammatory demyelinating polyneuropathy (AIDP), or subacutely (within 4 to 8 weeks). The weakness is usually symmetric, involving both distal and proximal muscles. If the distribution is asymmetric, the disease is called Lewis–Sumner syndrome or multifocal acquired demyelinating sensory and motor neuropathy (MADSAM). Sensory loss involves all modalities and is usually distributed in a "glove and stocking" fashion. Pain can be present in the sensory variants but is otherwise uncommon in CIDP. Similarly, autonomic findings and cranial nerve affection are much less frequent in CIDP than in AIDP. Tendon reflexes are reduced or absent early in the course of the disease in both upper and lower extremities.

CSF examination is also important for the diagnosis of CIDP: high protein (>1 g/L) is present in more that 90% of the cases with CIDP together with normal leukocyte content (<10 cells/mm^3). If pleocytosis is present, differential diagnoses such as Lyme disease, HIV infection or sarcoidosis should be considered.

Electrodiagnostic testing shows segmental demyelinating polyneuropathy with slowed nerve conduction velocities with conduction block, abnormal temporal dispersion, and prolonged distal and proximal (F-wave) latencies. These segmental abnormalities can usually differentiate CIDP from hereditary demyelinating polyneuropathies such as Charcot-Marie-Tooth type 1, which usually demonstrates a universal pattern of demyelination.

Magnetic resonance imaging (MRI) is usually not necessary for the diagnosis of CIDP, but gadolinium contrast enhancement can be detected in spinal roots and plexus. Hypertrophy of nerve roots may also be observed in CIDP of long duration.

Nerve biopsy is seldom necessary for the diagnosis. Nerve biopsy may help rule out a vasculitic neuropathy, and typical findings in CIDP are of a segmental demyelination with or without inflammation.

Immune electrophoresis of serum is a necessary examination for CIDP, as CIDP can be associated with M-protein IgM kappa is often associated with myelin-associated glycoprotein (MAG) antibodies. The most common form is the usually benign monoclonal gammopathy of unknown significance (MGUS), but M-protein may also be an expression of malignant disease such as multiple or solitary myeloma, lymphoma, and Waldenstr

öms disease. If M-protein is present, the usually presentation of CIDP is a slowly progressive predominately sensory affection of the distal limbs, also called distal acquired demyelinating symmetric (DADS) neuropathy. POEMS (polyneuropathy, organomegaly, endocrinopathy, M-protein, skin changes) may mimic CIDP but is usually not responsive to the standard CIDP treatment.

In rare cases, there may also be central nervous system (CNS) findings, and MRI may the reveal CNS demyelination. However, whether these findings represent associated diseases or coincidental occurrences is unclear.

Treatment and Prognosis

Most CIDP patients respond to immune-modulatory treatment. However, the treatment should be individualized and patients with mild disease may not require such immune therapy. Moderate to severely affected patients usually respond to steroids (prednisolone 60 mg daily with slowly tapering of the dose; azathioprine is usually added as a steroid-sparing agent). Alternatively, IVIg (2 g/kg) can be used. It is usual to start with IVIg and add prednisolone and azathioprine as necessary. A positive effect should be seen within the first 4 weeks. In relapsing CIDP, IVIg can for example be used monthly with a dose of 1 g/kg. Other medications like mycophenolate mofetil, rituximab, or ciclosporin may also be used (Figure 18.2). Mycophenolate mofetil is often used as the next alternative for CIDP treatment after IVIg and prednisolone/azathioprine. A randomized, multicenter study of fingolimod and an open-label study of alemtuzumab in CIDP have been started. Autologous stem cell treatment has been used in a few patients not responding to conventional immunosuppressive therapy. The clinical course, treatment effect, and possible side effects of the different medications require regular follow-up of the patients. Symptomatic treatment is also important and includes orthoses and sometimes antiepileptic drugs for paresthesias or pain.

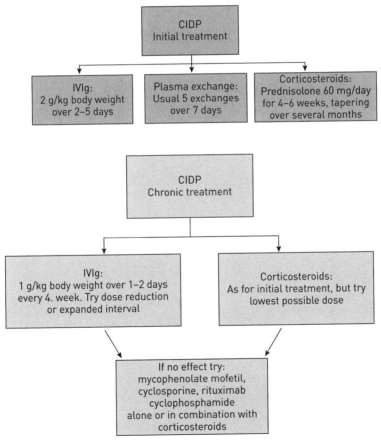

FIGURE 18.2
Algorithm for treatment of chronic inflammatory demyelinating polyneuropathy (CIDP).

The time course of CIDP is variable. The most favourable course is a mono-phasic illness with progression to nadir and complete recovery after treatment. A relapsing-remitting course with complete recovery between relapses can also be seen. The chronic progressive course usually leads to clinical deterioration and impair-ment, with less therapeutic response and risk of a secondary axonal loss. Subacute onset and presence of proximal weakness are usually good prognostic signs that cor-relate with a high rate of recovery, whereas distal accentuation or conduction slowing at presentation correlates with subacute onset and a relapsing course.

SUGGESTED READING

Mahdi-Rogers M, van Doorn PA, Hughes RA. Immunomodulatory treatment other than corticosteroids, immunoglobulin and plasma exchange for chronic inflammatory demyelinating polyradiculoneuropathy. Cochrane Database Syst Rev 2013;Issue 6. Art. No.: CD003280.

Vallat J-M, Sommer C, Magy L. Chronic inflammatory demyelinating polyradiculo-neuropathy: diagnostic and therapeutic challenges for a treatable condition. Lancet Neurol 2010;9:402–412.

van Doorn PA, Ruts L, Jacobs BC. Clinical features, pathogenesis, and treatment of Guillain-Barre syndrome. Lancet Neurol 2008;7:939–950.

Vedeler CA, Farbu E, Mellgren SI. Chronic inflammatory demyelinating polyneuropathy (CIDP). Acta Neurol Scand 2013;127(Suppl 196):48–51.

19 Neuromuscular Junction Disorders

Nils Erik Gilhus

INTRODUCTION

Clinical Picture

Neuromuscular junction disorders affect specifically transmission from motor nerve to skeletal muscle. Thus, skeletal muscle weakness is a hallmark for all these disorders. The disorders are generalized, but the symptoms and signs appear in some muscles, but not necessarily in all muscles. The weakness does not even need to be symmetric. Extraocular muscles and bulbar muscles represent frequently affected muscle groups. The asymmetry and selectivity implicate that safety factors in the target organ (muscle) are important.

Disease mechanisms for neuromuscular junction disorders are autoimmune where autoantibodies induce the muscle weakness, genetic with DNA mutations or toxic. Proteins near the junction are modified by one of these mechanisms, either presynaptically, postsynaptically, or in the synapse cleft. The disease-inducing factor may cross-react with and influence non–skeletal muscle organs, thereby giving additional symptoms and signs. Autoantibodies can in selected patients cross-react with the brain, heart muscle, the autonomic nervous system, and other organs.

With optimal treatment, the prognosis for most patients with neuromuscular junction disorders is good with little increased mortality risk. The major exception relates to the disorders that are paraneoplastic; Lambert-Eaton myasthenic syndrome (LEMS) with lung cancer and myasthenia gravis with an invasive thymoma. Some genetic disorders lead to severe muscle weakness. Respiratory function needs special attention in patients with neuromuscular junction disease, and heart muscle involvement is potentially a severe complication.

Neurophysiological examinations are important to diagnose neuromuscular junction disorders correctly. Specialized examination techniques such as testing of single nerve fibers and repeated stimulation at defined frequencies are often necessary and an appropriate selection of the muscles to be examined. Single-fiber examination is more sensitive, and repetitive stimulation more specific.

Myasthenia gravis (MG) is the most common neuromuscular junction disorder. The muscle weakness can be fluctuating in the form of fatigability or remain permanent and stable. The disease occurs because of a dysfunctional postsynaptic acetylcholine receptor (AChR). This dysfunction is caused by autoantibodies, either to AChR epitopes or to membrane molecules functionally related to AChR.

Lambert-Eaton myasthenic syndrome (LEMS) patients have in addition to muscle weakness an autonomic dysfunction. The weakness and the autonomic symptoms are caused by the same autoantibodies. The muscle weakness is proximal, often in the legs. Eye muscle weakness is usually not prominent. One half of LEMS patients have a small cell lung carcinoma, LEMS being a paraneoplastic disease. LEMS is mediated by antibodies against the presynaptic voltage-gated calcium channel (VGCC).

Neuromyotonia is a rare disorder where autoantibodies against voltage-gated potassium channels (VGKC) bind presynaptically, leading to a hyperexcitability of the motor nerve. Patients report muscle cramps, muscle twitching, and, rarely, muscle weakness.

Congenital myasthenic syndromes can be postsynaptic, due to either mutations in genes encoding AChR subunits or encoding key molecules involved in AChR clustering at the muscle endplate. DOK7, rapsyn, and lipoprotein receptor–related protein (LRP4) represent such molecules. Presynaptic and synaptic myasthenic syndromes occur as well but are rare. The exact mutation can be found in more than 60% of patients with congenital myasthenic syndromes. Symptoms are usually exercise induced, age of onset is typically before 2 years, and there is no response to immunosuppressive therapy. Ocular symptoms and signs are frequent.

Toxic neuromuscular disorders are caused by toxins binding presynaptically or postsynaptically. Such toxins occur in nature, paralyzing either prey (attack) or attacker (defense). Botulinum toxin binds irreversibly to SNARE proteins presynaptically and thereby prevents ACh release. Curare is widely used during anesthesia. This plant toxin binds and blocks the postsynaptic AChR. Alpha-bungarotoxin is a snake toxin that binds with high specificity to AChR and is used in diagnostic tests for AChR antibodies.

Disease Subgroups

Myasthenia Gravis

All the main neuromuscular junction disorders should be divided into distinct subgroups. Correct classification of every patient into subgroup is important when planning optimal therapy. Also, prognosis differs according to subgroup.

Early-onset MG patients have typically thymus hyperplasia and a therapeutic effect of thymectomy. This group has marked preponderance of females, and an *HLA-B7,-DR3* correlation. The patients do not have antibodies against intracellular muscle proteins such as titin and ryanodine receptor. Late-onset MG, in contrast, is characterized by an atrophic (normal) thymus, is equally common in the two sexes, and has no HLA correlation. Although MG incidence is bimodal with two age peaks, there is no absolute age of onset distinction between the two groups. Delayed-early onset can be used as a term for MG with the typical clinical characteristics of early-onset MG but with actual debut age above 50 years. Early-onset MG prevalence and incidence have been unchanged for decades, whereas late-onset MG has increased in the population, at least in part due to demographic changes. The distinction between early- and late-onset MG is linked to age at symptom debut, not to age at diagnosis or at follow-up. The AChR antibodies do not differ between early- and late-onset MG. In 10% to 15% of MG cases, the disease is paraneoplastic and caused by a lymphoepithelioma in thymus. Also, 30% of all patients with a thymoma develop MG, and an even higher proportion have AChR antibodies. This means that all MG patients should be examined for thymoma by computed tomography or magnetic resonance imaging of the mediastinum. They should also be examined for the presence of titin antibodies. Titin antibodies have a high sensitivity for thymoma, whereas the specificity is low in patients with MG debut after 50 years of age, much higher for early onset.

Ocular symptoms with ptosis and diplopia appear in nearly all MG patients, often as initial symptoms. In a minority of the patients, the symptoms remain confined to extraocular muscles only. Ocular MG is defined as having purely ocular symptoms more than 2 years after symptom debut. In half of ocular MG patients, no autoantibodies can be detected, most probably due to low test sensitivity.

MG patients can have antibodies against muscle-specific tyrosine kinase (MuSK). MuSK is a protein functionally linked to AChR in the postsynaptic muscle membrane. MuSK antibodies are detected in 1% to 50% of patients with generalized MG and no AChR antibodies; the prevalence has a marked geographical variation, being, for example, much higher in southern than in northern Europe. MuSK antibody MG tends to be more severe than AChR antibody MG. Muscles around eyes, mouth, and throat are frequently affected, and up to one-third of patients have at some time needed respiratory support. MuSK MG patients have a normal thymus.

Another MG subgroup has antibodies against lipoprotein receptor–related protein 4 (LRP4) in the postsynaptic muscle membrane. As for MuSK, this protein is functionally linked to AChR. LRP4 is also important for feedback from muscle to nerve terminal. LRP4 MG is less common than MuSK MG and counts for less than 10% of AChR antibody–negative MG. LRP4 MG and MuSK MG are clinically similar. There is at present no commercial test for the detection of LRP4 antibodies.

The antibody-negative group with generalized MG consists of two different types of patients. Some have AChR, MuSK or LRP4 antibodies that are not detected by routine assays due to low antibody affinity, low antibody concentration, or technical assay aspects. Other patients do not seem to have any of these antibodies as their symptom-inducing factor. Most probably they have antibodies against yet undefined postsynaptic proteins.

Lambert-Eaton Myasthenic Syndrome

Lambert-Eaton myasthenic syndrome (LEMS) can appear in a paraneoplastic form and in a nonparaneoplastic form. In half of the patients, the disease is caused by a small cell lung carcinoma. The VGCC antibodies are cross-reacting with tumor epitopes. The paraneoplastic and non-paraneoplastic patient groups do not differ for muscle weakness, neurophysiological pattern, autonomic dysfunction, or the VGCC antibody pattern. However, the prognosis differs markedly between the two groups due to the poor prognosis of small cell lung carcinoma. All LEMS patients should be checked for small cell lung carcinoma and regularly up to 2 years after LEMS debut. Positron emission tomography is necessary if other tumor tests are negative. Nonsmokers have a low risk for small cell lung carcinoma.

Treatment of Myasthenia Gravis

The treatment principles are summarized in Figure 19.1. The treatment components are symptomatic drug treatment, immunosuppressive drug treatment,

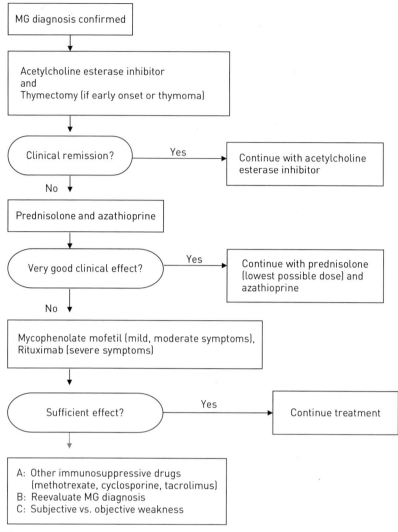

FIGURE 19.1
Treatment of generalized MG.

thymectomy, supportive therapy, treatment of MG crisis, and treatment of comorbidity. Symptomatic drug treatment consists of ACh esterase inhibitors. Pyridostigmine is usually the favored drug. Acetylcholine esterase inhibitors have as a rule much better effect for AChR antibody MG than for MuSK MG. In some patients, ACh esterase inhibitor alone leads to a full or near full pharmacological remission. Supportive therapy includes all types of health measures including lifestyle, weight control, and well-adapted exercise with a training program. The most relevant comorbidity disorders are infections, especially in the respiratory tract, lung disorders, and additional autoimmune disorders. Apart from thymoma cancers are not increased. Side-effects of drugs given for MG should be considered.

Early-Onset MG

In all early onset patients where ACh esterase inhibitors do not give full clinical remission, radical thymectomy should be performed, either by videoscopy-assisted technique or by sternum split. Thymectomy can be safely undertaken also in children tat age 5 years and older. The effect of thymectomy comes gradually for months and up to 2 years after thymectomy. The effect is better when undertaken early after MG debut.

The combination of prednisolone and azathioprine is chosen if further treatment is needed. Prednisolone is usually given on alternate days to minimize side effects. The lowest effective dose is used, especially important for prednisolone. Both drugs should be monitored for side effects, early bone marrow suppression of azathioprine being the most dangerous complication. The treatment can often be discontinued after a long-lasting remission, especially if thymectomy has been undertaken.

In the majority of patients, this treatment is sufficient. However, several additional drugs can be tried, including mycophenolate mofetil (mild cases), rituximab (more severe cases), methotrexate, cyclosporine, and tacrolimus.

Late-Onset MG

Thymectomy is usually not undertaken for this group. However, patients with thymic hyperplasia on CT/MR, no titin antibodies, and debut below 70 years probably have a delayed early-onset type of MG. Such patients should be considered for thymectomy even if older than 50 years.

Late-onset MG usually needs prednisolone and azathioprine. The treatment should in most patients go on for years, often life-long. Prednisolone can sometimes be given in very low doses, even discontinued. Titin antibodies indicate a more severe prognosis with a higher need for immunosuppression. Alternative and additional immunosuppressive drugs are the same as for early onset MG, and they are more commonly used.

Thymoma MG

MG with thymoma means a double treatment consideration; treatment of the neuromuscular deficit and treatment of the tumor. The MG should be treated as late-onset MG. This means ACh esterase inhibition and nearly always immunosuppressive drugs. MG with a thymoma tends to be generalized and moderate to severe, and long-term immunosuppression is required for most patients.

The thymoma is a lymphoepithelioma, hardly ever giving rise to distant metastasis. However, the tumor can be locally infiltrative and seed in the chest. Thus, a thymoma should if possible always be radically removed together with the thymus rest. If local spread either macroscopically or microscopically, supplementary anticancer treatment is required.

Ocular MG

Acetylcholine esterase inhibitor will usually improve diplopia and ptosis, but diplopia may persist and be troublesome even if eye muscle strength is markedly improved. Prednisolone will often further improve the condition. Azathioprine or other immuno-suppressants are usually not given. Early prednisolone treatment may reduce the risk for purely ocular symptoms to develop into generalized MG. Thymectomy is not indicated for ocular MG. The diplopia can be avoided by covering one of the eyes, and stable ptosis and diplopia sometimes improve after surgery on extraocular muscles.

MuSK MG

MG with MuSK autoantibodies is usually generalized and severe. Acetylcholine ester-ase inhibitor gives usually no marked improvement, and such drugs can in some patients even lead to increased muscle weakness. MuSK MG needs immunosuppres-sive treatment. If prednisolone and azathioprine in combination does not give suffi-cient improvement, rituximab is usually an effective drug. Thymus is normal in these patients, and thymectomy is not recommended for MuSK MG.

LRP4 MG

Treatment experience for this subtype is limited. Treatment as for MuSK MG is recommended.

Antibody-Negative MG

This subgroup is highly heterogeneous. Drug treatment should be similar to other gen-eralized MG subgroups. Thymectomy should be considered if thymus is enlarged on imaging. Thymoma MG "always" has AChR antibodies, so a thymoma is not suspected in this subgroup.

Severe MG Exacerbations

MG exacerbations need active treatment (Figure 19.2). The prognosis is generally good. Patients recover with optimal treatment and no mortality should be accepted. Most important is respiratory support and intensive care. Also cardiac function should be monitored during severe exacerbations with the need of respiratory support. Intravenous immunoglobulin (IVIg) and plasma exchange have a similar therapeu-tic effect. Plasma exchange is regarded as slightly faster but also with more frequent severe side effects. Respiratory infection is a common precipitating event and should be treated vigorously if present. Acetylcholine esterase inhibitors are temporarily with-drawn or given in a low dose when on respirator. Both IVIg and plasma exchange lead to good and fast improvement in 70% to 80% of the patients. The responders are not the same for the two treatments, so they can be given in sequence. High-dose cortico-steroids intravenously can be added, especially if protracted or insufficient improve-ment. For a minority of the patients, intensive care and respiratory support remains necessary for weeks. Active treatment should be continued with the highest intensity, also in elderly patients, as the weakness is always reversible.

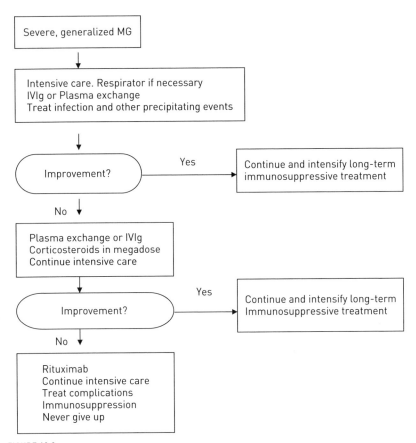

FIGURE 19.2
Treatment of severe MG exacerbations.

Pregnancy and Giving Birth

Pregnancy and giving birth is usually uncomplicated in MG. Young females will often prefer to become pregnant in a phase when they do not need immunosuppression. Pyridostigmine, prednisolone and azathioprine are all regarded as relatively safe during pregnancy. Breast-feeding should be recommended, also when on these drugs. From 10% to 15% of the newborn have a transient neonatal MG due to mother's IgG antibodies crossing the placenta. The children do not produce antibodies. Delivery should take place at a hospital with neonatal intensive care service. In rare cases, mother's AChR antibodies lead to so severe movement restriction in the fetus that it develops arthrogryposis. Any teratogenic potential of drugs given to females in reproductive age should always be considered.

Treatment of Lambert-Eaton Myasthenic Syndrome

For the half of LEMS patients with a small cell lung carcinoma, fast and effective treatment of the cancer is most important (Figure 19.3). For those with no carcinoma at the time of LEMS diagnosis, specialized diagnostic follow-up for the next 2 years is a crucial part of the therapy. Follow-up should include PET examination.

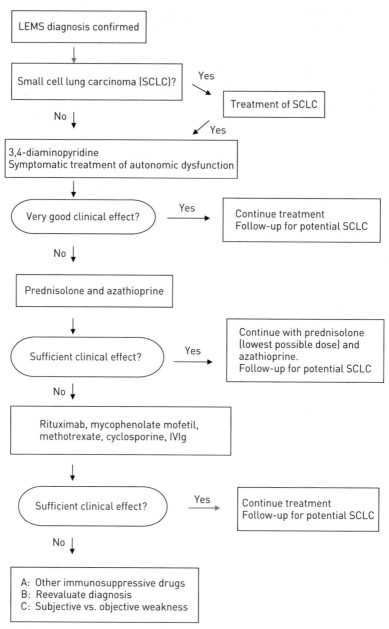

FIGURE 19.3

Treatment of Lambert-Eaton myasthenic syndrome (LEMS).

The decreased presynaptic release of ACh should be symptomatically treated with 3,4-diaminopyridine, which increases this release and prolongs the action potential. Acetylcholine inhibitors such as pyridostigmine increase the amount of ACh in the synaptic cleft and would be expected to have a positive effect in LEMS. However, it is usually much less effective than in MG and also less effective than 3,4-diaminopyridine.

In most patients with LEMS, the muscle weakness persists to such a degree that immunosuppressive drug treatment is needed in addition to cholinergic therapy. Prednisolone and azathioprine in combination is recommended and in doses similar to those for MG. Controlled studies are generally lacking. Drugs such as rituximab, mycophenolate mofetil, methotrexate, cyclosporine, and IVIg are listed as effective in LEMS. IVIg is the preferred treatment for acute or subacute exacerbations with severe symptoms. Plasma exchange represents an alternative.

Supportive therapy includes symptomatic treatment of autonomic symptoms such as dry eyes and mouth, constipation, and erectile dysfunction. Low-intensity physical training can be carried out safely in mild and moderate LEMS. Complicating disorders, including infections and overweight, should be treated. Drugs with a negative impact on neuromuscular transmission should be avoided. Potential side effects of any treatment given should be monitored and minimized.

Treatment of Neuromyotonia

Anticonvulsants including carbamazepine and phenytoin usually improve stiffness and muscle spasms. Immunosuppressive drugs such as prednisolone and azathioprine can give long-term relief. IVIg has usually a positive effect. A small proportion of cases have prominent symptoms of an autoimmune brain disorder (Morvan's syndrome). Such patients should be treated vigorously with IVIg, plasma exchange, and/or high-dose corticosteroids. Neuromyotonia can be paraneoplastic (thymoma or other cancer).

Treatment of Congenital Myasthenic Syndromes

The response to anticholinesterase treatment is usually only partial and moderate, but pyridostigmine and 3,4-diaminopyridine should be tried in these patients and in combination. In a minority of patients, the weakness becomes worse with such treatment. Ephedrine has sometimes a marked positive effect, including in patients with a mutation in the postsynaptic DOK7 protein. Salbutamol has a similar effect. The effect can be delayed for a couple of weeks. Fluoxetine has a therapeutic effect in slow-channel syndrome as this drug blocks the channel in the open state. Mutations that lead to loss of receptor function should respond to treatment increasing ACh availability, whereas cholinergic overstimulation of the endplate should have an alternative therapy. However, it is still not possible to tailor the treatment on the basis of a pathogenetic understanding. Treatment alternatives should be tried in all patients.

Treatment of Toxic Neuromuscular Disorders

Respiratory dysfunction needs immediate intensive care with respiratory support. The toxin effects are transient, even when the toxin binds irreversibly at the neuromuscular junction, as there is new synthesis of ACh receptor and other junction proteins. Botulism has a very low mortality rate. Antitoxin should be administered to speed up the recovery. Botulinum toxin is widely used as therapy, given locally in an optimally titrated dose to weaken spastic or dystonic muscles.

CONCLUSION

Neuromuscular junction disorders should have specific treatment that markedly improves the muscle weakness. From a previous high mortality rate, this is now very low for nearly all disorders. Function of respiratory muscles should always be evaluated. During acute deteriorations, respiratory function is crucial. Long-term therapy usually combines symptomatic treatment and treatment of underlying disease processes, most often immunosuppression. Long-term treatment and specialized follow-up are necessary.

SUGGESTED READING

Conti-Fine BM, Milani M, Kaminski HJ. Myasthenia gravis; past, present, and future. J Clin Invest 2006;116:2843–2854.

Farrugia ME, Vincent A. Autoimmune mediated neuromuscular junction deficits. Curr Opin Neurol 2010;23:489–495.

Gilhus NE. Myasthenia and the neuromuscular junction. Curr Opin Neurol 2012.

Gilhus NE. Lambert-Eaton myasthenic syndrome; pathogenesis, diagnosis and therapy. Autoimmune Dis 2011.

Gronseth GS, Barohn RJ. Thymectomy for autoimmune myasthenia gravis; an evidence-based review. Neurology 2000;55:7–15.

Guptill JT, Sanders GB, Evoli A. Anti-MusK antibody myasthenia gravis; clinical findings and response to treatment in two large cohorts. Muscle Nerve 2011;44:36–40.

Palace J, Beeson D. The congenital myasthenic syndromes. J Neuroimmunol 2008;201–202:2–5.

Higuchi O, Hamuo J, Motomura M, et al. Autoantibodies to low-density lipoprotein receptor-related protein 4 in myasthenia gravis. Ann Neurol 2011;69;418–422.

Skeie GO, Apostolski S, Evoli A, et al. Guidelines for treatment of autoimmune neuromuscular transmission disorders. Eur J Neurol 2010;17:893–902.

Spillane J, Beeson DJ, Kullmann DM. Myasthenia and related disorders of the neuromuscular junction. J Neurol Neurosurg Psychiat 2010;81:850–857.

Vrolix K, Fraussen J, Molenaar PC, et al. The auto-antigen repertoire in myasthenia gravis. Autoimmunity 2010;43:380–400.

20 Myopathies

Laurence Bindoff

INTRODUCTION

"Myopathy" is a descriptive term for any disease process affecting muscle, whereas the term "muscular dystrophy" is usually reserved for an "inherited" disease in which degenerative changes are seen in the muscle biopsy. Myopathy can be caused by a wide spectrum of disease processes ranging from metabolic disturbances to disruption of structural proteins, inflammatory or autoimmune-mediated damage, toxins, hormonal imbalance, and degeneration; myopathies may also be inherited or acquired. I will use the terms "myopathy" and "muscle disease" interchangeably. Classification of muscle disease has evolved and now reflects both mechanistic and genetic understanding together with features such as age of onset and distribution of involvement. A full review of the causes, classification, and diagnosis of these diseases is beyond the scope of this chapter, and readers are referred to standard myology texts for details (see "Suggested Reading").

Muscle is the effector element of the motor unit and as such is required either to facilitate movement, by shortening the distance between two points (usually across a joint), or, by being tonically active, to stabilize elements of the skeleton (i.e., maintain posture). Muscle is also a major source of the heat that helps maintain body temperature. Thus, it follows that the consequences of muscle disease include weakness, postural instability, and difficulty maintaining body temperature (Box 20.1). To these must be added the results of maladaptive responses such as the progressive shortening of sick or unused muscle (contracture formation), the secondary consequences of instability (pain and deformity), the mechanical disruption of ventilation (causing respiratory insufficiency), dysphagia, and fatigue. Symptoms due to disturbance of the electrical properties of the muscle membrane are a special case and are known as "myotonia."

Currently, no cure exists for the vast majority of myopathies, and there are few specific treatments. There is, however, much that can be achieved by knowing the correct diagnosis and therefore the expected complications, the appropriate use of physiotherapy and surgery, and the provision of aids and appliances. Detailed management protocols exist for several neuromuscular diseases including Duchenne muscular dystrophy (DMD), spinal muscular atrophy, congenital muscular dystrophies, and myotonic dystrophy, and examples of these can be found in English at the Treat NMD website (http://www.treat-nmd.eu/) and in Scandinavian languages (http://www.unn.no/referanseprogrammer/category27673.html).

> **Box 20.1** Symptoms of Muscle Disease
> Weakness
> Postural instability
> Difficulties maintaining body temperature
> Maladaptive responses
>   Contracture formation,
>   Instability causing pain and deformity
>   Mechanical disruption of ventilation
>   Dysphagia
>   Fatigue

MANAGEMENT OF MUSCLE DISEASE

General Comments

The management of a child with a severe, congenital myopathy will differ to that of an adult with a late-onset limb-girdle muscular dystrophy (Box 20.2). Furthermore, diseases with major systemic complications, such as myotonic dystrophy and DMD, generate "nonmuscle" problems (e.g., relating to cognitive development). Management of muscle disease generally requires a multidisciplinary focus; in our muscle clinic, the team includes a physiotherapist, occupational therapist, family care officer (*socionom*), nurse, and physician. Referral to other specialists such as speech therapist and respiratory and cardiac physicians is made separately as required.

Given the enormity of the subject "myopathy", this chapter will simply give an overview of the practical issues associated with muscle disease and deal with the management in general terms only. Those wishing to have a more detailed discussion of specific diseases are recommended to use the available references (see "Suggested Reading").

Consequences of Muscle Disease

Muscle disease may be diagnosed at an asymptomatic or very early stage by the coincidental finding of an elevated creatine kinase (CK) level or because of a known diagnosis

> **Box 20.2** Important Principles of Management
> Bone growth requires muscle activity.
>   Weakness in the growing child can lead to bone shortening and scoliosis.
>   Loss of ambulation leads to faster development of scoliosis.
>   Scoliosis can lead to mechanical disruption of ventilation.
> Contractures destroy functional movement.
> Inactive muscles atrophy (faster in those with muscle disease than in healthy individuals).
>   Patients should be encouraged to exercise.
>   Weak muscle must be stretched to maintain length and joint mobility.

in a family member. Elevated CK may not always reflect an underlying muscle disease, although there are many examples in which it is present long before the disease symptoms manifest (e.g., limb-girdle muscular dystrophy type 2L; LGMD2L).

Establishing the correct diagnosis is vital because this will indicate which complications must be considered and allow monitoring to be set in place (e.g., to detect the cardiac complications that can manifest before symptoms in several muscle diseases, including myotonic dystrophy, Bethlem myopathy, and others). Management of mild or asymptomatic disease will otherwise be influenced by factors such as age, disease type, and nature of the impact.

Weakness

The consequences of muscle weakness will differ depending on whether it develops during growth/development or later. The growing skeleton requires muscle activity to stimulate and maintain growth: muscle weakness will affect this and can lead to both bone shortening and deformity. Postdevelopment weakness leads to loss of function and, in some cases, deformity of joints or spine (hyperlordosis); in the absence of axial or appendicular growth, however, complications such as scoliosis do not usually occur, although worsening of preexisting spinal deformity can be seen.

The principles of managing weak muscles (Box 20.3) involve

- Maintaining regular use, within the functional capacity of the affected muscle/movement
- Stretching to maintain muscle length and avoid contracture development
- Optimizing function by strengthening affected muscles where possible, by recruiting other muscles to perform the function, or by using aids and appliances to as required

In asymptomatic or very mildly affected patients, it is important to establish regular exercise, such as walking and particularly swimming, as a part of their lifestyle. Patients often ask what and how much they should do. There is research that shows certain forms of high-intensity exercise may be beneficial (and not cause muscle injury,

---

Box 20.3 Managing Weakness

Early

Submaximal activity

    Level set according to patient's ability/desire

    Choice of exercise possibilities

Moderate

Continued activity possible

    Focused training (usually supervised by physiotherapist)

Severe

    Focus on maintaining muscle length and joint mobility

        Maintaining standing a vital goal

        Training in water helps reduce load on affected muscles

as is often feared), but this must be carefully monitored as excessive muscle loads can lead to injury. Since each individual differs, I suggest that patients take a form of exercise that they enjoy and that they can continue with over time. Further, I suggest that the exercise should involve both arms and legs (e.g., swimming, walking using ski poles): the degree to which they exercise should render them tired but not lead to such profound tiredness that lasts for longer than 1 to 2 hours. If they are still tired the next day, this strongly indicates overtraining. As weakness progresses, assisted training (i.e., together with a physiotherapist) should take a more central role. The weaker the patient becomes, the more critical it is that training is adapted to his or her needs and level of motor function.

Progressive loss of muscle function will eventually necessitate changes in the lifestyle. This should be considered before significant impediment exists, so as to prepare the patient psychologically for what is to come. It is easy to imagine that most patients will experience the need to use a wheelchair as a major defeat in their struggle to cope with their illness. Interestingly, it is apparent in my practice that most feel the same even about having to use a walking stick! Thus, both must be discussed early and planned properly for the patient to understand the need and enjoy the benefit these give. Even prior to developing significant muscle weakness, patients may experience increased fatigability and derive benefit from, for example, using an electric wheelchair for longer distances. Patients with significant weakness often keep pushing themselves to walk even when this exposes them to the considerable risk of falling. For those unlucky enough to fall and injure themselves, the effect of both the trauma and treatment, particularly any prolonged bed-rest, will often mean that motor function is lost. In cases with already marginal muscle function, this may also includes the ability to stand (not walk, just the capacity to rise and take weight through the legs). This can lead to a major loss of independence.

Spine and Joints

Managing children, and particularly the developing skeleton, demands greater focus on detail. The combination of paraspinal muscle weakness and skeletal growth leads to progressive deformity such as scoliosis. Scoliosis can in turn lead to a progressive mechanical disturbance of chest wall movement. All infants and children diagnosed with an early-onset, progressive muscle disease (e.g., DMD, congenital muscular dystrophies, etc.) can develop this complication, and it is vital, therefore, that measures be instituted to monitor the spine and prepare for intervention as required. Importantly, it is also clear that scoliosis develops faster in the nonambulant child (i.e., as soon as they become entirely wheelchair dependent). Measures that delay loss of ambulation also retard scoliosis development. Thus, physiotherapy, including the use of standing frames, and stretching to limit contracture development are vital. Surgery must be performed by a surgeon experienced in spinal surgery.

In the postdevelopment patient, proximal weakness in the lower limbs leads to pelvic changes, particularly a tendency for it to tilt forward; this can be accentuated by distal changes such as ankle contractures (see later). Forward pelvic tilt increases the normal curvature of the lumbar spine, resulting in hyperlordosis; this in turn can cause pain and, through abnormal movement and weight bearing, increases the rate of degenerative change in the lumbosacral spine. While sufficient strength remains to support body weight, it is important to focus on recruiting abdominal muscle function to stabilize the pelvis and prevent forward tilting. This also increases postural stability. If abdominal muscle strength is marginal, it is important to consider other ways of reducing the load such as the use of sticks or ski poles.

Immobile joints become stiff and painful. Maintaining joint movement is essential and, in the presence of profound weakness, this must be performed by others. As daily treatment by a physiotherapist is often difficult to obtain, carers can be trained to perform these movements as well as other maneuvers such as postural drainage for mobilization of sputum.

Immobility also leads to osteopenia/osteoporosis and an increased risk of bone fracture. This should be monitored with appropriate blood/urine tests and bone mineral density evaluation and treated as necessary.

Contractures

Contracture is the abnormal shortening of a muscle such that it impairs function. This can involve any and all muscles, including paraspinal muscles. Contracture development can be seen early in certain muscle diseases (e.g., Bethlem myopathy) and in these cases can occur even in the presence of good residual muscle function. Often, however, contractures develop late when muscle function is already significantly reduced. Immobility will increase the tendency for contracture development, which can even develop in otherwise healthy muscles that are immobilized by the use of plaster of Paris splints.

Contractures destroy function whether it is the movement through the affected joint or, in the case of muscles that no longer perform their function, the passive movement of the joint so as to improve posture, facilitate personal hygiene, improve ventilation, or reduce pain and stiffness. I will deal with two examples: Achilles contractures and rigid spine.

Achilles contracture will reduce dorsiflexion of the ankle. This will produce no major problems until it is no longer possible to achieve the 90-degree angle that allows both heel and forefoot to be placed comfortably on the ground at the same time as the axis of the body is perpendicular. Compensation for this involves hyperextension of the knee, which in turn drives forward movement of the pelvis. The latter accentuates the lordosis (Figure 20.1) and may indeed be a major factor in the process of whereby lordosis develops. Alterations in the lumbosacral spine also lead to adaptive responses in the thoracic and cervical spines, often with associated pain and discomfort. Achilles contracture can also result in loss of ambulation in a patient with such severe proximal weakness that cannot adjust to the postural adaptations these entail.

Contractures involving spinal muscles occur in a range of congenital muscle diseases including disease due selenoprotein N 1 deficiency and Ullrich congenital muscular dystrophies, calpainopathy, and Emery-Dreifuss muscular dystrophy. Spinal contractures usually limit forward flexion or, when acting laterally, lead to traction that bends the spine and generates scoliosis. Both will limit movement and, most importantly, both can affect the mechanics of ventilation leading to respiratory failure.

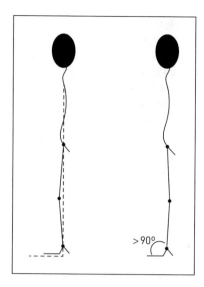

FIGURE 20.1

Normal posture and the effects of weakness and contracture. The left panel shows the relationship between the perpendicular and fixation points (joints) in the skeleton. The most energy efficient posture is for the head and body to be held directly over the pelvis and femoral heads. As proximal weakness occurs, there is a tendency for the pelvis to tilt forward increasing lumbar lordosis. Hyperextension of the knees as will occur if quadriceps are weak or Achilles contracture develops. In the latter, weakness will prevent the patient from walking on their toes (as patients with spasticity might), thus stability requires that the knees hyperextend to enable the heel to reach the ground.

Box 20.4 Management of Contractures

Contractures develop in all weak muscles that are not stretched.

Contractures can be an early feature of some diseases even in the absence of significant weakness.

The principle of management should be prevention.

Early contracture

    Stretching exercises either alone or supervised

    Patients can be taught how and perform stretching regularly in the daily activities.

Moderate nonfixed contracture

    Combination of physiotherapy and orthoses to maintain position

    Surgical correction if required

Fixed contracture that disturbs function (that cannot be treated with above)

    Surgical intervention—tendon lengthening; fixation

While the best treatment for contracture is prevention (see Box 20.4, *Management of contractures*), active therapy is based on early recognition, physiotherapy to maintain muscle length, the use of orthoses, and the careful application of surgery. There is much that the patient can achieve by awareness of the problem and stretching exercises that are tailored to everyday activities: for example, Achilles stretching can be achieved while either sitting or standing (Figure 20.2).

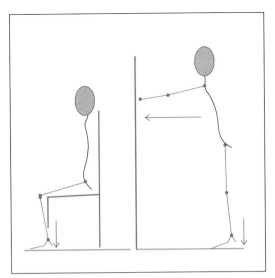

FIGURE 20.2

Simple exercises to counteract Achilles contracture. Placing the heels under the chair (or tilting the footrest of the wheelchair upward) will mean that the patient can press down his or her heels and stretch the Achilles. In patients who retain the ability to stand, they can use body weight to do this either leaning against a wall of bench (say in the kitchen or at work).

Ventilation

Muscle Weakness and Ventilation

Muscle contraction is the driving force behind respiration, and the most important of the muscles involved is the diaphragm. Respiratory insufficiency may manifest as exertional dyspnea, if exercise capacity is still good, or during sleep, as nocturnal hypoventilation, at any time during disease development. Respiratory drive (i.e., the central nervous system's control of breathing) is generally maintained in neuromuscular diseases, but in some cases, such as myotonic dystrophy, this too, may be affected. Diseases such as myotonic dystrophy type 1(DM1) and LGMD2I, Pompe, and nemaline myopathy may present with symptoms of respiratory insufficiency before weakness is manifest.

Hypoventilation during sleep leads to symptoms such as morning headache, poor daytime concentration, increased sleep requirement during the day, and tiredness (Box 20.5). If there is also an obstructive element, leading to snoring and sleep apnea, the patient may also experience poor sleep quality, frequent waking, and night sweats. If left untreated, chronic hypoventilation can lead to pulmonary hypertension and right heart failure.

The type of monitoring (Box 20.6) needed will depend on diagnosis; patients with DMD and many of the congenital muscular dystrophies will inevitably develop respiratory insufficiency, while patients with LGMD2I, fascioscapulohumeral muscular dystrophy (FSHMD), and many others are at risk but not destined to develop this complication. Forced vital capacity and forced expiratory volume in 1 second are simple and provide a sensitive way of monitoring ventilation. A progressive fall in forced vital capacity or values less than 60% of expected values should prompt further investigation by a respiratory physician. Patients must be asked specifically about symptoms associated with poor nocturnal ventilation and/or airway obstruction and, because

---

Box 20.5 Symptoms Suggestive of Nocturnal Hypoventilation

Daytime sleepiness

Morning headache

Poor daytime concentration

Tiredness/fatigue/poor appetite

Palpitations

Nocturia

With additional obstructive element (snoring; episodes of apnea)

    Poor sleep quality (repeated waking)

    Sweating

    Increased nocturnal movements (kicking/turning etc)

Recurrent infection may reflect either hypoventilation or aspiration.

---

they may not be aware of these symptoms, it is important also to ask the spouse or partner. In those with symptoms as well as those with disorders known to be associated with early respiratory involvement, such as myotonic dystrophy type 1, it is important to refer these patients early for monitoring of ventilation during sleep. Smoking should be discouraged and regular influenza vaccination is recommended.

Respiratory Tract Infection

Respiratory tract infection is an important cause of morbidity in muscle disease and may significantly accelerate the development of respiratory failure. In those with concomitant swallowing difficulties (see later), aspiration must be actively sought and treated. In those with adequate bulbar function, basal atelectasis due to poor ventilation offers a good substrate for bacterial colonization. In those with poor cough reflex, the inability to mobilize sputum can also lead to repeated infection. Other infections, particularly influenza, expose these patients to considerable risk

---

Box 20.6 Monitoring Respiratory Function

Symptoms (Box 20.5)

Signs such as:

    Tachypnea

    Accessory muscle use

    Paradoxical abdominal movement

    Elevated jugular venous pressure

    Edema

    Poor cough

Spirometry

    Appropriate for regular monitoring

        Forced vital capacity <60% refer for detailed investigation

Sleep studies

from both the original and secondary infection that follow. Patients or their carers should be trained in postural drainage techniques, and the threshold for initiating antibiotic treatment should be low. Where distance from medical services precludes easy access, patients can be given antibiotics to keep at home with instructions to use when symptoms arise.

Nutrition and Swallowing

Whether relating to weight reduction or just general health, questions concerning diet are among the commonest issues raised by patients with muscle disease. In my experience, overweight is a more common than underweight, but the latter does occur, especially in those with bulbar dysfunction. Being overweight will increase the demand on weak muscles and, in some cases, may mean the earlier-than-expected loss of ambulation. Poor nutrition affects well-being and, if extreme, can result in the loss of muscle protein.

It is important that patients with muscle disease eat a varied diet, including fat, carbohydrate, protein, and daily vitamin requirements, with a calorific content that does not exceed their requirement based on age and exercise capacity. Content will vary according to local dietary customs, and it may be necessary to obtain nutritional expertise in order to balance calorie requirement and activity. Treatment with steroids is often associated with weight gain (and an increased risk of diabetes), and this must be considered before starting treatment. In boys with DMD, for example, it has been shown that the benefits of treatment outweigh the risks of weight gain, but in other diseases, it may be necessary to consider other options.

Weight loss poses a major challenge in myopathy patients, making it vital that weight is an issue early in management, before obesity develops. The inability to exercise removes one of the most convenient adjuncts to weight reduction. Nevertheless, basic principles still hold true; as long as calorie intake is below requirement, weight will be lost. It is important, however, that this imbalance is not extreme as this will lead to mobilization of muscle proteins to fuel energy metabolism. In the seriously overweight, the question of surgery often arises: currently, there are no data concerning the safety of surgical intervention (gastric bypass and similar interventions) in patients with muscle disease and, based on the concerns aired earlier, I do not recommend this treatment.

Bulbar dysfunction occurs in several forms of muscle disease including the oculopharyngeal muscular dystrophies, inclusion body, and other forms of myositis and mitochondrial disease. Aspiration pneumonia is a danger in all cases, but especially in those who already have impaired ventilation. Early recognition of the problem is vital, and it may be necessary to perform functional investigations, such as video fluoroscopy, to identify what the problem is and specifically where the problem arises. Initial management may simply be referral to a speech therapist for advice and monitoring: subsequently, the patient may require parenteral feeding via a gastrostomy. In some cases, it is possible to offer surgical intervention such as cricomyotomy where such specific dysfunction is identified via barium swallow.

Dental health can have an impact on nutrition and can be a problem in diseases such as DM1 in which abnormalities of skull shape can also arise.

Loss of Heat-Generating Capacity

Since muscle is the major source of the heat we use to maintain body temperature, patients with significant atrophy experience problems with temperature control. Measures to counteract heat loss can be simple, such as appropriate clothing, or require the use of additional heating elements. Care to avoid complications such as burns must be exercised in nonambulant patents.

Problems Associated With Pedal Dependency

Edema

Once patients are entirely confined to the sitting position, diminished muscular activity reduces lymphatic return and edema can develop. Management includes passive stretching, if possible standing under controlled conditions (e.g., frame or adapted wheelchair), compression stockings, and mechanical compression such as the "Lympha Press" equipment.

Accelerated Contracture Formation

This can affect all three levels: hips, knees, and ankles. Prevention must be considered early, before contractures develop and treatment is necessary to help with personal hygiene, improve sleeping position, and provide pain relief.

Skin Problems

Pressure sores pose a serious health hazard for wheelchair-dependent patients. Attention to detail in evaluating sitting position is vital to avoid unnecessary skin ulceration. This is best managed by a team composed of occupational therapists, physiotherapists, and appliance experts.

Fatigue

Fatigue is a common symptom in muscle disease and has multiple causes. In some, it reflects the imbalance between functional capacity and workload; in others, it is part of the disease itself; and in yet others, it reflects nocturnal hypoventilation. Progressive loss of muscle dictates that a patient must use a larger fraction of residual strength to perform any desired function. Thus, the closer one comes to the threshold for function, the greater part of residual strength must be brought to bear and the quicker the muscle fatigues. Help in planning and prioritizing daily activities may improve coping with fatigue. In metabolic muscle disease such as McArdle disease, failure to mobilize glucose from stored glycogen during the initial phase of exercise can result in both pain and early fatigue. Nocturnal hypoventilation results in daytime tiredness that is often interpreted as fatigue.

Psychosocial and Family Issues

Any chronic disease will generate psychosocial problems for the affected individual and those close to them. Children experience isolation and a growing fear of what the future holds. Early psychosocial intervention and educational counseling may, however, prevent unnecessary loss of potential. Adults are affected by loss of employment, loss of independence, fears for their future, and fears for their offspring. Questions concerning risk of transmission of genetic muscle disease are common and should prompt referral for genetic counseling. Similarly, psychological distress among carers of patients can arise from the same concerns. It is vital that psychological health also be evaluated when managing patients with muscle disease and those who care for them.

ACKNOWLEDGMENTS

I am grateful to all the members of the muscle clinic in Bergen for all they have taught me about muscle disease and its management. Thanks also to Petter Sanaker for reading the manuscript and helping me to improve its content.

SUGGESTED READING

Abdel-Hamid, H., & Clemens, P. R. (2012). Pharmacological therapies for muscular dystrophies. *Current Opinions in Neurology*, *25*(5), 604–608 610.1097/WCO. 1090b1013e328357f328344c.

Bushby, K., Finkel, R., et al. (2010). Diagnosis and management of Duchenne muscular dystrophy, Part 1: Diagnosis, and pharmacological and psychosocial management. *The Lancet Neurology*, *9*(1), 77–93.

Bushby, K., Finkel, R., et al. (2010). Diagnosis and management of Duchenne muscular dystrophy, Part 2: Implementation of multidisciplinary care. *The Lancet Neurology*, *9*(2), 177–189.

Emery, A. E. H. (Ed.) (2001). *The muscular dystrophies*. Oxford, UK: Oxford University Press.

Karpati, G., Hilton-Jones, D., Bushby, K., & Griggs, R. C. (Eds.) (2010). *Disorders of voluntary muscle*. Cambridge, UK: Cambridge University Press.

Lilleng, H., Abeler, K., et al. (2011). Variation of serum creatine kinase (CK) levels and prevalence of persistent hyperCKemia in a Norwegian normal population. The Tromsø Study. *Neuromuscular Disorders*, *21*(7), 494–500.

Menezes, M. P., & North, K. N. (2012). Inherited neuromuscular disorders: Pathway to diagnosis. *Journal of Paediatrics and Child Health*, *48*(6), 458–465.

Mercuri, E., & Muntoni, F. (2012). The ever-expanding spectrum of congenital muscular dystrophies. *Annals of Neurology*, *72*(1), 9–17.

Nance, J., Dowling, J., et al. (2012). Congenital myopathies: An update. *Current Neurology and Neuroscience Reports*, *12*(2), 165–174.

Selcen, D. (2011). Myofibrillar myopathies. *Neuromuscular Disorders*, *21*(3), 161–171.

Sewry, C. A., Jimenez-Mallebrera, C., et al. (2008). Congenital myopathies. *Current Opinions in Neurology*, *21*(5), 569–575 510.1097/WCO.1090b1013e32830f32893c32837.

Udd, B., & Krahe, R. (2012). The myotonic dystrophies: Molecular, clinical, and therapeutic challenges. *The Lancet Neurology*, *11*(10), 891–905.

SECTION SIX
TOXIC AND METABOLIC NEUROLOGICAL DISORDERS

21 Toxic and Iatrogenic Neurological Disorders

Christina Ulane and Olajide Williams

INTRODUCTION

CLINICAL FEATURES

Toxic and iatrogenic neurological disorders manifest in a variety of clinical presentations, depending on the part of the nervous system that is affected. The range of potential neurotoxins that may distress the nervous system is quite broad and includes medications and environmental exposures. The effects on the nervous system are complex and clinical features may vary significantly depending on whether the exposure is acute or chronic and the level or degree of exposure. Many toxins do not cause unique clinical syndromes and establishing cause and effect can be challenging. Thus, toxic and iatrogenic neurological disorders should be considered in the differential diagnosis of all neurologic presentations.

The clinical history is often the most important element in determining whether there is a toxic or iatrogenic etiology is possible in a given neurological disorder. Specific and direct questioning is often necessary to elicit potential exposures, including duration and level of exposure in the case of environmental neurotoxins (Table 21.1).

Regarding neurological disorders attributable to toxins or adverse medication effects, it is important to perform a thorough review of systems. Effects of toxins and medications on the central nervous system (CNS) most often produce nonspecific symptoms, which can range from mild to severe. At the mild end of the spectrum, patients may exhibit mood changes, fatigue, memory complaints, and headache. In more moderate cases, confusion and attention deficits may be apparent, while in the most severe cases, seizures and coma can occur. Owing to the nonspecific nature of these signs and symptoms, the clinical context is crucial. In most cases, the general physical examination is not helpful, and the neurological examination often reveals only nonspecific and nonfocal findings, except for select situations where particular findings may indicate a particular toxic exposure (Table 21.1). Peripheral nervous system (PNS) toxicity usually manifests as peripheral neuropathy; however, myopathy and neuromuscular junction dysfunction can also occur.

DIAGNOSTIC EVALUATION

Laboratory testing can be done for a number of different toxins, but the typical urine toxicology screen that is rapidly and readily available identifies only a few commonly

Table 21.1 Clinical History for Toxic Exposures

Occupational		Recreational	Accidental	Dietary
Heavy metals	Welders, miners, smelters	Alcohol	Carbon monoxide	Seafood
	• Lead, manganese, arsenic Painters	Cocaine		• Arsenic
	• Lead, arsenic Electroplating/ batteries	Opioids		• Mercury
		Amphetamines		• Ciguatera
		Marijuana		• Shellfish
	• Manganese, lead Canning	Barbituates		Toxin
	• Tin	Phencyclidine		
Organophosphates	Insecticides	Hallucinogens		
Solvents	Varnish, rayon, textile and preservative manufacturing	Nitrous oxide		
	• Carbon disulfide paint, paint remover, degreasers, rubber solvents, glues			
	• Trichloroethylene, hexacarbons			

prescribed or abused drugs. Heavy metals can be tested for by 24-hour urine collection, which provides superior sensitivity than random spot testing given the diurnal excretion pattern of heavy metals. Some heavy metals can be tested for in the serum as well. If medication toxicity is suspected and laboratory testing for the agent is available, this, too, should be included in evaluation. Laboratory evaluation for suspected toxic and iatrogenic neurological disorders may include:

• Complete blood cell count and differential, comprehensive metabolic panel (including electrolytes, blood urea nitrogen, glucose, hepatic function), coagulation factor analysis, ammonia level
• Whole blood level of lead
• 24-Hour urine collection for heavy metal testing
• Arterial blood gas
• Urine toxicology screen
• Serum ethanol level
• Serum drug levels (e.g., lithium, antiepileptics, immunosuppressants)
• Electrocardiogram

Magnetic resonance imaging (MRI) of the brain and/or spinal cord can be helpful in some cases, although minimal abnormalities or nonspecific findings such as vasogenic edema are not infrequent. Most unique is the deposition of the heavy metals in the basal ganglia, an area also quite susceptible to hypoxemia. Electroencephalogram (EEG) may be helpful in some instances to eliminate nonconvulsive status epilepticus, although the majority of toxic encephalopathies demonstrate nonspecific EEG patterns. Nerve conduction studies (NCS) and electromyography (EMG) can provide useful information regarding whether a neuropathy is axonal or demyelinating, which can be helpful for differentiating possible toxic etiologies but will also identify whether a myopathy or neuromuscular junction abnormality is present.

TREATMENT

The guiding principle for treatment of any toxic or iatrogenic neurological disorder is removal of the offending agent. Thus, the accurate diagnosis of the underlying toxic exposure as the causative factor is essential for treatment but can be challenging. Further treatment and supportive care are guided by the particular neurotoxin and the severity of the neurological deficits.

Heavy Metals

Environmental or occupational exposure to heavy metals causes different acute and chronic syndromes. Identifying and eliminating the exposure can be difficult. The acute syndrome is most often marked by encephalopathy, which warrants more urgent and aggressive intervention. The mainstay of treatment for heavy metal intoxication is supportive, with judicious use of chelation therapy. Supportive therapy and treatment may require monitoring in the neurological intensive care unit. Chelation therapy functions by oral administration of an agent that binds the metal and passes through the gastrointestinal system, facilitating elimination and preventing systemic absorption (Table 21.2).

Medications

Numerous medications in common clinical use have untoward effects on the nervous system (Table 21.3). The major categories include immunosuppressive agents, chemotherapeutics, and cholesterol-lowering agents. In some cases, the neurotoxic effect is magnified by or uncovers a previously undiagnosed underlying neurologic condition. Temporal correlation between the development of symptoms and the initiation of the suspected agent, and resolution or halted progression of symptoms with discontinuation of the agent is considered evidence for causation.

Immunosuppressant Drugs

Immunosuppressive medications are used in a variety of medical conditions for primary autoimmune disorders and after organ transplantation. Post-transplantation, neurotoxicity may occur from opportunistic infections brought about by immunosuppression, direct neurotoxicity of the immunosuppressive medications themselves, or aberrant metabolic states induced by transplantation. Progressive multifocal leukoencephalopathy (PML), which is a life-threatening infection that affects the white matter of the brain, can be caused by several immunosuppressive drugs alone or in

Table 21.2 Heavy Metal Intoxication

Offending Agent	Clinical Features	Treatment
Lead	Blue gums Abdominal colic Encephalopathy Neuropathy Motor neuron disease–like syndrome Focal mononeuropathy (radial or fibular nerve) Serum lead level ≥40 µg/dL	Remove exposure Chelation therapy 1. Calcium ethylenediaminetetraacetic acid (EDTA) 30 mg/kg q24h 2. Dimercaprol/British anti-Lewisite (BAL) 4–5 mg/kg intramuscular 3. Dimercaptosuccinic acid (DMSA): safe, effective oral agent **calcium EDTA and dimercaprol have potential serious adverse effects such as cardiac arrhythmia and renal tubular acidosis*
Arsenic	Garlic/metallic taste Mees lines (white transverse lines on fingernails) Nausea, vomiting Encephalopathy Seizures Unilateral phrenic or facial nerve paralysis (rare) Peripheral neuropathy	Remove exposure Decontaminate patient, site Gastric lavage Supportive therapy for shock Chelation therapy 1. Dimercaprol/BAL 2. DMSA
Mercury	Acrodynia Cerebellar dysfunction Encephalopathy Sensory neuronopathy (particularly joint-position sense) Headache, weakness, visual changes Increased salivation Abdominal pain, metallic taste	Remove exposure Supportive therapy There is no antidote, but some patients may warrant chelation therapy Do not administer activated charcoal
Thallium	Alopecia Abdominal pain Peripheral neuropathy (painful, rapidly progressive, ascending) Distal weakness Cranial neuropathies Cerebellar signs Encephalopathy, seizures	Remove exposure, contaminated clothing Administer activated charcoal if within 1 h of ingestion

(continued)

Table 21.2 Continued

Offending Agent	Clinical Features	Treatment
Manganese	Extrapyramidal signs/ Parkinsonism Behavioral changes Weakness, incoordination	Remove exposure Chelation therapy may be helpful
Lithium	Cerebellar dysfunction Tremor Encephalopathy Seizures	Remove exposure Gastric lavage if within 1 h of presentation Whole-bowel irrigation with polyethylene glycol lavage Hydration, possibly dialysis

combination. Other complications include posterior reversible leukoencephalopa-thy (PRES)-like syndromes (even if serum drug levels within normal limits), central pontine myelinolysis (CPM), and post-transplant lymphoproliferative disorder (Table 21.3). PRES is discussed in more detail in the chapter on Metabolic Neurological Disorders.

Antiretroviral Therapy

Nucleoside analogs cause peripheral neuropathy as a result of mitochondrial tox-icity. Stavudine has been associated with a Guillain-Barré type of presentation. Non-nucleoside reverse transcriptase inhibitors also cause neurotoxicity, most com-monly seen as neuropsychiatric disturbances. Protease inhibitors were initially thought to cause peripheral neuropathy, but further study controlling for other factors and treatment found no increased risk (Table 21.3).

Chemotherapeutic Drugs

Neurotoxicity is often the limiting factor for chemotherapeutic drugs. Peripheral neuropathy from chemotherapy is cumulative and dose related. Most neurological effects are seen during treatment, but some effects (such as neurocognitive) may not be apparent for months to years after treatment. While several agents have been put forward as neuroprotective agents, clinical trials have generally failed to show benefits. Almost all chemotherapeutic drugs can cause acute encephalopathy with confusion, hallucinations, seizures, and lethargy (Table 21.3).

Statins

The use of 3-hydroxy-3-methylglutaryl-coenzyme (HMG-CoA) reductase inhibitors (statins) is widespread given that they are the most effective class of drugs for lowering serum low-density lipoprotein cholesterol concentrations and are a mainstay in the treatment and prevention of cardiovascular and cerebrovascular disease. Statins are generally well tolerated but can be toxic to muscle. The risk profile, clinical variants, and management of statin-induced myopathies are detailed in Figure 21.1.

Table 21.3 Selected Medication-Induced Toxicity

Offending Medication	Clinical Features	Treatment
Calcineurin inhibitors (tacrolimus, cyclosporine)	PRES (akinetic mutism, seizures, visual impairment, encephalopathy)	May improve with switching to the other agent
	Usually occurs early (within 1 mo, rarely after 1 y)	Discontinue medication (symptoms improve within days) Usually does not recur after restarting medication
	Axonal or demyelinating neuropathy	Consider changing to another agent
	CNS opportunistic infections (PML, fungal infections, toxoplasma, bacterial infections) Viral polyradiculitis (CMV, EBV)	Antimicrobials pertinent to infection
	CNS lymphoma	Oncological evaluation and treatment
	Drug-induced thrombotic microangiopathy (rare, petechial hemorrhages	Supportive, withdrawal of medication if severe
TNFα inhibitors (infliximab, adalimumab, etanercept)	Demyelinating neuropathy (usually within 8 mos after treatment onset)	Withdrawal of medication If mild may reduce dose Consider pulse IV steroids, IVIg, or PE
Platinum compounds (cisplatin, oxaliplatin)	Sensory neuropathy	Withdrawal of agent Duloxetine if painful
Ifosfamide	Encephalopathy Seizures Extrapyramidal signs	Prevent with methylene blue Often completely resolve
Vinca alkaloids (vincristine)	Peripheral neuropathy May uncover mild hereditary neuropathy (CMT)	Discontinue agent
Taxanes (paclitaxel, docetaxel)	Sensorimotor neuropathy	Discontinue agent Consider immunotherapy
Bortezomib, thalidomide	Demyelinating neuropathy	Discontinue agent Consider immunotherapy
Nucleoside analogs (didanosine, stavudine, zalcitabine)	Peripheral neuropathy (2-3 mos after initiation of treatment, involves hands earlier)	Discontinue agent (rarely used as other options available)
Non-nucleoside reverse transcriptase inhibitors	Neuropsychiatric disturbances (in >50% of patients starting efavirenz)	Resolve within 1 mo

TNF, tumor necrosis factor; CNS, central nervous system; PE, plasma exchange; PRES, posterior reversible encephalopathy syndrome; PML, progressive multifocal leukoencephalopathy; CMV, cytomegalovirus; EBV, Epstein-Barr virus; CMT, Charçot-Marie-Tooth.

SUSPECTED STATIN RELATED NEUROTOXICITY

Statins:

- <u>Highest risk:</u> Cerivastatin (withdrawn from market) and atorvastatin
- <u>Intermediate risk:</u> Simvastatin, lovastatin, pravastatin, red yeast rice (similar to lovastatin)
- <u>Lowest risk:</u> Fluvastatin

Additional history:

- Is the patient taking a CYP3A4 inhibitor? (most common: clarithromycin, verapamil, diltiazem, cyclosporine A)
- Is the patient taking a fibrate?
- Could the patient be an asymptomatic carrier for a metabolic myopathy or mitochondrial disorder?
- Is the patient taking a proton pump inhibitor ? (increased risk for polymyositis and dermatomyositis)

CLINICAL SYNDROMES :

1. Myalgias
2. Cramps
3. Asymptomatic hyperCKemia
4. *Rare: necrotizing myopathy, acute rhabdomyolysis/myoglobinuria/acute renal failure*

TREATMENT OF STATIN-INDUCED MYOPATHY:

- Asymptomatic or mild hyperCKemia
    - Can continue statin, monitor closely
- Drug cessation: most will resolve in 2–3 months
- Switch to a lower-risk statin
- If the symptoms persist or progress → muscle biopsy to look for underlying neuromuscular disorder or myositis
- Retrial with lower dose or less potent statin after period of recovery
- Acute rhabdomyolysis/myoglobinuria/renal failure: hospital admission, IV hydration, supportive measures, hemodialysis if needed
- Other:
    - Risk/benefit analysis regarding need for statin
    - Potential role for vitamin D, Coenzyme Q10

FIGURE 21.1
Treatment of Statin-related Toxicity.

Recreational Drugs

Recreational drugs and alcohol have numerous acute and chronic toxic effects on the nervous system. For example, acute alcohol intoxication has cerebellar and cognitive impairment, while the chronic overuse of alcohol can cause neuropathy, cerebellar degeneration, hepatic failure, metabolic abnormalities and nutritional deficiencies, each with their own effects on the nervous system. Table 21.4 shows the neurological effects of commonly used recreational drugs.

Table 21.4 Recreational Drugs

Drug	Clinical Features	Treatment
Alcohol	Acute Intoxication: – mild: euphoria, impaired concentration/judgement – moderate: dysarthria, ataxia, diplopia, nausea, tachycardia, labile mood – severe: stupor alternating with combativeness, coma, death Chronic Intoxication: – thiamine deficiency: Wernicke's (encephalopathy, ophthalmoplegia, ataxia), Korsakoff's (retrograde/anterograde amnesia) – peripheral neuropathy (predominantly sensory, axonal) – myopathy (acute or chronic; elevated CK, myopathic findings on EMG) – amblyopia – cerebellar degeneration – stroke – dementia – Marchiafava-Bignani disease (demyelination/necrosis of corpus callosum) Withdrawal: – "hangover": headache, malaise, nausea, diaphoresis – early: tremulousness, hallucinations, seizures, dysautonomia – late (48–72h): delirium tremens *alcohol withdrawal can be life-threatening*	Requires inpatient treatment if: – autonomic instability – cognitive impairment – history of DTs or seizures Early/mild withdrawal: – chlordiazepoxide 25–100 mg OR diazepam 5–20 mg q8h followed by taper over 3–6 days – thiamine 100 mg daily, multivitamin – may also use valproic acid or carbamazepine Severe withdrawal: – diazepam 10 mg IV OR lorazepam 2 mg IV, may repeat, for autonomic instability, agitation – refractory cases may require phenobarbital – thiamine 100 mg IV TID × 5 days, then PO (*must give prior to or with glucose to prevent precipitating Wernicke's or Korsakoff's*) – electrolyte and fluid management – prevent hypoglycemia – cooling if hyperpyrexia Chronic outpatient alcohol abuse treatment: – disulfuram – SSRIs – NMDA antagonists – cognitive-behavioral therapy – support groups/12-step programs
Opiates	Acute intoxication: – euphoria, analgesia, drowsiness – miosis, dry mouth, diaphoresis, constipation, urinary retention, nausea, vomiting	Acute intoxication: – naloxone 2 mg IV, repeat with 2–4 mg boluses up to total of 20 mg (rapid onset of 2–3 min with reversal of symptoms), may use IM or SQ if needed, caution: may precipitate withdrawal

(continued)

Table 21.4 Continued

Drug	Clinical Features	Treatment
	– respiratory depression, hypothermia, orthostatic hypotension Overdose: – coma with pinpoint but reactive pupils – respiratory depression/apnea – non-cardiogenic pulmonary edema Withdrawal (peaks at 24–72 h, may last 7–10 d): – craving, irritation/anxiety – weakness, lacrimation, rhinorrhea, diaphoresis, piloerection, mydriasis, nausea, vomiting, cramps, diarrhea, fever – muscle spasms	– may not respond to naloxone if concomitant BZD, barbiturate or alcohol use – respiratory and circulatory support Withdrawal: – methadone maintenance – clonidine for symptomatic treatment
Cocaine/ amphetamines	Acute intoxication: – alertness, euphoria, increased motor activity and endurance, overconfidence and impaired judgment – agitation, palpitations, systolic hypertension, reflex bradycardia, mydriasis – rapid tolerance development – with chronic use may develop dyskinesias and psychosis At higher doses: – tremor, dystonia, anorexia, diaphoresis, thirst, arrhythmias, difficulty urinating, hyperthermia, hallucinations – sympathetic overactivity leads to: headaches/migraines, seizures	Decrease agitation: – IV benzodiazepines – cardiorespiratory support as needed – calm environment – barbiturates may aggravate delirium – neuroleptics may precipitate seizures Hypertension: – alpha-blockers (phenoxybenzamine, phentolamine) OR – vasodilators (nitroprusside) *beta blockers increase the risk of unopposed alpha activity which may worsen hypertension* May require bicarbonate for acidosis

(*continued*)

Table 21.4 Continued

Drug	Clinical Features	Treatment
	Overdose: – all of the above plus: – acidosis, delirium, seizures, shock, stroke, hyperpyrexia, abnormal movements, coma, death Withdrawal: – hypersomnia, dysphoria, depression	
Marijuana	– Euphoria, paranoia/anxiety, relaxation, depersonalization, impaired cognition – conjunctival injection, decreased salivation, increased urination, tachycardia, increased appetite and thirst – analgesia	Supportive May use low dose BZDs or neuroleptics if agitated

CK = creatine kinase, BZD = benzodiazepine, IV = intravenous, SSRI = selective serotonin reuptake inhibitor, EMG = electromyography, DT = delirum tremens.

SUGGESTED READING

Brust, J. C. M. (2002). Neurologic complications of substance abuse. *Journal of Acquired Immune Deficiency Syndromes, 31*, S29–S34.

Cavaliere, R., & Schiff, D. (2006). Neurologic toxicities of cancer therapies. *Current Neurology and Neuroscience Reports, 6*, 218–226.

Dobbs, M. R. (2011). Toxic encephalopathy. *Seminars in Neurology, 31*, 184–193.

Feske, S. K. (2011). Posterior reversible encephalopathy syndrome: A review. *Seminars in Neurology, 31*, 202–215.

Harper, C. R., & Jacobson, T. A. (2010). Evidence-based management of statin myopathy. *Current Atherosclerosis Reports, 12*, 322–330.

22 Metabolic Neurological Disorders

Christina Ulane and Olajide Williams

INTRODUCTION AND CLINICAL FEATURES

Systemic disease is long known to affect the nervous system. Metabolic neurological disorders exhibit broad clinical presentations, depending on the part of the nervous system that is affected. The breadth of metabolic abnormalities that may distress the nervous system is quite wide and includes systemic diseases and conditions which perturb homeostasis. The effects on the nervous system are complex and clinical features may vary significantly depending on whether the metabolic abnormality is acute or chronic and the degree of dysfunction. Many metabolic abnormalities do not cause unique clinical syndromes and establishing cause and effect can be challenging. However, metabolic abnormalities as cause for neurological dysfunction should be considered in the differential diagnosis of all neurologic presentations.

The clinical history and selected diagnostic testing are important in determining whether a metabolic abnormality may be the cause of a neurological disorder, and a thorough review of past medical history and review of systems may provide clues to systemic disease relevant to the disorder. Metabolic abnormalities may be secondary to systemic medical disease, medication or toxin effects, or idiopathic. Identifying an underlying cause of a metabolic abnormality assists in treatment and correction. The effects of metabolic abnormalities on the central nervous system most often produce nonspecific symptoms, which can range from mild to severe. At the mild end of the spectrum, patients may exhibit mood changes, fatigue, memory complaints, and headache. In more moderate cases, confusion and attention deficits may be apparent, while in the most severe cases, seizures, coma, and irreversible damage can occur. Owing to the nonspecific nature of these signs and symptoms, the clinical context is crucial. In most cases, the general physical examination is not helpful, and the neurological examination often reveals only nonspecific and nonfocal findings, except for select situations where particular physical exam findings may signify a particular metabolic disorder. The peripheral nervous system effects of metabolic abnormalities usually manifest as peripheral neuropathy; however, myopathy can also occur.

DIAGNOSTIC EVALUATION

Laboratory testing can easily be performed to assess many metabolic disorders. Routine testing for electrolyte disturbances and endocrine abnormalities are readily available and can rapidly identify potentially reversible disturbances. Laboratory evaluation for suspected metabolic neurological disorders may include:

- Complete blood cell count and differential
- Comprehensive metabolic panel (including sodium, potassium, calcium, magnesium, blood urea nitrogen, creatinine, glucose, hepatic enzymes)
- Coagulation factor analysis
- Ammonia level
- Thyroid stimulating hormone, parathyroid hormone levels, hemoglobin A1c, 25-hydroxy vitamin D, thiamine, vitamin B12
- Arterial blood gas
- Urine porphobilinogens
- Electrocardiogram

Magnetic resonance imaging of the brain and/or spinal cord can be helpful in some cases, although minimal abnormalities or nonspecific findings such as vasogenic edema are not infrequent. Electroencephalogram (EEG) may be helpful in some instances to rule out nonconvulsive status epilepticus, although the majority of metabolic encephalopathies show nonspecific EEG patterns. Nerve conduction studies and electromyography can provide useful information regarding whether a neuropathy is axonal or demyelinating and identify whether a myopathy is present.

TREATMENT

The mainstay of treatment of metabolic neurological disorders is to correct the underlying metabolic abnormality in a manner that is safe and reduces the risk of permanent neurological damage. Thus, the accurate diagnosis of a metabolic abnormality and its underlying cause is essential for treatment. Further treatment and supportive care are guided by the particular metabolic abnormality and the severity of the neurological deficits.

Metabolic Abnormalities

Organ failure or dysfunction can lead to metabolic abnormalities and perturb homeostasis, which in turn can cause neurological dysfunction. Most well characterized are the neurological effects precipitated by liver dysfunction and renal dysfunction. In renal disease, the neurological effects may be direct or as the result of treatment with dialysis. The complexity of the neurological effects is underscored by the range in severity from subtle to fulminant neurological dysfunction. In addition, both acute and chronic effects are apparent (Table 22.1).

Disruption of electrolytes can have serious and life-threatening effects on the nervous system. These disruptions may be due to underlying endocrine dysfunction, such as hyperglycemia secondary to diabetes mellitus or hypercalcemia due to hyperparathyroidism. Correction of the electrolyte disturbance depends on the rapidity with which it initially developed and degree of departure from normal values (Table 22.2). Other endocrine disorders can have significant effects on the nervous system, in part mediated by hormonal effects. Thyroid dysfunction can also lead to neurological

Table 22.1 Neurological Disorders Caused by Selected Organ Dysfunction

Organ Dysfunction	Clinical Features	Treatment
Hepatic encephalopathy	Range: • Subtle personality/cognitive, tremor, insomnia, incoordination • Disorientation, amnesia, dysarthria, hyporeflexia, asterixis • Somnolence, hallucinations, hyperreflexia, weakness, nystagmus, rigidity • Coma, extensor/flexor posturing, cerebral edema, increased ICP EEG: diffuse slowing, triphasic waves, irregular delta (most useful in excluding NCSE) MRI: to exclude other causes, manganese deposition in the basal ganglia common in liver failure patients *Excluded if ammonia is normal	Lactulose Rifaximin Liver transplant If acute and severe, requires treatment in a neurological intensive care unit
Uremic encephalopathy	Acute or chronic (usually when GFR < 10%) Encephalopathy • Early: inattention, insomnia, hyperactivity, anorexia, nausea • Late: lethargy, impaired cognition, paranoia, vomiting • Severe: confusion, dysarthria, myoclonus, asterixis, seizures Chronic renal failure: • Neuropathy, restless legs syndrome *Severity not correlated with BUN/Cr	Dialysis Renal transplant
Dialysis disequilibrium	Headaches, altered mentation, seizures, cramps, nausea	Usually self-limited (begins within 24 h post-dialysis, resolves within 48 h) If severe: • Stop dialysis • Supportive • Consider rapidly raising plasma osmolality with mannitol, hypertonic saline, dextrose

Table 22.2 Selected Metabolic Neurological Disorders

Disorders of Sodium	Clinical Features	Treatment
Hyponatremia	Serum Na <135mEq/L (but depending on chronicity may be asymptomatic even at 125 mEq/L or less) Confusion, seizures, cramps, weakness Isotonic (hyperlipidemia, hyperproteinemia) Hypertonic (hyperglycemia, mannitol) Hypotonic (low cardiac output, SIADH, psychogenic polydipsia)	**if correct too rapidly, may precipitate osmotic demyelination syndrome* Hypovolemic hyponatremia: • Identify/treat underlying cause (GI loss, hemorrhage, renal salt wasting, excessive diuretics, adrenal insufficiency) • Isotonic saline Hypervolemic hyponatremia • Identify/treat underlying cause (CHF, cirrhosis, nephrotic syndrome) • Free water restrict Isovolemic hyponatremia • Identify/treat underlying cause (SIADH, hypothyroidism, reset osmostat) • If acute (<48 h) then can use 3% saline to raise Na by 4–6 mEq/L rapidly then by 10 mEq/L/24 h • Free water restrict • If chronic then raise Na slowly by <10 mEq/L/24 h • Free water restrict * Hyponatremia may worsen with saline in SIADH • If resistant, can use renal vasopressin receptor antagonists (i.e., conivaptan)
Hypernatremia	Serum Na >145 mEq/L, usually >160 mEg/L symptomatic Due to water deficit or inadequate ADH response Altered mentation, seizures, rigidity	Calculate water deficit Replace with water or 5% dextrose • Lower Na by no more than 2 mEq/L/h Central diabetes insipidus: • Deamino D-arginine vasopressin (DDAVP; ADH analog) Nephrogenic diabetes insipidus: • Salt restriction • Thiazide diuretics

Disorders of Calcium	Clinical Features	Treatment
Hypercalcemia	Weakness, headaches, encephalopathy Abdominal pain, constipation, polydipsia	Severe: • IV saline, calcitonin, bisphosphonate Asymptomatic/mild: • Avoid aggravating factors

(continued)

Table 22.2 Continued

Hypocalcemia	Paresthesias, cramps, carpopedal spasm, tetany, seizures, altered mentation, stridor, cardiac conduction defects (long QT), bradycardia Chvostek's/Trousseau's signs *Correct for low/high albumin levels or use ionized (free) calcium levels*	If rapid and/or severe: • Calcium gluconate 1–2 mg IV in 50 mL 5% Dextrose over 10–20 min, followed by continuous slower infusion • Correct hypomagnesemia Asymptomatic/mild: • Calcium carbonate or citrate 1500–2000 mg daily • Vitamin D if deficient
Disorders of Potassium	*Clinical Features*	*Treatment*
Hypokalemia	Serum K < 3.5 mEq/L Proximal weakness, hyporeflexia Can be severe with paralysis, life-threatening cardiac arrhythmias	Identify/treat underlying cause Sodium restrict (<80 mEq/d) to reduce renal K loss PO KCl If severe, IV KCl infusion with cardiac monitoring
Hyperkalemia	Serum K >5.5– 6.0 mEq/L Muscle weakness Cardiac conduction abnormalities usually appear before neuromuscular effects	*Identify/treat underlying cause* • Muscle injury • Medications (B2 antagonists, digitalis, succinylcholine) • Insulin resistance • Addison's • Aldosterone deficiency (ACEI, NSAIDs, heparin) • Aldosterone resistance (renal failure, RTA, K-sparing diuretics) *Severe:* Calcium gluconate 10% (20 mL IV) for cardioprotection Insulin 5 U IV q15min to promote cellular K uptake Albuterol 10–20 mg inh Kayexalate ±Furosemide

(*continued*)

Table 22.2 Continued

216

Toxic and Metabolic Neurological Disorders

Porphyria	Abdominal pain/crises (due to autonomic dysfunction)	• Pain (narcotic analgesics, chlorpromazine) • Anxiety/insomnia (low-dose short-acting BZDs) • Tachycardia/HTN (consider beta-blockers) • Slow correction of hyponatremia to prevent seizures (AEDs may worsen porphyria) • Carbohydrate load or hemin load • Liver transplantation considered in severe cases
Disorders of Glucose	*Clinical Features*	*Treatment*
Hyperglycemia	Encephalopathy Focal neurological deficits (rare) Continuous partial seizures	IV insulin infusion IV hydration/volume expansion
Hypoglycemia	Encephalopathy Seizures	IV D$_{50}$

ICP, intracranial pressure; NCSE, nonconvulsive status epilepticus; EEG, electroencephalogram; GFR, glomerular filtration rate; BUN/Cr, blood urea nitrogen/creatinine; GI, gastrointestinal; SIADH, syndrome of inappropriate antidiuretic hormone secretion; CHF, congestive heart failure; ADH, antidiuretic hormone; BZD, benzodiazepine; HTN, hypertension; AED, antiepileptic drug; PO, per os; IV, intravenous; KCl, potassium chloride; ACEI, angiotensin converting enzyme inhibitors; NSAIDs, nonsteroidal anti-inflammatory drugs; RTA, renal tubular acidosis; D50, 50% dextrose.

consequences, including Hashimoto's encephalopathy in severe hypothyroidism and tremor in hyperthyroidism.

Posterior Reversible Encephalopathy Syndrome

The posterior reversible encephalopathy syndrome (PRES) is a common underlying pathology associated with diverse toxic and metabolic conditions. It is also known as hypertensive encephalopathy, reversible posterior encephalopathy syndrome, which reflects the lack of understanding surrounding its precise pathophysiology. It affects white matter, often in the posterior hemispheres, and it is usually, but not always, reversible (both clinically and radiographically). The primary pathophysiology involves reversible cerebral edema due to disruption of the blood–brain barrier. Clinical features and treatment can be found in Table 22.3. Originally described in the setting of malignant hypertension, there are now many conditions associated with PRES (Table 22.4).

Table 22.3 Clinical Features and Treatment of Posterior Reversible Encephalopathy Syndrome

Clinical Features	Treatment
Sudden or gradual onset headache, cortical visual symptoms, encephalopathy, seizures, hypertension, brisk DTRs MRI (may be normal early in course): vasogenic edema, often hemispheric and symmetric bilaterally, hemorrhage (~15% focal hematoma or sulcal SAH), ischemia, minimal enhancement, petechial hemorrhage on GRE CSF: may have mild pleocytosis, elevated protein (mostly to exclude other causes)	1. Prompt reduction of blood pressure 　a. Often will require ICU level of care 　b. Initially reduce MAP by 20% (caution not to reduce cerebral or renal perfusion) 　c. IV is optimal, potential agents: nicardipine, labetalol, sodium nitroprusside, diazoxide, enalaprilat, hydralazine, nitroglycerin, fenoldopam, phentolamine, trimethaphan 2. Remove underlying cause (if identified) 　a. Eclampsia: fetus delivery, magnesium sulfate 　b. Discontinue/switch immunosuppressives 3. Treatment of seizures with AEDs or magnesium in eclampsia

DTRs, deep tendon reflexes; MAP, mean arterial pressure; MRI, magnetic resonance imaging; SAH, subarachnoid hemorrhage; CSF, cerebrospinal fluid; AED, antiepileptic drug; GRE, gradient echo.

Table 22.4 Related Conditions and Drugs Associated With Posterior Reversible Encephalopathy Syndrome

Reported Conditions/Drugs Associated With PRES		
Medical/ Systemic	Malignant hypertension	Renal, collagen vascular diseases, pheochromocytoma, acute glomerulonephritis, vasculitis, antihypertensive medication withdrawal, autonomic dysfunction
	Pregnancy	eclampsia
	Organ transplantation	Renal, cardiac, liver
	Hematologic	TTP
	Autoimmune/ inflammatory	SLE, PAN, HSP
	Systemic/infectious	Sepsis, SIRS
	Oncologic	Tumor lysis syndrome
	Electrolyte disturbances	Hypomagnesemia, hypercalcemia
	Trauma	TBI, dysautonomia from spinal cord injury
Medication	Neuropsychiatric	NMS, serotonin syndrome, TCAs, MAOI tyramine
	Cardiac/vascular	Midodrine, fludrocortisone, sympathomimetics
	Immunosuppressants	CSA, tacrolimus
	Infusions	IVIg, blood transfusion

(*continued*)

Table 22.4 Continued

Reported Conditions/Drugs Associated With PRES

	Chemotherapeutics	Cisplatin, cytarabine, gemcitabine, bevacizumab
	Antiretrovirals	Indinavir
Drug	Stimulants	Cocaine, ephedrine
	Withdrawal	Alcohol, other drugs

TTP, thrombotic thrombocytopenic purpura; SLE, systemic lupus erythematosis; PAN, polyarteritis nodosa; HSP, Henoch-Schönlein purpura; SIRS, systemic inflammatory response syndrome; NMS, neuroleptic malignant syndrome; TCA, tricyclic antidepressant; MAOI, monoamine oxidase inhibitor; CSA, cyclosporine A; IVIg, intravenous immunoglobulin.

SUGGESTED READING

Feske, S. K. Posterior reversible encephalopathy syndrome: A review. *Seminars in Neurology*, (2011) *31*, 202–215.

Frontera, J. A. Metabolic encephalopathies in the critical care unit. *Continuum Lifelong Learning Neurology*, (2012) *18*(3), 611–639.

Samuels, M. A., & Seifter, J. L. Encephalopathies caused by electrolyte disorders. *Seminars in Neurology*, (2011) *31*, 135–138.

SECTION SEVEN

INFECTIONS OF THE CENTRAL NERVOUS SYSTEM

23 Bacterial Meningitis

Miguel Valdes-Sueiras and Elyse J. Singer

INTRODUCTION

These chapters will aid the physician, nurse practitioner, or other healthcare provider in the recognition, diagnosis, and management of many infections affecting the nervous system. Some infections can result in meningitis, encephalitis, and myelitis or a combination of these processes (i.e., meningoencephalitis). Some infections may not result in a frank inflammatory process but nevertheless can cause encephalopathy and myelopathy. Some of these entities have been known since ancient times, while some are just being elucidated. Although the list of possible infectious agents can seem endless, we shall try to organize in a sensible manner the more commonly encountered infectious agents and by disease process. Some diseases are rare but treatable, and others may have regional predominance. In each section, the respective microbe will be discussed regarding its regional distribution, clinical presentation, imaging findings, diagnosis, and treatment available.

Knowledge of regional distribution of a disease along with a history and physical examination remain important tools in diagnosing infections of the nervous system. For example, recognizing the signs of endocarditis or the erythema chronica migrans of Lyme disease can aid tremendously in diagnosis. In each section, where possible, the salient clinical indicator will be highlighted.

Blood and urine testing should be routinely sought. Tests to consider include serum antigens, serum antibodies both acute and convalescent, and blood cultures. If indicated, respiratory cultures, fecal examination, and skin biopsies/cultures may also be helpful in diagnosis.

Imaging is an increasingly important modality in the management of infections of the nervous system. A magnetic resonance imaging (MRI) scan with contrast is almost invariably more helpful than a computed tomography (CT) scan. Reference in the chapter to imaging will be made and will always imply that contrast material has been administered. Emergency scans, however, normally do not have contrast administered, as the main point of these studies is to assess for space occupying lesions that will necessitate surgical intervention. In addition to identifying space-occupying lesions such as abscess, imaging can be highly suggestive of a diagnosis such as herpes encephalitis, neurocysticercosis and Creutzfeldt-Jakob disease.

Cerebrospinal fluid (CSF) testing remains the mainstay of diagnosis. The initial differential of the cell count along with the glucose and protein can lead the clinician along the right path to diagnosis with confirmation by CSF culture. The increasingly availability of polymerase chain reaction (PCR) tests, antigen and antibody tests have now made the need for brain biopsies in diagnosis much less frequent.

Electroencephalogram is an additional modality that can sometimes assist in diagnosis and will be mentioned in those agents that it is helpful such as subsclerosing pan-encephalitis and Creutzfeldt-Jakob disease.

MENINGITIS

Infectious meningitis is a diffuse inflammation of the meninges (pia and arachnoid) that can be caused by bacteria, fungi, viruses, and parasites. Meningitis can be accompanied by fever, headache and meningismus.

BACTERIAL MENINGITIS

Distribution is worldwide.

Presentation

Bacterial meningitis is an extremely serious illness; even with optimal treatment, mortality is estimated to be 15% and 20% of survivors will have one or more serious neurologic sequelae. Most patients with acute, community-acquired bacterial meningitis present within hours to a few days of symptom onset. However, bacterial meningitis should be considered in any patient who presents with unexplained fever, sepsis, or altered mental status.

The classic symptoms of bacterial meningitis are generally considered to be headache (which is typically severe, unrelenting, and generally unresponsive to analgesics), meningismus (stiff neck), fever, and altered level of consciousness. Likewise, only 44% of adults with bacterial meningitis will present with the complete triad of fever, neck stiffness, and altered mental status, but almost all will have two of the following four symptoms: headache, fever, altered mental status, and neck stiffness. In particular, very old, very young, or immunosuppressed patients may have atypical presentations. Infants may present with seizures, hypothermia, lethargy, irritability, poor feeding, vomiting, or bulging fontanelles. Immunosuppressed patients and the elderly may have minimal or no fever or neck stiffness.

Epidemiology

The majority of cases of acute, community-acquired bacterial meningitis are caused by these three organisms: *Haemophilus influenzae*, *Streptococcus pneumoniae*, and *Neisseria meningitidis*. The incidence of *H. influenzae* type b is rapidly declining in industrialized countries as increasing numbers of persons are vaccinated.

History and Physical Examination

The history and physical examination can provide important clues to the diagnosis, such as an antecedent pharyngitis, otitis media, sinusitis, pneumonia, rash, injection drug use, infectious endocarditis, head trauma, recent neurosurgery, placement of a cochlear implant, living in close quarters such as dormitories or barracks, or a history of immunosuppression (e.g., absence of a spleen, complement deficiency, immuno-globulin deficiency, some cancers, use of immunosuppressive drugs, or HIV/AIDS). It is important to ascertain whether the patient has received antibiotics prior to presentation as this may attenuate some of the findings and delay diagnosis.

Diagnosis

CSF examination remains the mainstay of diagnosis of bacterial meningitis. In developed countries where neuroimaging is widely available, it is common to perform brain imaging (usually a noncontrast brain CT scan) prior to CSF examination, due to concerns that a lumbar puncture (LP) may precipitate cerebral herniation in patients with increased intracranial pressure/mass effect. However, this practice has raised concerns because it may also delay diagnostic LP and early antibiotic treatment, thus increasing morbidity and mortality. Thus, in evaluating possible bacterial meningitis, both diagnosis and treatment must be performed in tandem.

Neuroimaging

The primary purpose of neuroimaging in the initial diagnosis of bacterial meningitis is to exclude clinical abnormalities that preclude safe performance of an LP. In most cases of bacterial meningitis, the CT imaging will be normal or there will be nondiagnostic abnormalities such as sulcal effacement, meningeal enhancement, or stroke. In such instances, any herniation that subsequently occurs is likely the result of the underlying disease. A prospective clinical study indicated that neuroimaging is most likely to detect a cerebral abnormality in patients with suspected meningitis who are over age 60, who are immunocompromised, who have new-onset seizures or signs of focal neurological lesions on examination, or who have altered mental status.

Blood

It is essential to obtain blood (and urine if possible) before beginning empiric antibiotic treatment, especially if the LP must be deferred or delayed. Blood cultures are diagnostic from 40% to 90% of the time depending on the type of organism and whether antibiotic treatment has been started.

Cerebrospinal Fluid

An LP is contraindicated in patients who have clinical and/or imaging evidence of incipient cerebral herniation, with localized infection at the lumbar puncture site, severe thrombocytopenia, untreated or bleeding diathesis and those who are taking anticoagulants. CSF bacterial cultures are likely to be useful in adults with bacterial meningitis up to 4 hours after antibiotics are initiated, if LP must be delayed by imaging. The use of serologic tests and PCR may still assist in diagnosis even after antibiotics are initiated.

All LPs performed to evaluate bacterial meningitis should minimally include a CSF opening pressure, CSF cell count and differential, CSF total protein, CSF glucose,

Gram stain, and cultures. Additional testing should be tailored as to availability, cost-effectiveness, and clinical suspicion.

CSF opening pressure is elevated (>180 mm H_2O in adults) in 90% cases of adult acute bacterial meningitis.

CSF cell count: The CSF WBC usually exceeds 1000 cells/mm^3 in untreated, non-immunosuppressed adult patients. Ninety percent (90%) of cases will have a polymorphonuclear (PMN) cell predominance at presentation, which will shift to lymphocytic predominance with treatment. In a few patients, primarily those who are immunosuppressed, the CSF WBC count will be normal, and this is associated with a poor outcome.

CSF glucose: The CSF glucose level is usually low in untreated acute bacterial meningitis. A more reliable measure is a CSF/concurrent plasma glucose ratio of 0.4 or less.

CSF total protein: Over 90% of cases of acute bacterial meningitis will have an elevated (>50 mg/dL, average >200 mg/dL) CSF protein at presentation.

CSF Gram stain: The sensitivity of the CSF Gram stain is 70% in uncentrifuged CSF and 90% in ultracentrifuged CSF sediment. Specificity approaches 100%.

CSF bacterial culture: Bacterial culture ranges from 70% to 90% sensitivity in untreated patients; however, this varies according to the individual organism, and local collection and laboratory practices.

CSF PCR: In one research study of bacterial meningitis caused by the common pathogens *S. pneumoniae, N. meningitidis,* and *H. influenzae,* CSF real-time PCR demonstrated a sensitivity of 95% versus 81% for bacterial culture. PCR was also less likely to be influenced by previous antibiotic exposure. However, PCR was not more sensitive than gram stain in this study.

CSF latex agglutination antigen testing: This test is available for several common causes of acute bacterial meningitis such as *H. influenzae* type B, *S. pneumoniae, Neisseria meningitidis,* group B *Streptococcus,* and *Streptococcus agalactiae.* The sensitivity of this test tends to be poor except for *H. influenzae,* and it does not exceed the sensitivity of the Gram stain in antibiotic-treated patients. Not routinely recommended for routine use.

CSF lactate: Elevated levels of lactate (>3. 5 mmol/L) are indicative of bacterial or fungal meningitis. However, these results may be confounded by seizures, hypoxia, or antibiotic use.

Serum procalcitonin levels can be elevated (>2 ng/mL) in bacterial meningitis compared with viral meningitis and will decline with successful antibiotic treatment. However, this test cannot exclude a meningitis diagnosis.

Treatment

All patients with suspected meningococcemia should be placed in respiratory isolation until meningococcus is ruled out. Those in contact with patients with *N. meningitides* should have prophylaxis with rifampin 600 mg PO bid × 2 days.

Presumptive empiric therapy is begun and then tailored to the specific agent once cultures and sensitivity return from laboratory. Delay in initiation of antibiotics, especially when over 6 hours, is associated with higher morbidity and mortality. Treatment should be initiated immediately after diagnostic specimen collection and if LP is to be delayed to obtain a CT, antibiotics should be administered first. Tables 23.1, 23.2,

Table 23.1 Commonly encountered bacterial pathogens by Risk Group

Group	Pathogen	Treatment
Neonate	Group B *Streptococcus*	Cefotaxime and ampicillin
	L. monocytogenes	
	S. pneumoniae	
Adult or child	*S. pneumoniae*	Ceftriaxone and vancomycin
	N. meningitides	
	L. monocytogenes	
	H. influenzae	
Immunocompromised	*S. pneumoniae*	Cephalosporin, vancomycin, and
	L. monocytogenes	ampicillin
	Gram-negative aerobes	

Table 23.2 Standard Dosages for commonly used Antibiotics in Meningitis

	Antibiotic/Dosing*	
	Adult	*Child (not infant)*
Ampicillin	2 g every 4 hours	400 mg/kg divided every 6 hours
Ceftriaxone	2 g every 12 hours	80–100 mg/kg divided every 12 hours
Vancomycin	30 to 45 mg/kg divided every 12 hours	60 mg/kg divided every 6 to 8 hours
Gentamycin	5 mg/kg divided every 8 hours	7.5 mg/kg divided every 8 hours

*Please note dosages are general guidelines that must be tailored to specific patient populations including age, weight, renal function. Divided doses mean total dose divided over a 24 hour period.

and 23.3 list the common agents by age group, treatment, and antibiotic doses for the respective bacterium.

Adjunctive Therapy

Corticosteroids are now recommended for the treatment of bacterial meningitis in industrialized countries to reduce rates of mortality, severe hearing loss, and neurological sequelae.

Dexamethasone 10 mg IV before first dose of antibiotics and every 6 hours for 4 days

Table 23.3 Duration of antibiotic usage in specific pathogens

Pathogen	Treatment Duration (minimum)
S. pneumoniae	10 days
N. meningitidis	7 days
H. influenzae	7 days
Gram-negative bacilli	21 days
L. monocytogenes	21 days

Duration of treatment varies according to pathogen. LP should be repeated to assess response.

ATYPICAL BACTERIAL MENINGITIDES

Tuberculous Meningitis (Mycobacterium Tuberculosis)

Distribution: worldwide

Presentation: Tuberculosis (TB) meningitis occurs in 7% to 12% of patients with untreated extrapulmonary TB. TB meningitis is more common and has a higher mortality in the developing world and in children, the elderly, and those with HIV infection. Mortality is high (20% to 50%) even with treatment and is the risk of neurologic sequelae is up to 30%.

Presentation: The clinical presentation is highly variable and may include a prodrome of weight loss and cough, fever, headaches, or anorexia. When compared with patients with bacterial meningitis, patients with TB meningitis are more likely to be symptomatic for a longer period of time (>5 days). Advanced cases frequently have nuchal rigidity and altered mental status. Cranial neuropathies occur in up to 30% of patients and are associated with poor outcome. Stroke occurs in up to 60% of patients.

Neuroimaging: MRI is preferable to CT in evaluating TB meningitis. While neuroimaging is not diagnostic, patients with TB meningitis are more likely to show hydrocephalus, basal meningeal enhancement, infarction, or tuberculoma (abscess) than patients with bacterial meningitis.

Diagnosis

Chest radiography: Up to 30% of patients may have no evidence of TB on routine chest radiography.

Mantoux or PPD (purified protein derivative) skin tests: These tests assess exposure to Mycobacterium tuberculosis. However, up to 20% of patients with TB may have a negative PPD. Patients may be anergic if they are HIV infected, take immunosuppressive drugs, are malnourished, or have advanced disseminated tuberculosis.

Interferon-gamma release assays (IGRA): These are blood tests are useful in the diagnosis of tuberculosis and are particularly useful in detecting infection in patients who have been previously vaccinated with bacilli Calmette-Guerin vaccination (BCG) and have a positive PPD on that basis. They are both more specific and more sensitive than the PPD. The QuantiFERON®-TB gold test measures how much interferon-gamma is released by the patient's T cells in response to three tuberculosis antigens, and is available within a few days.

CSF: When conmpared with patients with acute bacterial meningitis, patients with tuberculous meningitis are more likely to have a CSF WBC under 1000 cells/mm^3, to have over 30% lymphocytes in CSF, and to have a CSF total protein of over 100 mg/dL. However, HIV-infected patients may have less inflammation in their CSF.

A definitive diagnosis of tuberculous meningitis requires demonstration of MTB in CSF by acid-fast bacteria (AFB) smear (Ziehl-Neelsen staining) or culture.

CSF Profile

Cell count: elevated WBCs often mixed lymphocytic, monocytes
Protein: usually very elevated
Glucose: usually low to very low
AFB smears: 5% to 30% sensitivity
AFB culture: 45% to 90% sensitivity
CSF MTB PCR: 30% to 50% sensitive/98% specific

Treatment

Initially, treatment is a four-drug therapy followed by two-drug therapy, usually for 1 year of treatment.

Rifampin 5 mg/kg/day, maximum 300 mg†
Isoniazid 10 mg/kg/day, maximum 600 mg; give vitamin B6 (pyridoxine) in conjunction
Pyrazinamide 25 mg/kg/day*
Ethambutol or streptomycin 15 mg/kg/day*
*May require adjustment in renal insufficiency/failure.
†Interacts with HIV medications; will need to consider rifabutin.

According to a Cochrane Review, corticosteroids (dexamethasone or prednisolone) reduce the risk for death and severe neurological sequelae in HIV-negative persons with tuberculous meningitis. Inadequate information was available to make a recommendation in HIV-infected persons.

Spirochete Meningitis

Syphilitic Meningitis (*Treponema pallidum*)

Distribution: worldwide.

Presentation: Syphilitic meningitis can occur at any stage but often seen in secondary syphilis. Patients can have significant headaches, sometimes a low-grade fever, and cranial nerve involvement can be seen. Patients may have signs of secondary syphilis such as diffuse rash and may have a history of painless genital ulcer.

Imaging: Contrast-enhanced CT or MRI scans can show diffuse meningeal enhancement.

Diagnosis

Diagnostic suspicion begins with a serum nonspecific and specific treponemal tests (i.e., RPR [rapid plasmin reagin] or VDRL [venereal disease research lab]) followed by confirmation of infection with TPPA (treponemal pallidum particle agglutination assay) or FTA-ABS (fluorescent treponemal antibody-absorption). Once a serum etiology is established, LP should be completed to ascertain nervous system involvement. A definite diagnosis can be made with a reactive CSF VDRL test; however, a presumptive diagnosis is often made with reactive serum tests and an abnormal CSF profile.

CSF Profile

Cell count: elevated WBCs, usually lymphocytic

Protein: elevated

Glucose: normal

CSF VDRL if positive confirms diagnosis but sensitivity is low (10% to 70%)

CSF FTA-ABS: This is helpful if negative in CSF, making a diagnosis of neurosyphilis unlikely.

Treatment

Aqueous penicillin G 18 to 24 million units divided every 4 hours × 10 to 14 days

Or

Procaine penicillin 2.4 million units with probenecid 500 mg every 4 hours × 10 to 14 days

Follow-up: Patient should repeat CSF studies at 6 months to determine cleared cell count and at 2 years to confirm normalization of VDRL.

Neuroborreliosis, NeuroLyme (*Borrelia burgdorferi,* *B. garinii, B afzelii*)

Distribution is North America, Europe, and Central Asia.

Presentation: Patients with *Borrelia* meningitis may have fever, headaches, cranial nerve palsies (especially facial nerve palsy), and (particularly in Europe) painful radiculitis (Garin-Bujadow-Gannwarth syndrome). A history of characteristic rash, erythema chronica migrans, and tick bite are helpful clinical clues in establishing a diagnosis.

Imaging: MRI may demonstrate cranial nerve or radicular enhancement.

Diagnosis: A diagnosis of neuroborreliosis should be made on the basis of clinical, serological, and CSF findings.

Serum tests: Lyme's titer can be supportive of the diagnosis.

CSF Profile

Cell count: elevated WBCs, often lymphocytic but can be normal

Protein: normal or elevated

Glucose: normal or slightly depressed

CSF Lyme PCR: low sensitivity

CSF culture: difficult, require special media, long culture duration

CSF: CSF Lyme specific antibody concentration greater than 1.0 to serum Lyme titer

Treatment

There are various treatment strategies for the treatment of neuroborreliosis and several are mentioned here:

Ceftriaxone 2 g/d IV; children 50 mg/kg to 75 mg/kg IV every day

Penicillin G 3 to 4 million units every 4 hours IV; pediatric 200,000 to 400,000 units/ kg/day every 4 hours

Doxycycline 100 mg PO bid; pediatric 4 mg/kg/day bid (if >8 years of age)

SUGGESTED READING

Thigpen, M. C., Whitney, C. G., Messonnier, N. E., Zell, E. R., Lynfield, R., Hadler, J. L., et al. (2011). Bacterial meningitis in the United States, 1998–2007. *N Engl J Med.* *364*(21), 2016–2025.

Hasbun, R., Abrahams, J., Jekel, J., Quagliarello, V. J. (2001). Computed tomography of the head before lumbar puncture in adults with suspected meningitis. *N Engl J Med.* *345*(24), 1727–1733.

Brouwer, M. C., Tunkel, A. R., van de Beek, D. (2010). Epidemiology, diagnosis, and antimicrobial treatment of acute bacterial meningitis. *Clin Microbiol Rev.* *23*(3), 467–492. PMCID: PMC2901656.

Tunkel, A. R., Hartman, B. J., Kaplan, S. L., Kaufman, B. A., Roos, K. L., Scheld, W. M., et al. (2004). Practice guidelines for the management of bacterial meningitis. *Clin Infect Dis.* *39*(9), 1267–1284.

van de Beek, D., de Gans, J., McIntyre, P., Prasad, K. (2007). Corticosteroids for acute bacterial meningitis. *Cochrane Database Syst Rev.* *1*, CD004405.

24 Viral and Fungal Meningitis

Miguel Valdes-Sueiras and Elyse J. Singer

INTRODUCTION

In this section, nonbacterial causes of meningitis will be reviewed. Some nonbacterial causes include viruses and fungi.

VIRAL MENINGITIS

Presentation

Viral meningitis is the most common manifestation of viral central nervous system (CNS) infections, which can include meningitis, encephalitis, myelitis, and aspects of all three. Viral meningitis is more common than bacterial meningitis and typically has similar but less severe symptoms (such as headache, fever, meningismus, and altered mental status) and less morbidity and mortality. Patients may have associated upper respiratory infection, gastrointestinal illness, or a flu-like illness.

In the immunocompetent host, Enteroviruses are the most common cause of viral meningitis. The Enteroviruses include polio (now much diminished due to vaccination), enterovirus 71 (associated with "hand, foot, and mouth" disease), coxsackieviruses, and echoviruses. These enteric viruses are often spread via contaminated water and replicate in the gut, causing gastrointestinal symptoms and release of infectious virus in the stool.

Other causes of viral meningitis that should be considered given available treatment include some of the herpesviruses and HIV. There are many other viruses that can cause meningitis but no specific treatment is available. These viruses include adenovirus, arboviruses, paramyxoviruses, and togaviruses, to name a few.

Imaging

Imaging criteria are the same as for bacterial meningitis. Findings in viral meningitis are usually not specific but may show contrast enhancement on magnetic resonance imaging (MRI) and computed tomography (CT) scanning.

Diagnosis

Enterovirus 71 usually causes viral meningitis but may also cause brainstem encephalitis or severe flaccid paralysis (to be discussed in the section on encephalitis).

Enterovirus 71 can be detected with polymerase chain reaction (PCR) from cerebrospinal fluid (CSF), blood, or swabs of vesicular lesions. PCR is more sensitive than viral culture for enteroviruses.

CSF analysis is the mainstay of diagnosis. In addition to evaluating for viral etiologies, the CSF should be used to rule out other processes that can mimic viral meningitis such as bacterial, fungal, and atypical bacterial infections.

Serum screening for HIV, syphilis, and Lyme disease should be considered in every case of viral meningitis.

CSF Profile

Cell count: usually lymphocytic white blood cells (WBCs), although very early on can have polymorphonucleocytes (PMNs)
Glucose: usually normal
Protein: elevated
Viral cultures: low yield
CSF PCRs: herpes simplex virus (HSV), varicella zoster virus (VZV), enterovirus
CSF antibodies: VZV antibodies

Treatment

The treatment of viral meningitis is mostly supportive with the exception of HSV and VZV, in which case acyclovir is used.

HSV or VZV meningitis: acyclovir 10 mg/kg every 8 hours

FUNGAL MENINGITIDES

Fungal meningitides are encountered frequently in clinical practice, especially given the increased use of immunosuppressive therapy in organ transplantation as well as the immunosuppression from HIV infection.

Cryptococcal Meningitis (*Cryptococcus neoformans, C. gatii*)

Distribution is worldwide.

Presentation

Patients with cryptococcal meningitis usually present with headaches and fever, sometimes with altered mental status and cranial nerve palsies. Meningismus is uncommon. Rarely, blindness can occur. Some patients may have cutaneous manifestation of cryptococcosis or pulmonary involvement.

Patients with immunosuppression, whether it is from HIV infection, chemotherapy, or immunosuppression therapy, have increased susceptibility.

Imaging

CT or MRI result scan vary from that are normal, to showing diffuse enhancement, or sometimes showing enhancement in Virchow-Robin spaces, the last can be almost pathognomic of cryptococcal infection.

Diagnosis

CSF analysis is paramount in the diagnosis of cryptococcal meningitis, but a clear clinical picture with reactive serum tests can be highly suggestive.

Serum cryptococcal antigen 90% to 95% sensitivity

CSF Profile

Cell count: elevated WBCs but can be normal, especially in immunosuppressed patients
Glucose: low or normal
Protein: elevated, less often normal
India ink: about 50% positive in immunosuppressed, 75% sensitive in immunocompetent
CSF Cryptococcal Antigen (CrAG): elevated titer
CSF fungal culture: 90% sensitive

Treatment and Management

AmphotericinB (0.7 mg/kg/day) with flucytosine (100mg/kg/day) induction followed
 by fluconazole

If elevated pressure on lumbar puncture, patient will need serial lumbar punctures until CSF pressures normalize.

Patients with HIV infection will need long-term suppressive therapy until immune reconstitution occurs, usually defined as two consecutive T-cell/CD4 counts of 200 or greater separated by a 6-month interval.

Neurococcidiodmycosis (*Coccidiodes immitis*)

Distribution is the southwestern United States (California/Arizona) and South America.

Presentation

Patients with neurococcidiodmycosis (cocci) can present with headaches, fevers, altered mental status, and neurological deficits, particularly radiculitis. Patients may have concomitant pulmonary disease and/or be immunosuppressed.

Imaging

CT and MRI with contrast are often abnormal and can show diffuse enhancement, hydrocephalus, and even vasculitis and infarction. Nerve root enhancement can be seen when radicular involvement occurs.

Diagnosis

This often requires various approaches including serologies in blood along with CSF analysis in either immunocompromised patients or patients from endemic areas.

Serum: cocci titers

If there is pulmonary involvement, sputum culture should be sought.

CSF Profile

Cell count: elevated WBCs (can have eosinophils)
Glucose: normal to low glucose
Protein: elevated
Cocci antibody titers: 70% to 90% sensitivity
Fungal cultures: low yield about 15% sensitivity

Treatment

Fluconazole 400 to 800 mg daily followed by chronic suppressive therapy of 200 to 400 mg day

Histoplasmosis (*Histoplasma capsulatum*)

Distribution is the central United States and Central America.

Presentation

Patients with *Histoplasma* meningitis may present with headaches, fevers, altered mental status, and cranial neuropathies. It is usually seen in association with HIV infection and is an AIDS-defining illness. Patients may have concomitant pulmonary disease and/or skin manifestations.

Imaging

CT and MRI scans may show meningeal enhancement and/or hydrocephalus.

Diagnosis

This often requires various approaches including serologies in blood and urine along with CSF analysis.

Serum: histoplasmosis antigen or positive culture
Urine: *Histoplasma* antigen 60% sensitivity

CSF Profile

Cell count: elevated WBCs, lymphocytic
Protein: elevated

Glucose: normal to low
CSF cultures: about 50% sensitive
CSF *Histoplasma* antigen up to 50% to 80% sensitive
CSF *Histoplasma* antibody 60% to 80% sensitive

Treatment

Liposomal amphotericin B 5 mg/kg/day for 4 to 6 weeks followed by itraconazole 200 mg 2 or 3 times per day for 1 year

Blastomycosis (*Blastomycosis dermatidis*)

Distribution is the southern United States.

Presentation

Patients with CNS blastomycosis often present with altered mentation and less often with fevers, headaches, or meningismus; up to 60% of patients can have cutaneous or pulmonary manifestations.

Imaging

MRI and CT scan may show meningeal enhancement.

Diagnosis

This often requires various approaches including serologies in urine along with CSF analysis.

Urine *B. dermatidis* antigen: greater than 90% sensitivity

CSF Profile

Cell count: early PMNs, followed by lymphocytosis
Glucose: low
Protein: elevated
CSF *B. dermatidis* antigen can be sent with variable sensitivity reported.
CSF *B. dermatidis* antibody can be sent with variable sensitivity reported.
CSF culture can be positive in 40–65% of cases, usually about 1 week for growth

Treatment

Liposomal amphotericinB 5 mg/kg for 4 to 6 weeks followed by fluconazole 800 mg PO every day; or itraconazole 200 mg 2 or 3 times per day; or voriconazole 200 mg 2 or 3 times per day; all for at least 1 year

Aspergillosis (*A. fumigatus, A. flavus, A. niger*)

Distribution is worldwide.

Presentation

Patients with CNS Aspergillosis meningitis can headaches, fevers, focal neurological deficits, altered mentation. Patients are often immunosuppressed or may have had surgical procedures.

Imaging

CT or MRI may show solitary mass lesion, multiple abscesses, cavernous sinus thrombosis, basilar meningitis, vasculitis with possible hemorrhages or infarction, and myelitis.

Diagnosis

Overall, establishing a diagnosis with aspergillosis is difficult. This often requires various approaches including antigen testing, imaging, and cultures from various sites along with CSF analysis.

Chest radiograph or chest CT: may see abnormalities; halo sign in 40% to 60% but evanescent

Bronchial alveolar lavage (BAL) culture: 50% for pulmonary lesions

Serum galactomannan ELISA: about 80% sensitivity, 89% specificity in diagnosis

CSF Profile

Cell count: early PMNs followed by lymphocytosis

Glucose: low

Protein: elevated

CSF PCRs: limited study and availability

CSF culture: low yield

CSF galactomannan has been obtained in patients with CNS aspergillosis.

Treatment

Voriconazole 6 mg/kg IV every 12 hours for 2 doses followed by 4 mg/kg IV every 12 hours with possible benefit to adding caspofungin

Candida (*Candida albicans*)

Distribution is worldwide.

Presentation

Patients with *Candida* meningitis can present with headaches, fever, stiff neck, and altered mental status over days to weeks, sometimes acute. It is often seen in association with immunosuppression, especially neutropenia.

Imaging

CT or MRI can show meningeal enhancement, multiple enhancing abscesses or granuloma, rare hydrocephalus and infarcts.

Diagnosis

This often requires various investigative approaches, especially blood and urine cultures.

CSF Profile

Cell count: elevated PMNs evolving to lymphocytic predominance; may be mildly elevated
Protein: mildly elevated
Protein: often reduced
CSF gram stain: up to 40% of smears reported positive
CSF culture may yield candida species.

Treatment

Liposomal amphotericinB 3 to 5 mg/kg daily and 5-flucytosine for several weeks followed by fluconazole 400 to 800 mg daily until clinical, radiological, and cerebrospinal resolution

Zygomycosis (*Especially Mucormycosis*)

Distribution is worldwide.

Presentation

This is often seen in diabetics and often begins as sinusitis or pneumonia, with contiguous spread through the sinuses to the brain. Patients can have facial pain, ophthalmoplegia, proptosis, and blindness. An eschar may be visualized on inspection of the nose.

Imaging

CT or MRI can demonstrate area of contiguous spread of infection.

Diagnosis

This is usually only made with biopsy and stain with culture.

CSF Profile

CSF is rarely obtained due to direct nature of infection and spread.

Treatment

Surgical debridement and IV amphotericinB, preferably liposomal; second-line posaconazole; adjunctive hyperbaric oxygen may be considered

Penicillium marnefeii

Distribution is southeast Asia.

Presentation

Often seen in patients with AIDS, patients can present with altered mentation, fever, confusion, agitation, and skin lesions similar to molluscum.

Imaging

Reports of imaging findings are sparse but have ranged from normal to diffuse edema, with at least one case report of ring-enhancing lesion.

Diagnosis

This is important to consider in endemic areas. Blood cultures are 75% sensitive in systemic disease.

CSF Profile

Cell count: may be acellular to mildly WBCs
Protein: may be normal to mildly elevated
Glucose: may be normal to mildly decreased
CSF culture: sensitivity not available but there are case reports of isolation of penicillium.

Treatment

AmphotericinB has been suggested in case reports.

Brancusi, F., Farrar, J., Heemskerk, D. (2012). Tuberculous meningitis in adults: a review of a decade of developments focusing on prognostic factors for outcome. *Future Microbiol.* 7(9), 1101–1116.

Fishman, R. (1992). *Cerebrospinal Fluid in Diseases of the Nervous System*, 2nd edition. WB Saunders company.

Halperin, J. (2010). A Tale of Two Spirochetes: Lyme Disease and Syphilis. *Neurologic Clinics* 28(1), 277–291.

Rauchway, A., Husain, S., Selhorst, J. (2010). Neurologic Presentations of Fungal Infections *Neurologic Clinics* 28(1), 293–309.

Sheld, W., Whitley, R., Marra, C. (2004). *Infections of the Central Nervous System*, 3rd edition. Lippincott Williams & Wilkins.

25 Infectious Encephalitis and Myelitis

Miguel Valdes-Sueiras and Elyse J. Singer

INTRODUCTION

Encephalitis is inflammation within the brain parenchyma, in contrast to inflammation of the meninges. Infectious etiologies are most often viral, but occasionally other microbes can be involved, including atypical bacteria and parasites. Not all infections result in inflammation, and infectious agents can cause an encephalopathy and myelopathy that will be included in this section.

VIRAL ENCEPHALITIS AND MYELITIS

Numerous viruses can cause encephalitis and myelitis, yet very few have treatment. It can be difficult to distinguish between meningitis and encephalitis and sometimes both occur. Clinical practice usually requires empiric coverage for both processes until ancillary data lead to a definitive diagnosis.

HERPESVIRUSES

Herpes Simplex Encephalitis (Herpes Simplex 1, Less Commonly Herpes Simplex 2)

Distribution is worldwide.

Epidemiology

Herpes simplex virus (HSV) is the most common cause of acute, sporadic encephalitis. It has no animal reservoir and is transmitted by human-to-human contact. It may occur after a primary herpes infection or after reactivation of a latent infection, presumably from the trigeminal ganglion or olfactory bulb. HSV1 is more common in adults and teenagers, whereas HSV2 occurs primarily in neonates.

Presentation

HSV encephalitis can present with headaches, fever, photophobia, altered mental status, cognitive impairment, psychiatric symptoms, focal neurologic signs, seizures, or any combination of these. The course of disease may be slower in those who are immunosuppressed. If untreated, the mortality rate approaches 70%. Survivors almost uniformly have significant neurological sequelae.

Imaging

HSV causes extensive cortical edema, hemorrhage, and necrosis. It particularly targets the inferior and medial temporal lobes, followed by the frontal and parietal regions. A contrast-enhanced magnetic resonance imaging (MRI) study is preferable to computed tomography (CT) scanning in demonstrating the lesions of HSV infection (Figure 25.1).

Diagnosis

CSF: There are usually abnormalities but 10% of cases may be normal in early disease.

CSF WBC count: this is usually elevated, averaging about 100 cells; lymphocytes predominate. Red blood cells can be seen in a nontraumatic lumbar puncture (LP) but are not diagnostic of HSV.

CSF protein: usually elevated

CSF glucose: usually normal

CSF HSV PCR: This is the diagnostic method of choice, with sensitivity of 94% and specificity of 98%.

Electroencephalography (EEG): Focal changes in the EEG such as spike and slow wave activity or periodic lateralized epileptic discharges (PLEDs) arising from the temporal lobes may occur but are not specific for HSV.

Brain Biopsy

This was the gold standard for diagnosis prior to the development of PCR. The tissue shows intranuclear and intracytoplasmic inclusion bodies that contain viral antigen.

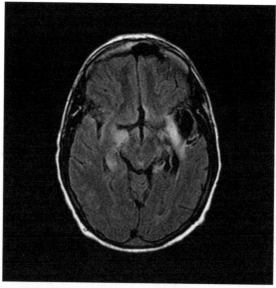

FIGURE 25.1
MRI brain FLAIR hyperintensity in a patient with recurrent HSV encephalitis.

Treatment

HSV encephalitis is a treatable disease, and delay in therapy may worsen prognosis. For that reason empiric treatment with acyclovir should be considered even in cases where the pathogenic etiology of encephalitis is uncertain. The recommended therapy is acyclovir 10 mg/kg IV every 8 hours for 14 to 21 days. Currently, there is insufficient evidence to support a role for corticosteroids in HSV management.

Varicella Zoster Encephalitis

Distribution is worldwide.

Presentation

Classically, patients will have associated trigeminal zoster, headaches, fevers, occasionally vision and hearing involvement, and facial nerve palsy. A higher incidence of varicella zoster is found in immunosuppressed patients, diabetics, and older age.

Imaging

MRI or CT with contrast may show stroke, contrast enhancement, and white matter T2 hyperintensity.

Diagnosis

This can be made with a clear clinical picture and appropriate CSF analysis.

CSF Profile

Cell count: elevated WBCs, lymphocytic predominance
Glucose: usually normal
Protein: usually elevated
CSF PCR: VZV variable sensitivity
CSF antibodies: IgG or IgM VZV should be sought as VZV PCR can be negative

Treatment

Acyclovir 10 mg/kg every 8 hours for at least 2 weeks

Cytomegalovirus Encephalitis

Distribution is worldwide but most often in immunocompromised people.

Presentation

Usually, cytomegalovirus (CMV) encephalitis occurs in the setting of concomitant immune suppression such HIV infection or immunosuppressive therapy. Patients will present with altered mentation, sometimes cranial nerve abnormalities, less often seizures; patients usually have evidence of CMV infection elsewhere such as the eyes (retinitis) or gastrointestinal tract (colitis).

Imaging

MRI and CT may be normal, be nonspecific, or classically will demonstrate a ventriculitis.

Diagnosis

CSF is the gold standard for diagnosis but should be highly considered in patients with immune suppression and evidence of CMV in another organ system such as CVM retinitis.

CSF Profile

Cell count: can have early PMN WBCs followed by lymphocytic WBCs
Glucose can have low glucose
Protein: elevated
CSF PCR for CMV greater than 70% sensitivity

Treatment

Ganciclovir 5 mg/kg bid $\times$ 2 to 3 weeks
Foscarnet 60 mg/kg every 8 hours $\times$ 2 to 3 weeks

Therapy should continue thereafter with maintenance valganciclovr until patient stabilizes, immune system improves, and in the setting of HIV at least greater than CD4/T-cell count of 100.

Herpesviruses: Human Herpesviruses 6 and 7, Epstein-Barr Virus

Distribution is worldwide.

Presentation

Uncommon infections, usually found in immunosuppressed adults or children. Patients can present with altered mental status, fever, and seizures. In EBV-related encephalitis, patients may have preceding sore throat and lymphadenopathy. Children can present with metamorphopsia (Alice in Wonderland syndrome).

Imaging

Although data are sparse, MRI scans demonstrating mesial temporal lobe hyperintensity have been reported in HHV-6. MRI scans demonstrating demyelination have been reported for EBV infection of the brain.

Diagnosis

CSF analysis is the gold standard for diagnosis.

Serum: Heterophile antibody test can be suggestive of EBV infection. EBV antibody serologies can also assist in diagnosis of EBV infection.

CSF Profile

Cell count: elevated WBCs, usually lymphocytic

Protein: normal to low

Glucose: normal

CSF PCRs: qualitative PCRs should be sought if available; however a quantitative PCR for EBV is suggested when available especially in immune suppression to distinguish benign EBViremia

Treatment

HHV-6: Ganciclovir has been used but is not approved for this use.

EBV: Ganciclovir has been used by various authors but is not approved for this use.

RETROVIRUSES

HIV1 and HIV2

Distribution is worldwide.

Epidemiology

HIV-associated neurological syndromes can be classified as primary HIV neurological disease (in which HIV is both necessary and sufficient to cause the illness), secondary or opportunistic neurological disease (in which HIV interacts with other pathogens, resulting in opportunistic infections and tumors), and treatment-related neurological disease.

HIV-Associated Viral Meningitis or Meningoencephalitis

Presentation

This syndrome can occur during primary infection (seroconversion) or anytime thereafter. It may also be a symptom of viral rebound when a patient stops cART (combined antitretroviral therapy).

It is indistinguishable from other viral meningitides. In one series, the average CD4$^+$ cell count was in the 400+ range.

Imaging

Normally, imaging is nonspecific but may show meningeal enhancement.

Diagnosis

Serum antibody testing is necessary, although it may be negative at seroconversion. If suspected, serum HIV viral load can be helpful

CSF Profile

CSF analysis is used mostly to rule out any opportunistic infection.

Cell count: elevated WBCs, lymphocytic
Protein: usually mild elevation
Glucose: normal.

Treatment

Data are limited to case reports, but most cases require supportive care. Case reports have suggested that the symptoms of HIV meningitis usually respond to cART, preferably a regimen composed of drugs with good central nervous system penetration, but there are no controlled studies.

HIV-Associated Neurocognitive Disorders

Presentation

It is now accepted that chronic HIV-1 infection can result in neurodegenerative brain disease clinically manifested by gradually progressive neurocognitive impairments. The severity of HIV brain disease, now renamed HIV-associated neurocognitive disorder (HAND), is recognized to range from an asymptomatic neurocognitive impairment (ANI), to a mild neurocognitive disorder (MND), to a full-blown HIV-associated dementia. Nonetheless, even milder forms of neurocognitive impairment may be associated with problems such as medication adherence. As the HIV-infected population ages, these impairments must be distinguished from common age-associated neurodegenerative diseases.

HIV neurocognitive deficits may be subclinical (apparent only after careful neuropsychological testing) or present with decreased attention/concentration, psychomotor speed, reduced short-term memory, learning, information processing, and executive function. Central motor abnormalities, including slowing of movements, incoordination, and tremor, can also be seen but these are not invariable findings in early disease. Patients with advanced HIV may still progress to develop disabling upper-motor type weakness, spasticity, or extrapyramidal movement disorders. Bilateral paraparesis, when it occurs, is often due to a concurrent HIV-associated myelopathy. Behavioral effects such as apathy, irritability, and psychomotor retardation (associated with damage to the frontostriatal systems) are relatively common in HAND. A new-onset psychosis that is associated with advanced HIV and cognitive impairment has been reported but has become relatively rare in cART-treated patients.

Imaging

Most HAND patients have a grossly normal brain MRI or CT scan, or have varying degrees of central and global atrophy, or periventricular white matter disease, but these findings are not specific for HAND. Research neuroimaging studies such as MR spectroscopy (MRS) and diffusion tensor imaging (DTI) are more sensitive to the changes associated with HAND but are not available outside academic centers (Figure 25.2).

Diagnosis

Similar to HIV meningitis, CSF analysis should be done to rule out any opportunistic or neoplastic process. Serum tests to evaluate for syphilis and b12 should be checked.

CSF Profile

Cell count: mildly elevated, if greater than 20 WBCs other etiology should be sought
Protein: mildly elevated
Glucose: normal

CSF PCRs and cultures should be sent to rule out other causes such as CMV, EBV, cryptococcal infection, syphilis.

Treatment

cART should be initiated in all patients with confirmed HANDs regardless of CD4$^+$ count.

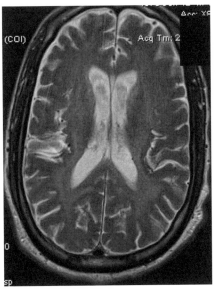

FIGURE 25.2
MRI brain T2 in patient with HAND.

HIV-Associated Myelopathy

Presentation

Vacuolar myelopathy is the most common spinal cord disease in AIDS, found in up to 30% of autopsies in the pre-cART era.

Clinical symptoms include lower extremity weakness, which may initially be asymmetric, ataxia, spasticity, paresthesias (often painful). and. in advanced stages, incontinence.

Neuroimaging

CT is not helpful for the diagnosis but does help in evaluating for tuberculosis of the spine. MRI of spine can occasionally show matter changes.

Diagnosis

In a patient with HIV infection and spinal cord disease, it is often a diagnosis of exclusion. CSF should be analyzed for evidence of opportunistic infection. Serum tests for B12 deficiency and syphilis should be checked.

CSF Profile

Cell count: normal to mildly elevated lymphocytes; if above 20 suspicion for another etiology should sought
Protein: mildly elevated
Glucose: normal

CSF PCRs and cultures should be sent to rule out other causes such as CMV, EBV, cryptococcal infection, and syphilis.

Human T-Lymphotrophic Virus Type 1 (HTLV-1)

Distribution is worldwide but endemic in Japan and the Americas.

Presentation

Those who are symptomatic from HTLV-1 can develop a slowly progressive myelopathy, with rare brain involvement.

Imaging

MRI of the spine may be normal or white matter changes have been reported.

Diagnosis

Serum HTLV-1 positive.

CSF Profile

Cell count: mild to moderate elevation
Protein: mild elevation
Glucose: normal

CSF HTLV-1 antibody.

Treatment

Supportive. Various authors have used interferons and glucocorticorticoids with variable success.

PAPOVAVIRUSES

Progressive Multifocal Leukoencephalopathy (JC virus)

Distribution is worldwide.

Presentation

Usually presents in patients with immune suppression either from HIV infection or immunosuppressive therapy. There have also been notably cases associated with the use of the multiple sclerosis medication natalizumab. Patients present with focal neurological deficits such as vision loss, hemiparesis, ataxia, or dementia-like picture. Patients usually do not have significant headaches or fevers.

Imaging

CT scan can show hypodensity; MRI of the brain will usually show hypointense lesion on T1, hyperintense lesions on T2 and these lesions are usually nonenhancing. However, enhancement can occur in the setting of immune reconstitution syndrome (25.3A, B,).

Diagnosis

CSF analysis is the mainstay of diagnosis.

CSF Profile

Cell count: usually normal or mild elevation of WBCs, lymphocytic
Protein: usually normal or mild elevation
Glucose: normal

CSF JC virus PCR: about 70% sensitivity.

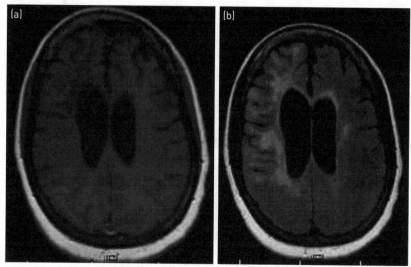

FIGURE 25.3

MRI brain T1 (A) and T2 (B) in a patient with PML.

Treatment

There is no specific treatment in HIV-associated PML but patients should be treated with cART. In patients with natalizumab-related PML, plasmapheresis has been used. Mirtazapine has been reported to have anti–JC virus activity and has been used in the treatment of patients with PML. It is unclear if it is of any benefit.

FLAVIVIRUSES

West Nile Encephalitis

Distribution is Africa, Europe, and North America.

Presentation

Patients with West Nile encephalitis may have headaches, fevers, depressed mentation, and occasionally weakness. The weakness although uncommon can be either a myelitis-type presentation or Guillain-Barre–like picture.

Imaging

CT scan is usually normal. MRI can be abnormal in up to 35% of cases with leptomeningeal enhancement or parenchymal hyperintensity.

Diagnosis

CSF analysis is the gold standard for diagnosis.

CSF Profile

Cell count: Patients can have elevated WBCs, both PMNs and lymphocytic are reported, sometimes acellular

Glucose: normal

Protein: elevated

PCR: WNV pcr in CSF about 50% sensitivity

Antibodies: acute and convalescent antibodies useful or CSF IgM West Nile

Treatment

Treatment is supportive.

Japanese Encephalitis (JE), St. Louis Encephalitis (SLE), Murray Valley (MV), and Powassan and Tick-Borne Encephalitis (TBE)

Distribution is regional distribution for JE (Eastern Asia, India, and Australia), SLE (the Americas), MV (Australia), Powassan (United States, Canada, and Asia), and tick-borne (Russia and Eastern Asia).

Presentation

Patients can have nonspecific encephalitis with headaches, fever, and altered mental status; children more at risk (JE, MV), movement disorder/parkinsonism (JE), urinary symptoms (SLE), and poliomyelitis (JE, TBE).

Imaging

MRI can show high signal in basal ganglia and brainstem. CT scan can be normal.

Diagnosis

Serologies: acute and convalescent antibodies

CSF Profile

Cell count: Patients will have elevated WBCs, lymphocytic predominant.

Protein: elevated or normal

Glucose: normal or low

CSF antibodies and PCR, when available.

Treatment

Treatment is supportive with a possible role for interferon in SLE.

PICORNAVIRUSES

Enterovirus Encephalitis

Distribution is worldwide.

Presentation

Patients with enterovirus-71 infection usually present with meningitis but encephalitis and myelitis can also occur. Patients may have associated hand/foot/mouth disease or herpangina and will often have an antecedent diarrheal illness.

Imaging

CT scan is often normal. MRI with contrast can be normal or abnormalities in brainstem, cerebrum, or hippocampi have been reported.

Diagnosis

CSF analysis is the gold standard for diagnosis.

CSF Profile

Cell count: usually elevated WBCs lymphocytic, sometimes PMNs
Protein: elevated
Glucose: normal

Treatment

Treatment is supportive. Pleconaril is used but is not available in the United States.

Echoviruses, Coxsackieviruses, Polio

Distribution is worldwide, although poliovirus is now mostly in Africa and Asia.

Presentation

Echovirus and coxsackievirus are most often associated with meningitis but can cause encephalitis and myelitis. Patients may present with headache, altered mental status, and seizures. Patients may have rash and herpangina, and most often children and adolescents are affected. Cardiac involvement can occur, especially with coxsackievirus infection. Poliovirus causes a change in mentation, seizures, and myelitis.

Imaging

There are sparse data on imaging with these entities, but there are reports of basal ganglia, brainstem, and spinal cord abnormalities on MRI.

Diagnosis

Stool and throat cultures can be suggestive.

CSF Profile

Cell count: elevated WBC, lymphocytic or PMNs (30%)
Protein: normal to mild elevation
Glucose: normal to mildly decreased

CSF PCRs: 60% to 90% sensitivity; culture 30%.

Treatment

Treatment is supportive.

Rabies

Distribution is worldwide.

Presentation

Patients present with altered mental status and evidence or history of bite.

Imaging

There are a few case reports of imaging. Mostly, MRI can show nonspecific white matter lesions and brainstem hyperintensity.

Diagnosis

A history of bite or contact with bats or raccoons can be highly suggestive.
Saliva: culture and PCR
CSF: antibody and PCR in nonvaccinated individuals

Autopsy identification, Negri bodies.

Treatment

No specific treatment, but reports of survival with prolonged induced coma state with ketamine, midazolam, and phenobarbital
Prevention is key with postbite vaccination.

Lymphocytic Choriomeningitis (LCMV)

Distribution is worldwide.

Presentation

Patients often have had contact with infected mice and feces. Patients will present with altered mental status, headaches, fever, and, rarely, myelitis.

Imaging

Sparse data are available but a CT report was noted to be normal.

CSF Profile

Cell count: elevated WBCs, lymphocytic
Glucose: can have **low** glucose
Protein: elevated

Treatment

Treatment is supportive but there is some evidence for the use of ribavirin.

PARAMYXOVIRUSES

Measles, Mumps, Hendra, and Nipah viruses

Distribution is worldwide (measles, mumps) and India, Southeast Asia, and Australia (nipah/hendra).

Presentation

Other than the headaches, altered mental status, seizures, and fevers, the different viruses can have some additional suggestive clinical clues. They are most commonly seen in unvaccinated individuals (measles, mumps), patients with parotitis or orchitis (mumps), and patients with exanthems (measles).

Nipah virus is associated with abattoir workers. Hendra virus is associated with horse workers.

Imaging

MRI can show abnormalities of gray and white matter.

Diagnosis

Serum: elevated amylase in mumps

CSF Profile

Cell count: elevated WBCs, lymphocytic
Protein: elevated
Glucose: normal

CSF antibodies, PCR when available for suspected virus.

Treatment

No proven treatment but ribavirin has been used in small case reports for measles encephalitis with reduction in duration and severity and in cases of Nipah virus.

SUBSCLEROSING PANENCEPHALITIS

This is a rare, slowly progressive encephalitis usually seen in adolescents or young adults. This occurs in patients with a history of measles. It is characterized by seizures, altered mental status, myoclonus, and, ultimately, death. Diagnosis relies on clinical syndrome, elevated CSF measles antibodies, and suggestive EEG with high-voltage, repetitive, periodic sharp and slow wave complexes. These patients can be treated with interferon and ribavirin combination if the disease is diagnosed early enough.

TOGAVIRUSES

Rubella, Eastern Equine, Western Equine, and Venezuelan Equine Encephalitis

Distribution for rubella is worldwide; that for Eastern, Western, and Venezuelan is in the Americas.

Presentation

Rubella (rash, unvaccinated individuals) followed by altered mental status, headaches, seizures, and neurological deficits. Equine encephalitides have variable severity with Eastern Equine being most severe with altered mental status, headaches, seizures, coma, and death.

Imaging

There is sparse reporting of imaging in equine encephalitides, but MRI results with white matter disease, basal ganglia involvement, and diffuse edema as well as normal scans have been reported.

Diagnosis

Diagnosis especially relies on serologies in both serum and CSF, during the acute and convalescent phases of infection.

CSF Profile

Cell count: elevated WBCs lymphocytic; can be very high in Eastern Equine encephalitis
Protein: elevated
Glucose: usually normal

CSF antibodies IgM for respective microbe.

Treatment

Treatment is supportive.

ORTHOMYXOVIRUS

Influenza Virus

Distribution is worldwide.

Presentation

Patients will present with altered mental status, headaches, fevers, and seizures usually in association with respiratory tract infection. Most commonly affected are children.

Imaging

MRI scans have shown thalamic hyperintensity, diffuse edema, necrotizing encephalopathy, and PRES (posterior reversible encephalopathy syndrome).

Diagnosis

Respiratory isolate PCR
Viral culture

CSF Profile

Cell count: can have elevated WBCs, lymphocytic
Protein: elevated
Glucose: normal

CSF PCR low yield.

Treatment

Oseltamivir can be considered.

BUNYAVIRUSES

LaCrosse, California Encephalitis Virus

Distribution is North America.

Presentation

Patients can often have subclinical infection but can cause altered mental status, headaches, seizures, and paralysis; usually children are at higher risk. Patients can have a significant peripheral leukocytosis.

Imaging

Few reports are available regarding imaging, but there are various reports of normal CT brain scans or scans demonstrating focal or diffuse edema.

Diagnosis

Diagnosis relies on serologies on both serum and CSF in acute and convalescent phases of infections.

CSF Profile

Cell count: elevated WBCs, lymphocytic
Glucose: normal
Protein: elevated

CSF IgM

Treatment

Treatment is supportive.

ADENOVIRUS

Adenovirus

Distribution is worldwide.

Presentation

Patients usually have associated upper respiratory infection, and children and immunocompromised are more likely develop encephalitis with fevers, altered mental status, and seizures.

Imaging

Data are sparse regarding imaging findings in adenovirus encephalitis, but reports of thalamic hyperintensity and rhombencephalitis are noted.

Diagnosis

This can be a difficult diagnosis to make given limitations of laboratory testing. Respiratory isolate PCR and culture.

CSF Profile

Cell count: mild elevation in WBCs, lymphocytic
Protein normal to mild elevation
Glucose normal

CSF viral culture and PCR for adenovirus can be sought.

Treatment

Treatment is supportive.

BACTERIAL ENCEPHALITIS AND MYELITIS

Bacteria are a much less frequent cause of encephalitis. However, they are often treatable and thus remain important to consider when evaluating and treating patients with encephalitis and myelitis.

Listeria monocytogenes

Distribution is worldwide.

Presentation

Patients are often immunosuppressed or age extremes. In addition to headaches, fevers and focal neurological deficits involving the brainstem can occur.

Imaging

MRI or CT can demonstrate meningeal enhancement, and MRI is more likely to demonstrate brainstem rhombencephalitis.

Diagnosis

CSF analysis is the gold standard for diagnosis. Blood cultures are 60% sensitive.

CSF Profile

Cell count: elevated WBC, PMNs or lymphocytic
Protein: elevated
Glucose: normal to low
CSF cultures about 40% sensitive
Listeria antigen

Treatment

Ampicillin 1 to 2 g IV every 3 to 4 hours

Neurosyphilis (*Treponema pallidum*)

Distribution is worldwide.

Presentation

Patients can present acutely or subacutely with progressive signs and symptoms, including cognitive impairment, abnormal pupils, headaches, seizures, strokes, myelopathy, radiculopathy, blindness, and deafness. Syphilis is the great mimicker and can present as almost any neurological disease.

Imaging

MRI or CT can demonstrate infarcts, space-occupying lesions (gumma), meningeal enhancement, and even temporal lobe involvement mimicking herpes encephalitis.

Diagnosis

CSF VDRL is the gold standard for diagnosis. Serum is TPPA positive and RPR positive.

CSF Profile

Cell count: mild to markedly elevated WBC, lymphocytic
Protein: elevated protein
Glucose normal
VDRL: diagnostic if positive but poor sensitivity (10–70%)
CSF FTA-Abs: if negative, a diagnosis of neurosyphilis is very unlikely

Treatment

PCN 20 million units IV every day × 10 days; otitic and ocular syphilis may require longer treatment and concomitant corticosteroids.

Mycoplasma pneumoniae

Distribution is worldwide.

Presentation

Patients can present with altered mental status, seizures, and focal neurological deficits.

Imaging

There is a dearth of data regarding imaging in these patients. Most cases reported are in association with a postinfectious ADEM (acute disseminated encephalomyelitis).

Diagnosis

This is a challenging and for some a controversial diagnosis. Multiple investigative approaches may be needed for confirmation. Chest radiography may be helpful.

Acute and convalescent serologies

CSF Profile

Cell count: elevated WBCs, lymphocytic
Glucose: normal
Protein: elevated

CSF PCR and antibodies

Treatment

Doxycycline 100 mg PO bid × 21 days and children 2.2 mg/kg bid

RICKETTSIOSES/ERLICHIOSES

Rickettsia rickettsii (Rocky Mountain Spotted Fever [RR]), Erlichia chaffeensis (EC), Anaplasma phagocytophilum (AP), and Coxiella burnetii (Q Fever [CB])

Distribution is North America (RR, EC, AP, CB), Europe (CB, AP), and Central and South America (RR).

Presentation

All patients can present with altered mental status, headaches, and seizures. There is an important seasonal variation with these diseases, usually in summer and fall. Exposures are an important consideration in considering these entities. Tick vector

(AP, EC, RR) and contact with cats, sheep, and goats (CB) can have associated rash (RR) and thrombocytopenia (CB, RR).

Imaging

Often normal, MRI or CT may show infarcts, edema, or meningeal enhancement.

Diagnosis

Clinical suspicion and seasonal occurrence along with multiple investigations are often needed to confirm diagnosis.

Blood smears for morulae 20% sensitivity (AP, EC)
Skin biopsy PCR and staining (RR)
Whole blood PCR (AP, EC)
Serologies for respective microbe: all

CSF Profile

Cell count: usually elevated WBCs, lymphocytic
Protein: mild elevation
Glucose: usually normal
CSF PCRs: low yield

Treatment

Doxycycline 100 mg PO bid (AP, EC, RR)
Doxycycline 100 mg bid + fluoroquinolone + rifampin (CB)

Neuro-Whipple's Disease (*Trophyrema whipplei*)

Distribution is unclear, mostly reported in North America and Europe.

Presentation

CNS Whipple's disease has mostly been reported in white male adults, usually associated diarrheal illness (80%) and arthralgias/arthropathy. Patients may have classic oculomasticatory myorhythmia. Whipple's disease can present with dementia, ophthalmoplegia, myoclonus, hypothalamic dysfunction, headache, and seizures.

Imaging

Reports of MRI findings in Whipple's disease have shown subcortical white matter disease and basal ganglia abnormalities.

Diagnosis

Duodenal biopsy.

CSF Profile

Cell count: normal to mild elevation lymphocytosis
Protein: normal to mild elevation
Glucose: usually normal
CSF PAS staining: suggestive
CSF PCR sensitivity: 80%

Treatment

Procaine penicillin G 1.2 million units IM daily and streptomycin 1 g IM daily for 14 days followed by bactrim 160/800 PO bid for 1 year

CNS Bartonellosis (*Bartonella henselea*)

Distribution is worldwide.

Presentation

Patients usually have a preceding history of cat scratch/bite and lymphadenopathy. CNS bartonellosis symptoms include headaches, seizures, retinitis, and encephalopathy. Patients may have concomitant endocarditis.

Imaging

Sparse data exist on CNS *Bartonella* findings, but reports of MRI findings include enhancing cortical lesions, positive signal changes of pulvinar nucleus on DWI (diffusion weighted imaging)

Diagnosis

Serum antibody titers, acute and convalescent

CSF Profile

Cell count: mild to moderate elevated WBCs, lymphocytic; can be normal
Protein: mild to moderate elevation
Glucose normal
CSF *Bartonella* antibody and PCR testing, where available

Treatment

Doxycycline 100 mg PO/IV bid with consideration of rifampin 300 mg PO bid

Neuroborreliosis (*Borrelia burgdorferi, Borrelia garinii*)

Distribution is North America, Europe, and central Asia.

Presentation

Patients with Lyme disease will rarely have encephalitis with altered mental status and fevers. A history of characteristic rash (erythema chronica migrans) is suggestive or involvement elsewhere such as joint disease or heart disease.

Imaging

There are reports of MRIs that have shown demyelinating disease–type presentation and rare tumor-like presentations. Some may have concomitant meningeal enhancement.

Diagnosis

A definitive diagnosis is similar to *Borrelia* meningitis. Serum Lyme antibody may aid in diagnosis.

CSF Profile

Cell count: normal or elevated WBCs, usually lymphocytic
Protein: normal or elevated
Glucose: normal
CSF Lyme PCR: low sensitivity
CSF culture: difficult, require special media, long culture duration
CSF: CSF Lyme-specific antibody concentration greater than 1.0 to serum

Treatment

Ceftriaxone 2 g/day IV; children 50 mg/kg to 75/kg IV daily
Penicillin G 3 to 4 million units every 4 hours IV; pediatric 200,000 to 400,000 units/
    kg/day to every 4 hours
Cefotaxime 2 g every 8 hours IV; pediatric 150 to 200 mg/kg/day IV tid

PARASITIC ENCEPHALITIS AND MYELITIS

Neurocysticercosis (*Taenia solium*)

Distribution is Central and South America, Sub-Saharan Africa, India, and southeast Asia.

Presentation

Patients may be asymptomatic or have seizures, headaches, focal neurological deficits, and altered mental status.

Imaging and Diagnosis

CT or MRI can have various findings depending on stage and location of the cysts and is very important in the diagnosis of neurocysticercosis.

Parenchymal Neurocysticercosis (NCC)

Vesicular stage: well-demarcated round cystic lesion with little or no edema
Colloidal stage: less-defined lesions with edema and contrast enhancement
Nodular stage: much less defined, less edema, persistent contrast enhancement
Calcified: may be missed on MRI, hyperintense on CT, no contrast enhancement

Ventricular Cysticercosis

MRI or CT: often hydrocephalus* and cyst usually identified with MRI but not with
   CT scan of the brain

Subarachnoid Cysticercosis

MRI or CT may reveal cysts within cortical sulci, sylvian fissures, CSF cisternae, and hydocephalus; cysts can be large and multilobulated.
   Hydrocephalus can be seen in association with any of the parenchymal imaging findings.

CSF Profile

Unlike most infectious disease processes, CSF analysis is not the mainstay of diagnosis and is often not sampled. The commonly reported pattern of CSF is:

Cell count: elevated with occasional eosinophilia reported
Protein: elevated
Glucose: normal to low
CSF cysticercal antibody: sensitivity is highly variable depending on stage of disease

Treatment

Parenchymal lesions

Vesicular Cysts

Single cyst: albendazole 15 mg/kg/d ×3 days, corticosteroids as needed
Mild to moderate infection: albendazole 15 mg/kg/d × 1 week, corticosteroids as needed
Heavy infection: albendazole 15 mg/day × 1 week and corticosteroids

Colloidal Cysts

Single cyst: albendazole 15 mg/kg/day × 3 days, corticosteroids as needed
Mild to moderate infection: 15 mg/kg/day × 1 week and corticosteroids
Heavy infection: treatment contraindicated
Granular and calcified cysticerci: treatment is unnecessary

Subarachnoid Cysticercosis

Small cysts over convexity of cerebral hemispheres: albendazole 15 mg/kg/day × 1 week, corticosteroids as needed
Large cysts in sylvian fissures or basal cisternae: albendazole 15/mg/day × 15 to 30 days and corticosteroids
Hydrocephalus: ventricular shunt; if ventricular cyst endoscopic resection of cyst should be performed and shunt if ependymitis is present

CNS Toxoplasmosis (*Toxoplasma gondii*)

Distrubution is worldwide.

Presentation

Patients more commonly present with headaches, fevers, focal neurological deficits, seizures, and altered mental status. Rarely, spinal cord involvement can be seen. It is most often associated with HIV co-infection.

Imaging

CT or MRI can show multiple or solitary ring enhancing lesions (Figure 25.4).

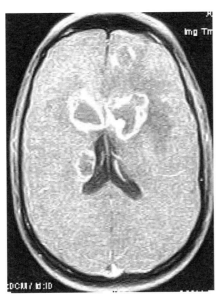

FIGURE 25.4
MRI crain T1 with contrast in patient with CNS toxoplasmosis.

Diagnosis

Diagnosis is often made by response to antitoxoplasma medications. However, serum antibody tests, suggestive neuroimaging in a susceptible patient are used to diagnose a patient with toxoplasmosis.

Serum: *Toxoplasma* antibody IgG or IgM are suggestive
If safe to do, CSF analysis:

CSF Profile

Cell count: elevated WBCs, lymphocytic
Protein elevated
Glucose: normal
CSF *Toxoplasma* PCR: reported sensitivity of 83%

Treatment

Pyrimethamine with sulphadiazine, folinic acid
Alternative treatments include pyrimethamine and clindamycin; occasionally high-dose bactrim can be used
Corticosteroids can be used if significant edema is found

In HIV-infected individuals, continued suppressive therapy is recommended until the patient has had immune reconstitution marked by at least two consecutive CD4/Tcell counts of 200 or greater separated by 6-month interval.

Plasmodium falciparum (Cerebral Malaria)

Distribution is Sub-Saharan Africa, Central and South America, India, and Southeast Asia.

Presentation

Patients can present with fevers, headaches, and depressed level of consciousness. Children more commonly affected.

Imaging

CT or MRI can be normal or demonstrate diffuse edema.

Diagnosis

A clinical picture in conjunction with identification of parasite is often used to diagnosis cerebral malaria.

Serum antigen RDT (rapid diagnostic test) is available but is not as sensitive as smears.
Serum parasite smears (variable sensitivity due to parasite load and microscopist)

CSF Profile

CSF analysis is often normal but occasionally CSF lymphocytosis; elevated protein with normal glucose has been observed.

Treatment

For severe malaria, treatment involves quinidine and either doxycycline, tetracycline, or clindamycin.

Quinidine: 6.25 mg base/kg (=10 mg salt/kg) loading dose IV over 1 to 2 hours, then 0.0125 mg base/kg/min (=0.02 mg salt/kg/min) continuous infusion for at least 24 hours; (duration 3 to 7 days and switch to oral quinine when possible)
Doxycycline dosage is 100 mg IV/PO bid; if child less than 45 kg then 2.2 mg/kg IV every 12 hours (duration usually 7 days)
Tetracycline 250 mg PO qid (7 days)
Clindamycin: 10 mg base/kg loading dose IV followed by 5 mg base/kg IV every 8 hours. Switch to oral clindamycin (oral dose as above) as soon as patient can take oral medication. For IV use, avoid rapid administration (7 days)

Amebic Meningoencephalitis

Distribution is worldwide.

Presentation

Variable presentations respective to ameba involved.
Primary amebic meningoencephalitis (PAM) *Naegleria fowleri*: high fever, severe headache, stiff neck, seizures, and rapid progression to death
Granulomatous amebic encephalitis (GAE) *Acanthamoeba* species and *Balamuthia mandrillaris*: can present with chronic meningitis, brain abscess, low-grade fever, cranial nerve palsies, focal neurological deficits, seizures, and coma
Cerebral amebiasis *Entamoeba histolytica*: similar to GAE clinical presentation but usually abscess formation; often will have abscesses elsewhere such as liver

Imaging

Although reporting has been sparse, CT scans have shown diffuse edema, meningeal enhancement, and abscess.

Diagnosis

Unfortunately, this is often only diagnosed post-mortem. However, CSF analysis can sometimes yield a diagnosis.

CSF Profile

The findings vary as to the infecting agent.

PAM: elevated PMNs, low glucose, elevated protein, trophozoites may be visualized
GAE and cerebral amebiasis: elevated lymphocytes, no trophozoites visualized, biopsy
    or culture

Treatment

No proven therapy; amphotericinB intrathecal can be tried

African Trypanosomiasis/African Sleeping Sickness (*T. ambiense, T. rhodesiense*)

Distribution is Sub-Saharan Africa.

Presentation

Patients often have lymphadenopathy, Winterbottom's sign, headache, joint pain, back pain, abnormal sleep, and subsequent progressive deterioration of consciousness.

Imaging

CT and MRI can show cerebral edema and white matter changes.

Diagnosis

A diagnosis is made in patients from endemic areas and various investigations including serum and CSF analysis.

Serum *T. b. gambiense* antibody screening available
Blood smear for trypanosomes

CSF Profile

Varies by stage of disease
Cell count: normal to elevated lymphocytic pleocytosis
Protein: normal to elevated
Glucose: low
CSF Mott cells: plasma cells with PAS-positive inclusions
CSF antibody testing available
Direct visualization of parasite

Treatment

First stage: pentamidine and suramin
Second stage (neurological): melarsoprol 2.2 mg/kg daily $\times$ 12 days
Alternate: nifurtimox, eflorthinine

Schistosomiasis

Distribution is Africa, South America, Caribbean, and Asia.

Presentation

Patients with schistosomiasis are either from endemic areas or have traveled to these areas. Patients may have a history of hematuria and can present with focal neurological deficits, particularly myelopathy.

Imaging

MRI or CT may show enhancing lesions in brain and spinal cord.

Diagnosis

A diagnosis is made in patients from endemic areas and various investigations including serum, urine, fecal, and CSF analysis. Urine and stool examination are used for schistosoma. Serum serologies are helpful if patient is not from an endemic area.

CSF Profile

Cell count: elevated WBCs, rarely eosinophilia
Protein: elevated
Glucose: low to normal
CSF antibody and PCR available

Treatment

Praziquantel and corticosteroids should be considered.

PRIONS

Prions, the word derived from *pro*tein and infec*tion*, are infectious agents lacking nucleic acids. The prions lead to a neurodegenerative process mimicking encephalitis.

Creutzfeldt–Jakob Disease (CJD)

Distribution is worldwide.

Presentation

Patients with CJD present with a rapidly progressive dementia (typically less than 1 year's duration), myoclonus, and ataxia; can be familial 10% to 15% of cases.

Imaging

MRI DWI sequence can show cortical hyperintensity and basal ganglia hyperintensity (Figure 25.5).

Diagnosis

Diagnosis relies on a clinical picture, neuroimaging, EEG and CSF findings, or some combination thereof.

CSF Profile

Cell count: may be normal or mild elevation WBCs, lymphocytic
Protein: normal or mild elevation
Glucose: normal
CSF Tau and 14-3-3 protein, variable sensitivity and specificity reported; improved in patients with rapidly progressive dementia
EEG: The EEG can show periodic sharp wave complexes.

Treatment

Treatment is spportive and palliative.

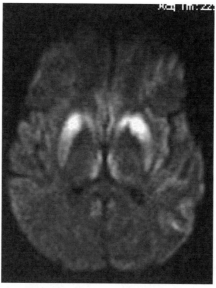

FIGURE 25.5
MRI brain DWI in patient with biopsy proven Creutzfeldt-Jakob disease.

SUGGESTED READING

Fishman, R. (1992). *Cerebrospinal Fluid in Diseases of the Nervous System*, 2nd edition. WB Saunders company.

Miller, A., Ed in Chief. (2012). *Infectious Disease*. 1255–1416.

Sheld, W., Whitley, R., Marra, C. (2004). *Infections of the Central Nervous System*, 3rd edition. Lippincott Williams & Wilkins.

Singer, E., Valdes-Sueiras, M., Commins, D., Levine, A. (2010). Neurologic Presentations of AIDS. *Neurologic Clinics 28*(1), 253–275.

Steiner, I., Budka, H., Chaudhuri, A., Koskiniemi, M., Sainio, K., Salonen, O., et al. (2010). Viral meningoencephalitis: a review of diagnostic methods and guidelines for management. *Eur J Neurol. 17*(8), 999–e57.

Tunkel, A., Glaser, C., Bloch, K., Sejvar, J., Marra, C., Roos, K., et al. (2008). The Management of Encephalitis: Clinical Practice Guidelines by the Infectious Diseases Society of America CID. *47*(1 August), 303–327.

SECTION EIGHT
MULTIPLE SCLEROSIS AND RELATED DISORDERS

26 Multiple Sclerosis

Kjell-Morten Myhr

INTRODUCTION

Multiple sclerosis (MS) is an immune-mediated disease of the central nervous system (CNS). Onset of the disease is usually between 20 and 40 years of age, and it is the leading nontraumatic cause of nervous system disability in young adults. MS is clinically characterized by repeated subacute episodes (relapses) of nervous system symptoms and signs followed by remission, relapsing-remitting MS (RRMS) (80–90% of cases) or insidious progression from onset, primary progressive MS (PPMS) (10–20% of cases). An increasing proportion of people with RRMS develop a secondary progressive course (SPMS) later during the disease course, initially with superimposed relapses but later steady progression without relapses and no remission. The pathological characteristics of the disease are focal inflammatory demyelinating white matter lesions in the CNS with probably secondary axonal damage, but central and cortical grey-matter lesions are also seen. The causes of MS are largely unknown, but the current hypothesis is that the disease evolves among genetically susceptible individuals as an infrequent response to environmental factors. The disease is most prevalent in northern Europe and North America, and in Scandinavia the prevalence rates approach 180–200/100 000 inhabitants.

No single clinical feature or diagnostic test is sufficient for diagnosing MS. The diagnosis is therefore based on careful evaluation of the disease history, clinical examination, as well as paraclinical examinations aiming to document disseminated disease in both time and space. No curative treatment for MS is available, but corticosteroid infusion during acute relapses and increasingly effective disease-modifying therapies are available.

DIAGNOSIS

The diagnosis is based on objective evidence of dissemination in time and space of CNS lesions typical of MS and on excluding other more plausible explanations for the clinical features. Diagnostic criteria define the clinical and paraclinical evidence of the disease. However, a typical busy neurological practice may overemphasize magnetic resonance imaging (MRI) and other paraclinical examinations compared with clinical examination. In this context, it is important to emphasize that MS cannot be diagnosed without carefully clinically evaluating the patient and classifying symptoms and signs as either monofocal (indicating a single lesion) or multifocal (indicating more than one lesion) to define disseminated disease in space and time.

Clinical Presentation

RRMS presents typically with recurrent episodes (relapses) of nervous system symptoms, followed by remissions. A relapse is defined as patient-reported symptoms or objectively observed signs typical of an acute inflammatory demyelinating event in the CNS, current or historical, with duration of at least 24 hours, in the absence of fever or infection. A new attack should be documented by contemporaneous neurological examination, but in a typical clinical context, historical events with symptoms and evolution characteristic for MS in the absence of objective neurological findings can provide reasonable evidence of a prior demyelinating event.

Repeated paroxysmal episodes (such as a tonic spasm) occurring for more than 24 hours are considered a relapse. At least 30 days should separate the onset of a first relapse from the onset of a second relapse.

To define a definite diagnosis of MS, at least one attack must be corroborated by findings on neurological examination, visual evoked potential (VEP) response in patients reporting prior visual disturbance, or MRI consistent with demyelination in the area of the CNS implicated in the historical report of neurological symptoms. A diagnosis of MS on purely clinical evidence remains possible if there is objective evidence of lesions separated in time and space.

PPMS presents typically with insidious progression of nervous system impairment without relapses or remissions.

Paraclinical Examinations

The diagnostic evaluation for MS should include MRI, cerebrospinal fluid (CSF), and in some cases also visual evoked response (VER) examinations.

Magnetic Resonance Imaging

MRI shows hyperintensive white matter T2 lesions in typical areas such as periventricular including corpus callosum, juxtacortical, infratentorial or the spinal cord. New active lesions often enhance gadolinium contrast indicating active inflammation and blood–brain barrier disruption. MRI may provide evidence of dissemination of lesions in both time and space (Table 26.1). MRI support for dissemination of lesions in space requires at least one demyelinating T2 lesion in at least two of four defined typical locations for MS; periventricular; juxtacortical; infratentorial or spinal cord, with lesions within the symptomatic region excluded in patients with brainstem or spinal cord syndromes. MRI supports disseminated disease in time when a new T2 lesion is detected on a new examination irrespective of the timing of the baseline MRI, or when silent gadolinium-enhancing and silent non-enhancing lesions are seen at any time (Table 26.1).

Cerebrospinal Fluid (CSF)

A positive CSF is defined as the presence of oligoclonal immunoglobulin G (IgG) bands, preferably based on isoelectric focusing with immunofixation, differing from those in serum, or an increased IgG index. Lymphocytic pleocytosis is usually less than $50/mm^3$ and total protein concentration less than $1 g/mm^3$. Positive CSF findings can support the inflammatory demyelinating nature of the underlying condition and

Dissemination in space:

At least one T2 lesion in at least two of the following four areas characteristic for MS

- Periventricular
- Juxtacortical
- Infratentorial
- Spinal cord

Note: If a subject has a brainstem or spinal cord syndrome, the symptomatic lesions are excluded from the Criteria and do not contribute to lesion count.

Dissemination in time—one of the following:

- A new T2 and/or gadolinium-enhancing lesion(s) on follow-up MRI, with reference to a baseline scan, irrespective of the timing of the baseline MRI
- Simultaneous presence of asymptomatic gadolinium-enhancing and non-enhancing lesions at any time

---

is also important to evaluate alternative diagnoses, and to predict conversion from clinical isolated syndrome (CIS; first clinical episode) to clinical definite MS (CDMS; second clinical episode/relapse).

Visual Evoked Response (VER) Abnormal VER, typical of MS, is delayed but with well-preserved wave form and can provide objective evidence of demyelination in the visual pathways.

Diagnostic Criteria

A diagnosis of MS is based on objective evidences for disseminated disease in time (≥ 2 relapses) and space (≥ 2 lesions). The most straightforward situation is therefore two attacks and clinical evidence of two or more lesions. When the evidence indicates less than two relapses and/or two CNS lesions, supportive evidence from MRI examinations is increasingly needed (Table 26.2). The most difficult situation is often insidious nervous system progression, suggesting PPMS (Table 26.2). Thus, the additional criteria needed to diagnose MS become more stringent as the clinical evidence on presentation becomes weaker.

TREATMENT

No curative treatment is available for MS, but corticosteroid treatment for relapses and immunomodulatory and immunosuppressive therapies are important to modify the disease course. In addition, it is also important to evaluate people with MS for symptomatic treatment for various symptoms such as spasticity, pain, depression, and bladder dysfunction. All available disease-modifying therapies have mainly anti-inflammatory effects. Clinical relapses and gadolinium-enhancing lesions are the clinical and MRI correlates for inflammatory disease activity in MS. Thus, RRMS with present clinical relapse and/or MRI disease activity, and SPMS with inflammatory disease activity with superimposed relapses and/or MRI disease activity, may benefit from the anti-inflammatory disease-modifying therapies.

Table 26.2 McDonald Diagnostic Criteria for Multiple Sclerosis

Clinical presentation	Additional data needed for MS diagnosis
≥ 2 attacks and objective clinical evidence of ≥ 2 lesions; or objective clinical evidence of 1 lesion with reasonable historical evidence of a prior attack	• None. *But* MRI and CSF examinations should be done to exclude other diagnoses. If these tests are *negative,* extreme caution needs to be taken before making a diagnosis of MS.
≥ 2 attacks and objective clinical evidence of 1 lesion	• Dissemination in space, demonstrated by: MRI *or* Await a further clinical attack implicating a different CNS site
1 attack and objective clinical evidence of ≥ 2 lesions	• Dissemination in time, demonstrated by: MRI *or* Await a further clinical attack
1 attack and objective clinical evidence of 1 lesion (CIS)	• Dissemination in space, demonstrated by: MRI *or* Await a further clinical attack implicating a different CNS site—*and* • Dissemination in time, demonstrated by: MRI *or* Await a further clinical attack
Insidious neurological progression suggestive of MS (PPMS)	• One year of disease progression (retrospectively or prospectively determined) *and* two of the three following criteria: 1. Dissemination in space, demonstrated by brain MRI; ≥ 1 T2 lesions in at least one area characteristic for MS (periventricular, juxtacortical, or infratentorial) 2. Dissemination in space, demonstrated by spinal cord MRI; ≥ 2 T2 lesions 3. Positive CSF

Treating Relapses in MS

Relapses are the dominant clinical feature of relapsing-remitting MS but also occur in the initial phase of SPMS with superimposed relapses. The onset of a relapse is usually subacute and appears as either new nervous system deficits or worsening of previous ones lasting for at least 24 hours. Recurrent episodes of paroxysmal symptoms, such as trigeminal neuralgia occurring over at least 24 hours, may also constitute a relapse. It is also important to rule out a pseudo-relapse related to an increase in body temperature or infection. Although most relapses improve somewhat, incomplete remission is an important determinant of irreversible nervous system impairment and disability progression in MS.

Intravenous infusion of methylprednisolone (MP) in a dose of at least 500–1000 mg daily for 5 days is first-line treatment of MS relapses. There is also some support for intravenous infusion of 1000 mg of MP for 3 days with or without an oral tapering dose. The treatment speeds up the recovery, but there is no evidence for long-term effects on the degree of recovery or risk of new relapses. No major differences have been reported in the clinical efficacy or side effects of intravenous or oral MP, but it is argued that prolonged oral treatment may be associated with a higher prevalence of side effects. The treatment is usually well tolerated, and typical side effects are dyspepsia, a feeling of well-being or euphoria, facial flushing, disturbance of taste, insomnia, and mild weight gain. However, psychosis, pancreatitis, and anaphylactoid reactions to intravenous MP have been reported, and the risk of osteoporosis should be considered when repeated treatment is needed.

Some patients with severe relapses who have been refractory to treatment with high-dose MP may be treated with plasma exchange.

Disease-Modifying Therapies in MS

Although a few people with RRMS may have a temporary benign disease course with minimal disease activity and impairment, most eventually accumulate increasing disability over time and convert to SPMS. Thus, disease-modifying therapies in MS should aim to minimize disease activity to prevent the progression of disability. Since the early 1990s, eight different disease-modifying compounds have been registered and become available for MS therapy: interferon-beta, glatiramer acetate, teriflunomide, dimethyl fumarate, natalizumab, fingolimod, alemtuzumab and mitoxantrone.

Interferon-beta

Interferon-beta is a polypeptide naturally produced predominantly by human fibroblasts. The mechanisms by which it exerts its therapeutic effect in MS are not fully understood. Nevertheless, its anti-inflammatory effects are largely believed to result from the inhibition of T-lymphocyte proliferation, shifting the cytokine response from an inflammatory response to a favorable anti-inflammatory profile and reducing the migration of inflammatory cells across the blood–brain barrier. Interferon beta is available in recombinant forms for MS treatment as interferon beta-1b (Betaferon˚, Extavia˚) or interferon beta-1a (Avonex˚, Rebif˚). Betaferon˚ and Extavia˚ are identical formulations and are given 250 µg subcutaneously every other day, Avonex˚ 30 µg intramuscularly once weekly and Rebif˚ subcutaneously 22 or 44 µg three times a week.

Relapsing-Remitting MS Pivotal trials of the preparations in RRMS have shown beneficial effects by reducing the annual relapse rate by about 30–34% and MRI disease activity by 60–80% depending on MRI-modality and study design, and reducing the progression of disability. The treatment is usually well tolerated, but most patients experience side effects when therapy starts. Most frequent are flu-like symptoms (50–75%), including muscle aches, fever, chills, headache, and back pain that usually appear 2–8 hours after an injection and resolve within 24 hours. Injection at bedtime, gradual titration of dose over the first 3–4 weeks of therapy and prophylactic paracetamol or nonsteroidal anti-inflammatory medication can reduce the incidence and intensity of these side effects. Injection-site reactions (pain, erythema and inflammation) are also frequent and more common in regimens with frequent subcutaneous administration. There may also be isolated cases of severe injection-site reactions involving infection or necrosis. Rotating injection sites and carefully using a sterile technique are important to limit the problem of injection-site reactions. Liver enzymes may be elevated and bone marrow depressed, which warrants periodic surveillance of liver function and blood counts before starting therapy and every 6 months thereafter. The dose may need to be adjusted or therapy changed in case of severe deviation. Severe cases of acute liver failure and pancreatitis during IFNB therapy have been reported.

Clinically Isolated Syndromes A clinically isolated syndrome (CIS) is an initial demyelinating event suggestive of MS. These typically include optic neuritis, partial transverse myelitis or brainstem lesions. People with CIS who have evidence of clinically silent MRI lesions have a high risk of developing new clinical relapses (40–45%) and MRI lesions (90%) within 2 years from the onset of the initial symptom. Studies of all interferon beta preparations have reported a reduced risk of new disease activity among people with CIS (with clinically silent MRI lesions) as shown by significant prolonged time to a second relapse and reduction in new MRI lesions as well as in some cases also progression of disability.

Secondary Progressive MS Patients with RRMS may eventually develop SPMS with irreversible, steady progression of nervous system disability with or without superimposed relapses. Since the relapse frequency drops during conversion to SPMS and later disappears, it is believed that the inflammatory component of the disease is reduced and that degenerative processes of axonal loss dominate disease progression. Thus, anti-inflammatory therapies are less likely to have major effects in these stages of the disease. All the interferon beta preparations have been evaluated in the treatment of SPMS. The first interferon beta-1b study showed efficacy of the treatment as measured by both relapse rate and disability progression, but later studies of both interferon beta-1b and interferon beta-1a could only detect some treatment effects on the relapse rate. Thus, it is generally believed that only SPMS patients with superimposed relapses may benefit somewhat from interferon beta treatment.

Primary Progressive MS Interferon beta therapy has not shown significant benefit in PPMS.

Neutralizing Antibodies Against Interferon beta Interferon beta treatment may induce an immune response, with the formation of neutralizing antibodies (NAB) against the preparation (~2–20%). The NAB appear usually within 6–18 months of treatment, and evidence is accumulating that bioavailability, biological response, and efficacy of treatment are reduced in the presence of NAB. Accordingly, it is recommended to test all patients for the presence of NAB every 6 months during the first 2 years of therapy. Testing can be discontinued in patients who remain NAB-negative. In patients with sustained high titers of NAB at repeated analysis, treatment should be switched to alternative disease-modifying therapy other than interferon beta.

Glatiramer Acetate

Glatiramer acetate is a pool of synthetic peptides, resembling sequences of myelin basic protein, randomly composed of four amino acids (tyrosine, glutamic acid, alanine, and lysine) with an average length of 40 to 100 residues. The mechanisms of action for its therapeutic effect in MS have not been fully clarified but are probably largely related to anti-inflammatory effects by promoting Th2 deviation under the development of Th2 glatiramer acetate-reactive CD4+ T cells that can accumulate in the CNS and promote bystander suppression, releasing anti-inflammatory cytokines. Glatiramer acetate is available as Copaxone® and is given once daily as subcutaneous injections of 20 mg.

Relapsing-Remitting MS The pivotal trial in RRMS showed significant reduction in the annual relapse rate (30%) similar to IFNB, and a later study also showed reduction in gadolinium-enhancing MRI activity. Glatiramer acetate is usually well tolerated, but most patients (65%) experience injection-site reactions (pain, erythema, swelling and pruritus). About 15% report a transient self-limited systemic reaction (immediate after injection) of facial flushing and chest tightness, accompanied at times by palpitation, anxiety and dyspnoea. Other reported side effects are lymphadenopathy, dyspnoea and lipoatrophy.

Clinically Isolated Syndromes Glatiramer acetate has been tested in a randomized, double-blind, placebo-controlled trial of CIS patients with silent MRI lesions. The treatment resulted in a reduced risk of new disease activity among people with CIS as shown by significant prolonged time to a second relapse and reduction in new MRI lesions.

Progressive MS Glatiramer acetate has not been investigated for the treatment of SPMS and has not shown significant benefit in PPMS patients.

Teriflunomide

Teriflunomide is an immunomodulatory agent with anti-inflammatory properties that selectively and reversibly inhibits the mitochondrial enzyme dihydroorotate dehydrogenase (DHO-DH), required for the de novo pyrimidine synthesis. As a consequence teriflunomide reduces the proliferation of dividing cells that need de novo synthesis of pyrimidine to expand. The exact mechanism by which teriflunomide exerts its therapeutic effect in MS is not fully understood, but this is mediated by a reduced number of lymphocytes. Teriflunomide is available as Aubagio® and is given orally 14 mg once daily.

Relapsing-Remitting MS Two phase III trials in RRMS showed that teriflunomide 14 mg once daily, compared to placebo, reduced the annual relapse rate by 31–36%, the rate of disability progression by 26–29%, and MRI gadolinium-enhancing lesions by about 80%. Another phase III trial of teriflunomide 14 mg once daily, compared to interferon beta-1a 44 µg subcunaneously three times weekly, showed similar effects on annual relapse rate (0,26 and 0,22 respectevely) and the time to a new relapse or termination of treatment.

Teriflunomide is in general, well tolerated, but common adverse events include upper respiratory tract infection, urinary tract infection, paraesthesia, diarrhoea, nausea, hair thinning, alanine aminotransferase (ALT) increase, reduction in white blood cells, and some patients experienced increase in blood pressure. It is therefore recommended relatively frequent (every second week) alanine aminotransferase (ALT) screening during the first six months of treatment and thereafter every second month. Regularly measurements of blood pressure and white blood cells and platelets counts are also recommended.

Clinically Isolated Syndromes Teriflunomide 14 mg once daily has been tested in a randomized, double-blind, placebo-controlled trial of CIS patients with silent MRI lesions. The treatment resulted in a reduced risk of new disease activity among people with CIS as shown by significant prolonged time to a second relapse and reduction in new MRI lesions.

Progressive MS No data on treatment with teriflunomide in patients with progressive MS has been presented.

Dimethyl Fumarate

Dimethyl fumarate is an immunomodulatory agent with anti-inflammatory properties, but the mechanism of action in MS is not fully understood. Preclinical studies indicate that dimethyl fumarate responses appear to be primarily mediated through activation of the Nuclear factor (erythroid-derived 2)-like 2 (Nrf2) transcriptional pathway. Dimethyl fumarate has also been shown to up regulate Nrf2-dependent anti-oxidant genes in patients. Dimethyl fumarate is available as Tecfidera® and is given orally 240 mg twice daily.

Relapsing-Remitting MS Two phase III trials of RRMS showed that dimethyl fumarate 240 mg twice daily, compared to placebo, reduced the annual relapse rate by 45–53%, the rate of disability progression by 24–41%, and MRI gadolinium-enhancing lesions by about 75–94%. Glatiramer acetate was also included as an active comparator in one of the trials. This study was not powered to detect statistical significant differences, but dimethyl fumarate 240 mg twice daily reduced (statistical non-significant) the annual relapse rate by 24%, and the rate of disability progression by 19%, and reduced (statistical significant) the number of new and enlarging MRI T2 by about 36%.

Dimethyl fumarate is in general, well tolerated, but common adverse events include flushing, nausea, diarrhoea, and abdominal pain. The treatment may also reduce white blood cell counts and elevations of hepatic transaminases, and regularly blood tests are therefore recommended.

Clinically Isolated Syndromes and Progressive MS No data on treatment with dimethyl fumarate fingolimod in patients with CIS or progressive MS has been presented.

Natalizumab

Natalizumab is a monoclonal antibody against α4-integrin, blocking the interaction with its ligands. The mechanism of action of its therapeutic effect in MS is largely through preventing adherence of activated leucocytes to inflamed endothelium, thus inhibiting the migration of inflammatory cells into the CNS. Natalizumab is available for MS treatment as Tysabri® and is given as 300-mg intravenous infusions every 4 weeks.

Relapsing-Remitting MS The pivotal trial of RRMS showed that natalizumab monotherapy reduced the annual relapse rate by almost 70%, the rate of disability progression by 42–54% and MRI gadolinium-enhancing lesions by more than 90%. Although natalizumab is well tolerated, the treatment is associated with increased risk of developing progressive multifocal leucoencephalopathy (PML). This is a potentially life-threatening central nervous system infection of oligodendrocytes by the JC polyoma virus (JCV). Therefore it is recommended that all patients receiving natalizumab should be screened for previous JCV infection. The risk for PML in JCV-negative patients is low (<0.09/1000) and is probably associated to recent seroconversion (estimated to

2–3% each year) or a false negative test. Among the JCV-positive patients the risk of developing PML is influenced by treatment duration, and previous immunosuppressive treatment. The risk is low during the first 2 years of treatment, increases thereafter, and the highest risk is among JCV-positive patients after 2 years of treatment, that previously also have received immunosuppressive treatment (~1/60). Based on this knowledge, it is recommended to retest JCV-negative patients every sixth month and JCV-positive patients should be carefully informed about the risk for PML at initiation and after 2 years of treatment. JCV-positive patients that previously have received immunosuppressive treatment should, if possible, be recommended for other treatment options. Due to the risk of PML, natalizumab is a second-line treatment in RRMS patients with high disease activity despite adequate first-line therapy or in some cases of naïve RRMS with very high disease activity, and careful patient selection and monitoring is needed.

Clinically Isolated Syndromes and Progressive MS Natalizumab has not been included in the treatment trials of patients with CIS or progressive MS.

Neutralizing Antibodies Against Natalizumab Natalizumab treatment may induce an immune response, with the formation of persistent NAB (~4–6%) against the preparation. NAB usually appear within the first 12 months of treatment, reduce the efficacy of the treatment and are associated with higher rates of infusion-related adverse events. Accordingly, patients should be tested for NAB at 6 and 12 months of therapy and in case of infusion-related adverse events or treatment failure. Testing can be discontinued in patients who remain NAB-negative during the first year of therapy. NAB-positive patients should be re-tested after 1–3 months, and if this is sustained, treatment should be switched to alternative disease-modifying therapy. Patients with significant infusion-related adverse events should immediately terminate treatment.

Fingolimod

Fingolimod is an oral sphingosine 1-phosphate receptor (S1PR) modulator that subsequent to its phosphorylation binds with high affinity to S1PR, which in turn leads to an internalization and degradation of the receptor on different tissues and cell types, including lymphocytes. As a consequence, fingolimod inhibits the ability of autoaggressive lymphocytes to egress from the lymph nodes towards the CNS, thereby limiting inflammatory and neurodegenerative processes in MS. Fingolimod is available as Gilenya® and is given orally 0,5 mg once daily.

Relapsing-Remitting MS Two phase III trials of RRMS showed that fingolimod 0.5 mg once daily, compared to placebo, reduced the annual relapse rate by 48–55%, the rate of disability progression by 13–25%, and MRI gadolinium-enhancing lesions by more than 80%. Another phase III trial of RRMS showed that fingolimod 0.5 mg once daily, compared to interferon beta 1a 30 µg intramuscularly once weekly, reduced the annual relapse rate by 52% and MRI gadolinium-enhancing lesions by more than 50%.

Fingolimod is in general, well tolerated, but common adverse events include upper respiratory tract infection, headache, cough, diarrhoea, and back pain. Fingolimod may also cause a transient bradycardia and might be associated with atrioventricular block. It is therefore recommended to monitor patients continuously with an electrocardiogram for six hours after the first dose, and extending the monitoring of patients who developed any clinically relevant heart symptoms. Rare adverse events of elevated liver enzymes and macular oedema may occur, and regular blood sampling and in addition a routine eye examination after three months of treatment are recommended. One death due to a fulminant primary varicella zoster infection was reported in one of the phase III trials. Therefore a blood sample for screening of a previous varicella zoster infection is advised, and in case of negative screening test, vaccination is prior to initiation of treatment is recommended.

Clinically Isolated Syndromes and Progressive MS No data on treatment with fingolimod in patients with CIS or progressive MS has been presented.

Alemtuzumab

Alemtuzumab, is a recombinant, humanised monoclonal antibody directed against CD52 that is a cell surface antigen present at high levels on especially T and B lymphocytes. Alemtuzumab acts through antibody-dependent cellular cytolysis and complement-mediated lysis following cell surface binding to T and B lymphocytes. The mechanism by which alemtuzumab exerts its therapeutic effects in MS is not fully elucidated. But, studies suggest immunomodulatory effects through the depletion and repopulation of lymphocytes that reduce the potential for relapses, and thereby delays disease progression. Alemtuzumab is available as Lemtrada®, and is administered by intravenous infusion for 2 treatment courses. The initial treatment course is 12 mg/day for 5 consecutive days (60 mg total dose), and the second treatment course is 12 mg/day for 3 consecutive days (36 mg total dose) administered 12 months after the initial treatment course. If new disease activity appears, additional courses (similar to the second course) may be given 12 months after the latest treatment course.

Relapsing-Remitting MS Two phase III trials of RRMS showed that alemtuzumab 12 mg, compared to interferon beta-1a 44 μg subcunaneously three times weekly, reduced the annual relapse rate by 50–54%, the rate of disability progression by 27–35%, and MRI gadolinium-enhancing lesions by 61–63%.

Alemtuzumab is in general well tolerated, but patients commonly experience infusion associated reactions including flushing, nausea, headache, tachycardia, urticaria, rash, pruritus, pyrexia and fatigue. Oral prophylaxis with aciclovir 200 mg twice daily (or equivalent) for herpes infection should also be administered to all patients starting on the first day of each treatment course and continuing for a minimum of 1 month after the last dose. Alemtuzumab treatment is also associated with increased risk of upper respiratory tract infection, urinary tract infection, and may also result in the formation of autoantibodies and increases the risk of autoimmune mediated conditions including thyroid disorders, immune thrombocytopenic purpura (ITP), or, rarely, nephropathies (e.g. anti-glomerular basement membrane disease). Caution should therefore be exercised in patients with previous autoimmune conditions other than MS, although available data suggests there is no worsening of pre-existing autoimmune conditions after alemtuzumab treatment. Based on the risk of autoimmune mediated conditions that may appear after several years, monthly blood and urine analyses are recommend for 4 years after the last dosing of alemtuzumab.

Clinically Isolated Syndromes and Progressive MS No data on treatment with dimethyl fumarate fingolimod in patients with CIS or progressive MS has been presented.

Mitoxantrone

Mitoxantrone is a synthetic anthracenedione derivative and is mostly used in treating various malignancies such as breast cancer and advanced prostate cancer, lymphoma and leukaemia. It interacts with nuclear DNA and is a potent immunosuppressive agent targeting proliferating immune cells, inhibiting proliferation and inducing apoptosis of T lymphocytes, B lymphocytes, macrophages and other antigen-presenting cells. Mitoxantron is available as Novantrone® (but is not approved for MS therapy in all countries), and is most often administered by intravenous infusion every third month at a dose of 12 mg/m^2 of body surface. Other dosing regimens, such as induction with monthly infusion the first 3 months, followed by every third month infusions may be used. The dose may be reduced according to efficacy and side effects. Importantly, due to potential cardiotoxicity, the maximum cumulative dose is restricted to 120–140 mg/m^2 of body surface and carefully monitoring is therefore important. Thus maximum the treatment period is usually limited to about 3 years.

Relapsing-Remitting and Secondary Progressive MS Limited efficacy data are available, but controlled studies of highly active RRMS have shown significant efficacy of the treatment, as shown by a 60–70% reduction in the relapse rate (compared with placebo or intravenous MP) as well as reduced disability progression and MRI disease activity. The largest Phase III investigator-blinded study randomized patients with worsening RRMS and SPMS (n = 194) for 5 or 12 mg of mitoxantrone per m^2 of body surface or placebo every 3 months for 2 years. The treatment showed a 60–70% reduction in the relapse rate in the high-dose arm compared with placebo and reduced disability progression and MRI disease activity. Side effects such as transient nausea, fatigue, mild hair loss (for days to a week) and menstrual disturbances were frequent (60–70%). Additional side effects were urinary tract infection (about 30%) as well as elevated liver enzymes and leukopenia (about 15–20%). The treatment induces transient leukopenia, with a nadir after about 10 days, and thus follow-up blood control is needed. Although not in the phase III trial, lethal congestive heart failure and therapy-related leukaemia have been reported, even years after treatment ends. Due to the potential cardiotoxicity, the maximum cumulative dose is restricted to 120–140 mg/m^2 of body surface, and echocardiograms should be done before and during treatment. Due to this risk of lethal congestive heart failure and therapy-related leukaemia, follow-up evaluation with echocardiography and blood control is highly recommended. Mitoxantrone treatment should accordingly be restricted to only RRMS patients with very high disease activity and insufficient response to available first- and second-line treatments, or SPMS patients experiencing rapid progression. The use of mitoxantrone is rapidly decreasing due to the complication rate of heart failure and leukaemia, and the increasing number of highly effective treatment options.

Clinically Isolated Syndromes and Progressive MS Mitoxantrone has not been included in treatment trials of patients with CIS or primary progressive MS.

Strategy for Disease-Modifying Therapy in MS

The first-line disease-modifying therapy for RRMS include interferon beta, glatiramer acetate, teridlunomide or dimethylfumarate. Treatment should be initiated early for people with active MS disease with evidence of relapses during the past year. Patients with CIS with severe deficit or multifocal presentation and multiple MRI lesions should also be initiated for treatment (interferon beta, glatiramer acetate). Patients must clearly be informed of the potential efficacy and possible side effects of the treatment, and should be followed at regular outpatient clinic visits every 6 months for evaluating efficacy, safety and compliance. Efficacy evaluation should include recording disease activity as measured by relapses and disability progression, as well as MRI. In case of suboptimal compliance or evidence of suboptimal efficacy, adjusting treatment or switching therapy should be considered.

Choosing Among the First-Line Preparations

The pivotal placebo-controlled trials indicate numerically higher efficacy on relapse reduction from dimethyl fumarate (about 45–50%) compared to the other first line preparations (about 30–35%). Head-to-head comparison between dimethyl fumarate and glatiramer acetate indicated numerically (although not statistically significant) better effect from dimethyl fumarate. Head-to-head comparison between teriflunomide and high-frequency interferon beta-1a showed comparable effects on the annual relapse rate. Head-to-head comparisons between intramuscular low-dose and low-frequency interferon beta-1a and subcutaneous high-dose and high-frequency interferon beta-1a and interferon beta-1b have shown that high-dose and high-frequency interferon beta regimens have short-term benefits on the relapse rate and MRI activity. Limitations in the design of these studies have been widely discussed, however, and the long-term differences in efficacy may be reduced by a significantly lower frequency of NAB formation with low-dose and low-frequency interferon beta-1a. Head-to-head comparisons of glatiramer acetate and subcutaneous high-dose and high-frequency interferon beta-1a and interferon beta-1b have also been performed. The results showed identical clinical benefit from the treatments, with some MRI parameters in favour of the interferon beta preparations. Thus, dimethyl fumarate may be preferred first among the first-line preparations (Figure 26.1). In case of intolerability or unacceptable side effects from dimethyl fumarate, one of the other first line preparations should be chosen (Figure 26.1). The efficacy of interferon beta, glatiramer acetate and teriflunomide are comparable. It is therefore most important to carefully evaluate the patient for a treatment regimen, aiming for optimal compliance, considering the administration form and side-effect profiles.

Suboptimal Effect or Compliance In cases of suboptimal efficacy, unacceptable side effects and reduced compliance, switching therapy should be considered. If the treatment effect on interferon beta therapy is suboptimal, NAB analysis should be performed, and NAB-positive patients should be considered for switching to one of the other first line preparations.

Treatment Failure—RRMS In case of breakthrough disease activity on first-line therapy, second-line therapy with natalizumab, fingolimod or alemtuzumab therapy

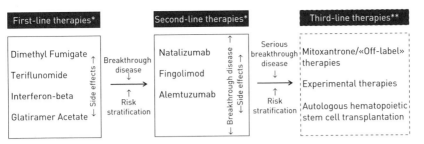

FIGURE 26.1

Treatment algorithm for relapsing–remitting multiple sclerosis.

*Second-line therapy should be considered in case of patients with rapidly evolving severe relapsing–remitting multiple sclerosis.

**Third-line therapy may be considered in some cases with serious and highly active inflammatory disease with breakthrough disease activity on second-line therapies.

is indicated (Figure 26.1). Although the alemtuzumab has an indication in active relapsing-remitting MS, many European neurologists would use this drug as a second line preparation. Natalizumab, fingolimod or alemtuzumab should be considered for RRMS patients who have failed to respond to a full and adequate course (normally at least one year of treatment) of a first-line preparation. Patients should have had at least one relapse in the previous year while on therapy, and have typical MS lesions on cranial MRI. A nonresponder could also be defined as a patient with an unchanged or increased relapse rate or ongoing severe relapses, as compared to the previous year. Second-line therapy may also be considered in case of patients with rapidly evolving severe RRMS defined by two or more disabling relapses in one year, and with gadolinium-enhancing lesions on brain MRI or a significant increase in T2 lesion load as compared to a previous recent MRI. All patients should have a definite MS diagnosis and must undergo risk stratification, and carefully be informed of the potential efficacy and side effects of the treatments. Detailed recommendations have been published on selecting patients, evaluating the effect and monitoring potential side effects, especially PML.

If patients experience breakthrough disease activity on natalizumab treatment, PML has to be ruled out by clinical and MRI examinations and JCV-analysis of the CSF may also be needed. A 3-month washout period has usually been recommended when switching to fingolimod or alemtuzumab, but this may be shortened in JCV-negative patients, and if PML is excluded (by MRI and/or CSF analyses) in JCV-positive patients. In case of disease activity on fingolimod treatment, a two-month washout period is usually recommended before switching to natalizumab or alemtuzumab.

Mitoxantrone may be considered in certain situations when patients experiencing serious breakthrough disease activity on second-line treatments (Figure 26.1). However the use of mitoxantrone has become less frequent due to the effective second-line preparations and the relatively high risk of serious side effects. The risk of PML in JCV-positive patients that previous has received natalizumab must also be included in a risk-benefit evaluation. If mitoxantrone therapy is chosen, the patients must carefully be informed of the potential efficacy and side effects of mitoxantrone (especially the risk of cardiotoxicity and leukaemia). Regular echocardiography with estimation of the left ventricular ejection fraction is mandatory, and continual evaluation of treatment effect, dosage and side effects is important. Patients experiencing serious breakthrough disease activity on second-line treatments, may also be considered for other off-label or experimental therapies, and in some cases also autologous hematopoietic stem cell transplantation (Figure 26.1).

Emerging Therapies Several compounds have shown promising results in modifying the disease course in MS. These include monoclonal antibodies targeting immune molecules such as CD25 (daclizumab) and CD20 (ofatumumab, ocrelizumab) as well as oral preparations such as laquinimod and new sphingosine 1-phosphate modulators. Thus, the treatment options and complexity are increasing, giving hope for improved and individualized therapy in the near future.

CONCLUSION

The diagnosis of MS is based on defining an inflammatory demyelinating disease in the CNS, disseminated in time and space, by clinical examination, supported by MRI and some cases also CSF analyses. Early and accurate diagnosis is important for initiating early treatment. No curative therapy is available, but corticosteroid treatment for relapses, symptomatic treatment and increasingly more effective disease-modifying therapies are available. Disease-modifying therapies should be initiated early, but continuous and careful monitoring is needed for evaluating potential side effects, treatment response and indications for escalating the therapy.

SUGGESTED READING

Compston A, Coles A. Multiple sclerosis. Lancet 2008;372:1502–1517.

Polman CH, Reingold SC, Banwell B et al. Diagnostic criteria for multiple sclerosis: 2010 revisions to the McDonald criteria. Ann Neurol 2011;69:292–302.

Miller DH, Weinshenker BG, Filippi M, et al. Differential diagnosis of suspected multiple sclerosis: a consensus approach. Mult Scler 2008;14:1157–1174.

Myhr KM, Mellgren SI. Corticosteroids in the treatment of multiple sclerosis. Acta Neurol Scand Suppl 2009;(189):73–80.

McGraw CA, Lublin FD. Interferon beta and glatiramer acetate therapy. Neurotherapeutics 2013;10:2–18.

Chataway J, Miller DH. Natalizumab therapy for multiple sclerosis. Neurotherapeutics 2013;10:19–28.

Pelletier D, Hafler DA. Fingolimod for multiple sclerosis. N Engl J Med 2012;366:339–347.

Marriott JJ, Miyasaki JM, Gronseth G et al. The efficacy and safety of mitoxantrone (Novantrone) in the treatment of multiple sclerosis: Report of the Therapeutics and Technology Assessment Subcommittee of the American Academy of Neurology. Neurology 2010;74:1463–1470.

Sørensen PS, Bertolotto A, Edan G, et al. Risk stratification for progressive multifocal leukoencephalopathy in patients treated with natalizumab. Mult Scler 2012;18:143–152.

Baldwin KJ, Hogg JP. Progressive multifocal leukoencephalopathy in patients with multiple sclerosis. Curr Opin Neurol 2013 [Epub ahead of print] PubMed PMID: 23493158.

27 Neuromyelitis Optica

Kjell-Morten Myhr

INTRODUCTION

Neuromyelitis optica (NMO) is a chronic demyelinating disorder with a predilection for the optic nerves and spinal cord that in most cases is associated with autoantibodies to aquaporin-4 (NMO antibodies) water channels. It is distinct from multiple sclerosis (MS), with a higher female preponderance and onset usually above 30 years of age. Most cases have a relapsing-remitting form (80–90%), a monophasic disease is seen among 10–20%, and progressive courses are rare. Untreated, NMO may cause severe disability with visual and motor impairment. The NMO antibodies are probably involved in pathogenesis, and the disease is characterized by focal inflammatory lesions in the CNS with complement-mediated astrocyte damage, followed by granulocyte infiltration, oligodendrocyte death, and ultimately neuronal cell death. Since the lesions are characterized by necrosis of these major CNS cell types, the clinical relapses may often be severe with limited recovery. NMO is, like MS, probably caused by a complex interplay between genetic and environmental factors, although only about 3% of patients with NMO have relatives with the disease compared with about 20% in MS. The distribution of the disease is also different from MS, as it account for only 1–2% of the demyelinating diseases in white people from Europe, North America, or Australia, but higher (20–50%) among people from the West Indies and Asia. The prevalence of neuromyelitis is estimated at 0.5–5.0 per 100,000 inhabitants. The diagnosis is based on a history optic neuritis and myelitis supported by paraclinical and laboratory examination. No curative therapies for NMO is available, but corticosteroid treatment for acute relapses and immunomodulatory or immunosuppressive therapies to prevent new relapses are available

DIAGNOSIS

The diagnosis as based on careful evaluation of the disease history, clinical examination as well as magnetic resonance imaging (MRI) and cerebrospinal fluid examinations, in addition to serological testing for NMO antibodies.

Clinical Presentation

Optic neuritis. NMO is typical associated with manifestation of bilateral simultaneous or sequential optic neuritis, with clinical features of visual loss, pain, and occurrence of positive visual phenomena such as movement-induced phosphenes. The visual loss may be more severe and the remission poorer than seen MS.

Myelitis. Spinal cord involvement in NMO usually presents in a form of complete transverse myelitis with para- or tetraparesis, often with a symmetrical sensory level and sphincter dysfunction. Myelitis in MS is usually milder and asymmetric and caused by acute partial transverse myelitis. Associated radicular pain, paroxysmal tonic spasms, and Lhermitte's may develop. Also signs of nausea, hiccups, and brainstem symptoms may develop due to cranial expansion of the lesion.

Other manifestations have been reported in about 15% of the patients including encephalopathy, hypothalamic dysfunction and cognitive impairment.

Paraclinical and Laboratory Examinations

The diagnostic evaluation for NMO should include MRI and cerebrospinal fluid (CSF) examinations, visual evoked response (VER), as well as NMO antibody analysis.

Magnetic Resonance Imaging

Optic nerve MRI examination shows hyperintensiveT2-weighted lesion, especially in the acute phase, but less often during remission. Acute lesions are also associated gadolinium enhancement on T1-weighted sequences, indicating inflammation and blood–brain barrier disruption.

Spinal cord MRI lesions extending over three or more vertebral segments are typical in NMO, but normal appearances or shorter lesions can be found very early during relapse or in residual atrophic stage. Lesions are most often located in the cervical and thoracic cord. Acute spinal cord lesions involve typical most of the cross-sectional area of the affected segment and are associated with swelling and gadolinium enhancement.

Brain MRI is usually normal in the initial phase, but nonspecific cerebral white matter lesions are to be expected over the course of the disease. Distribution of the less frequent NMO typical brain lesions correspond to structures with high aquaporin-4 expression such as ependymal cells, hypothalamus and brainstem.

Cerebrospinal Fluid

CSF abnormalities include pleocytosis, usually consisting of monocytes and lymphocytes, but neutrophils can also been seen. Pleocytosis is reported more frequent in patients with myelitis than those with optic neuritis. Increased protein levels are present in up to 75% of cases, but oligoclonal bands are less frequent (~0–40%), and can also be transient in contrast to MS.

Visual Evoked Response (VER)

VER is less studied in NMO, but abnormal finding indicating demyelination with delayed conduction is often (>80%) present.

Serum NMO (Aquaporin-4) Antibodies

NMO antibodies may be seen in about 75% of patients with NMO, but may also be seen in patients with longitudinally extensive transverse myelitis (LETM) and recurrent isolated optic neuritis (RION). The presence of NMO antibodies in these conditions seems to be associated with poorer remission and predict new clinical episodes

Table 27.1 Diagnostic Criteria for Neuromyelitis Optica

Two absolute criteria:
- Optic neuritis
- Myelitis

At least two of three supportive criteria:
- The presence of a contiguous spinal cord MRI lesion extending over three or more vertebral segments
- MRI criteria not satisfying the diagnostic criteria for multiple sclerosis
- NMO antibodies in serum

and conversion to NMO. NMO antibodies have been reported to have a sensitivity of about 75% and specificity of more than 90% in NMO.

Diagnostic Criteria

The most widely used diagnostic criteria of NMO (Table 27.1) include the two absolute criteria of a history/presence of optic neuritis and myelitis, in addition of at least two of three supportive criteria including the presence of a contiguous spinal cord MRI lesion extending over three or more vertebral segments; MRI criteria not satisfying the diagnostic criteria for multiple sclerosis; and NMO antibodies in serum.

Conditions not fulfilling the diagnosis of NMO is classifies as NMO spectrum disorders, and include spatially limited forms of the syndrome, such as recurrent longitudinally extensive transverse myelitis (LETM), recurrent inflammatory optic neuritis (RION), bilateral optic neuritis (BON), or atypical presentations associated with serum NMO antibodies.

TREATMENT

No curative treatment is available for NMO, but corticosteroid treatment for relapses and immunomodulatory and immunosuppressive therapies to prevent new relapses are essential. In addition, it is also important to evaluate people with NMO for symptomatic treatment and rehabilitation for various symptoms such as motor weakness, spasticity, pain, and bladder dysfunction.

Treating Relapses

Relapses are the dominant clinical feature of relapsing-remitting NMO with a subacute onset of optic neuritis or myelitis. More rare symptoms like nausea or hiccups may also be the initial symptoms of a new relapse. As in multiple sclerosis, it is important to rule out a pseudo-worsening related to an increase in body temperature or infection.

Intravenous infusion of methylprednisolone (MP) in a dose of 1000 mg daily for 5 days is first-line treatment of NMO relapses. Corticosteroid poorly responsive relapses should be treated with plasma exchange. Some would argue that plasma exchange should be started as early as within five days of starting methylprednisolone in cases of there is no response, and within 10 days if there is only a partial but inadequate response. However, marked improvements can occur even several weeks later. Tapering with oral prednisolone (1 mg/kg) for 2–3 months is also recommended.

Preventing Relapses

Long-term treatment to prevent new relapses and thereby reducing the risk for developing permanent disability should be initiated as soon as the diagnosis of NMO. Seronegative NMO is treated in the same way as seropositive NMO. There are no randomized controlled trials that have evaluated the effect from treatment, and therefore the evidence for favoring specific therapies is weak.

Azathioprine at maintenance doses of 2.5–3.0 mg/kg (divided in two doses) is usual recommended as a first-line therapy. This should be combined with oral prednisolone for 2–3 months until azathioprine becomes effective. Rituximab starting with two doses of 1000 mg intravenous infusions 2 weeks apart and repeated every 6 months would be an alternative. Mycophenolate mofetil can be an effective second-line therapy, and may be quicker acting than azathioprine. A typical starting dose is 500 mg daily that is titrated by 500 mg weekly to a maintenance dose of 1000 mg twice daily. All the suggested therapies need carefully monitoring for potential side effects such as bone marrow depression, infections, gastrointestinal symptoms, and elevated liver enzymes.

NMO spectrum disorders including recurrent LETM, RION, and BON should also receive relapse treatment with methylprednisolone (MP) in a dose of 1000 mg daily for 5 days. Whether these conditions also should receive treatment to prevent new relapses is ccurrently not clear. However, such treatment is often recommended in case of the presence of NMO antibodies and/or severe relapses with poor remission.

CONCLUSION

NMO is usually a chronic relapsing demyelinating disorder with a predilection for the optic nerves and spinal cord, often associated with NMO antibodies, and a high risk of developing severe visual loss and walking disability. Early diagnosis and active relapse treatment, in addition to long-term treatment to prevent new relapses and disability progression is important.

SUGGESTED READING

Lennon VA, Wingerchuk DM, Kryzer TJ, et al. A serum autoantibody marker of neuromyelitis optica: distinction from multiple sclerosis. Lancet 2004;364:2106–2112.

Palace J, Leite MI, Jacob A. A practical guide to the treatment of neuromyelitis optica. Pract Neurol 2012;12:209–214.

Papadopoulos MC, Verkman AS. Aquaporin 4 and neuromyelitis optica. Lancet Neurol 2012;11:535–544.

Sellner J, Boggild M, Clanet M, et al. EFNS guidelines on diagnosis and management of neuromyelitis optica. Eur J Neurol 2010;17:1019–1032.

Wingerchuk DM, Lennon VA, Pittock SJ, et al. Revised diagnostic criteria for neuromyelitis optica. Neurology 2006;66:1485–1489.

Wingerchuk DM, Hogancamp WF, O'Brien PC, et al. The clinical course of neuromyelitis optica (Devic's syndrome). Neurology 1999;53:1107–1114.

SECTION NINE
MOVEMENT DISORDERS AND DEMENTIA

28 Parkinson's Disease

Carlo Colosimo and Luca Marsili

INTRODUCTION

Clinical Picture

Parkinson' disease (PD) is a degenerative disease of the central nervous system clinically characterized by bradykinesia, rigidity, tremor, and postural instability (the latter is a late symptom). These symptoms and their response to dopaminergic agents constitute the basis for a clinical diagnosis of PD. The pathological hallmark of PD is a severe degeneration of the catecholaminergic neurons of the substantia nigra pars compacta and other pigmented nuclei of the brainstem, such as the locus ceruleus and the dorsal motor nucleus of the vagus. In the surviving neurons of these nuclei characteristic intracytoplasmic inclusions, called the Lewy bodies, are observed. The loss of nigrostriatal fibers and the consequent dopamine deficit in the neostriatum constitutes the basis for the use of dopamine replacement therapy in PD. This disease is one of the commonest causes of neurological disability, affecting around 1% of the population over the age of 55 years. The prevalence of the disease in the industrialized countries is 150–200 per 100,000, with a male-to-female ratio of 3:2. This is disease of the presenile age, with a mean age at onset of 58 years and a slowly progressive disorder over the following 15–20 years. The age at onset has a normal distribution, with a minority (8%) of patients starting before the age of 45; this group (young-onset PD) has some peculiar features in term of genetic background, progression of the disease, and response to therapy.

It is mandatory to refer a patient with suspected PD (or parkinsonism) for diagnosis and treatment to a neurologist, preferably to somebody with expertise in movement disorders. Although there is no cure for PD, a number of symptomatic treatments are available for managing both the motor and nonmotor symptoms of this condition. Research is also under way to assess the disease-modifying ability of both standard and newer treatments. The modern treatment of patients with PD and its related disorders implies a multidisciplinary collaboration of the neurologist, other specialists, PD nurse, and general practitioner. In addition to recognizing and treating PD-associated symptoms, the neurologist has a major role in supporting and counseling the patient and their partner or caregiver.

Main Classes of Antiparkinsonian Drugs

Levodopa (and Aromatic Amino Acid Decarboxylase Inhibitors) Levodopa remains the drug with the best therapeutic index for symptomatic antiparkinsonian medication. This compound is the natural precursor of dopamine and is activated

Table 28.1 Synoptic Table of Antiparkinsonian Drugs

Name	Dosage Unit	Daily Dose (mg)	Mechanism of Action
Selegiline	(5–10 mg)	5–10	IMAO-B
Rasagiline	(1 mg)	1	IMAO-B
Trihexyphenidil	(2 mg)	6–8	Anticholinergic
Benzatropine	(0.5; 1; 2 mg)/ampules 2 mL (1 mg/mL)	0.5–8	Anticholinergic
Biperidene	(2 mg; 4 mg CR ; 5 mg/1 mL ampules)	1–12	Anticholinergic
Orphenadrine	(50; 60; 100 mg; 100 mg CR;) ampules 10; 30 mg/mL	60–300	Anticholinergic
Procyclidine	(5 mg)	5–10	Anticholinergic
Amantadine	(100 mg)	200–300	Mixed (Dopamine release enhancer, Anticholinergic, NMDA Antagonist)
Levodopa/ Carbidopa	(100/10 mg; 100/25 mg; 200/50 mg; 250/25 mg) (200/50 mg CR; 100/25 mg CR)	200/50–2000/250	Dopamine precursor/Dopa decarboxylase inhibitor
Levodopa/ Benserazide	(100/25 mg; 200/50 mg) (100/25 mg CR) (100/25 mg dispersible)	200/50–2000/250	Dopamine precursor/Dopa decarboxylase inhibitor
Levodopa/ Carbidopa/ Entacapone	(50/12.5/200 mg; 100/25/200 mg; 150/37.5/200 mg; 200/50/200 mg)	1200/300/1200	Dopamine precursor/Dopa decarboxylase inhibitor/COMT inhibitor
Levodopa/ Carbidopa (intraduodenal)	Intestinal gel (1 mL 20/5 mg)	1–10 mL/hr	Dopamine precursor/Dopa decarboxylase inhibitor
Bromocriptine	(2.5; 5; 10 mg)	7.5 –40	Dopamine agonist
Cabergoline	(0.5; 1; 2 mg)	2–10	Dopamine agonist
Pergolide	(0.05; 0.25; 1 mg)	1.5–6	Dopamine agonist
Dihydroergo-cryptine	(20 mg)	20–120	Dopamine agonist
Ropinirole	(0.25; 0.5; 1; 2; 5 mg)	4–24	Dopamine agonist
Ropinirole ER	(2; 4; 8 mg)		
Pramipexole	(0.18; 0.7 mg)	3–4.5	Dopamine agonist
Pramipexole ER	(0.26; 0.52; 1.0 mg)		Dopamine agonist
Piribedil	(20 mg; 50 mg CR)	20–100	Dopamine agonist
Rotigotine (trasdermal)	Patch (2; 4; 6; 8 mg)	4–8	Dopamine agonist

(continued)

Table 28.1 Continued

Name	Dosage Unit	Daily Dose (mg)	Mechanism of Action
Apomorphine (subcutaneous)	Ampules (30 mg/3 mL; 50 mg/5 mL)	10–100	Dopamine agonist
Entacapone	(200 mg)	400–1200	COMT inhibitor
Tolcapone	(100 mg)	300–600	COMT inhibitor

through its decarboxylation by the cytosolic aromatic amino acid decarboxylase (AADC). As AADC is not rate-limiting, the higher the concentration of levodopa administered, the greater is the production of dopamine. Since 1975, combinations of levodopa with the AADC peripheral inhibitors (decarboxylase inhibitors [DCIs]) carbidopa and benserazide have been used for symptomatic replacement therapy, thereby allowing the administration of levodopa at doses that are approximately four times lower than levodopa alone and reducing dopaminergic side effects (Table 28.1). In commercially available preparations, levodopa is combined in a single tablet with carbidopa at a 1:10 or 1:5 ratio (Sinemet˙) or with benserazide at a 1:4 ratio (Madopar˙). The usual initial dosage of levodopa is 50–100 mg twice daily to three times daily; it can progressively be titrated up to an individual's optimal dosage (100–250 three or four times daily). In advanced and very severe cases, the total levodopa daily dose may reach 1.5–2 g, divided in 6–8 administrations. Levodopa is a very effective drug, but its long-term use is classically associated with motor complications (fluctuations and dyskinesia): these complications develop in the vast majority of PD patients, with an approximate rate of 10% per year. Since standard levodopa has a very short half-life (~90 minutes), controlled-release formulations of levodopa/carbidopa in a polymer matrix (Sinemet CR˙) have been specifically studied to produce delayed enteric absorption (with a 3- to 4-hour half-life) and possibly reduce long-term complications; unfortunately, the onset of the effects is slower occurring after 40–60 minutes, and often inconsistent. A similar controlled-release preparation of Madopar˙ has been marketed in Europe. The use of controlled-release formulations of levodopa is not recommended in early PD, whereas they may be considered in patients with mild fluctuations of the wearing-off type or in cases with significant nocturnal problems. When switching between levodopa preparations, it should be remembered that bioavailability of CR preparations is 70–80% of the immediate-release ones. Soluble levodopa preparations are also available; designed for faster onset of symptomatic effects, they are an useful adjunct in kick-starting immediately on wakening or in case of sudden "offs" during the day.

Possible side effects of levodopa, which include gastrointestinal adverse reactions such as nausea, vomiting and constipation, may be treated with the peripheral dopamine receptor blocker domperidone 10–20 mg three times daily. Orthostatic hypotension, hallucinations and mental confusion have also been described during levodopa therapy. Dopamine-induced hallucinations are most often visual, though they may also present under other sensory forms. The occurrence and severity of hallucinations increase in many patients over time and may eventually develop into full-blown psychosis with delusions.

In selected cases of advanced PD patients, levodopa may be administered continuously under the form of a gel called Duodopa˚, through a nasogastric tube or percutaneous gastrostomy connected to a portable pump. Complications of the duodenal infusion of levodopa/carbidopa gel are not infrequent, and usually related to the gastrostomy or to the dislocation or occlusion of the intestinal tube. The duodenal infusion of Duodopa˚ has also been linked to elevated plasmatic homocysteine levels and vitamin deficiency (B6 and B12), with consequent reversible metabolic axonal neuropathy or encephalopathy.

Dopamine Agonists Dopamine agonists (DA) are synthetic drugs that act directly on striatal postsynaptic dopamine receptors. They are divided in two main classes: ergot-derived and non–ergot-derived. Ergot-derived drugs, such as bromocriptine, cabergoline, lisuride, dihydroergocryptine and pergolide, are all second-line drugs because of their possible severe side effects, which include retroperitoneal, pleuropulmonary and valvular heart fibrosis. Nonergot compounds, such as pramipexole (D2-D3 agonist), ropinirole (D2-D3-D4 agonist), piribedil (D2-D3 agonist and α2 antagonist), and rotigotine (D1-D2-D3 agonist), are widely used for initial monotherapy of PD, or as adjunctive therapy to levodopa. Apomorphine, the first agonist to be synthesized, is also part of this class and has been the object of renewed interest in recent years. Apomorphine acts powerfully on D1 and D2 dopamine receptors and has the most complete pharmacological profile of all clinically available DA. Unfortunately, because of is poor oral bioavailability, apomorphine has to be administered subcutaneously.

To find the optimum dose and to avoid side effects, all agonists must be progressively titrated during the first 3–4 weeks of therapy. Classical formulations are usually given three times daily, though extended-release formulations given once daily are now available for ropinirole and pramipexole (oral preparations) as well as for rotigotine (the only one marketed as transdermal formulations). DA monotherapy induces fewer long-term motor complications, such as dyskinesia or wearing-off, than levodopa monotherapy. The motor benefit (i.e., reduction in the Unified PD Rating Scale score) when a DA is used alone is less marked than that achieved by using levodopa, and this difference increases as the disease progresses. Consequently, the vast majority of the patients requires add-on levodopa after some years. The adverse effects of dopamine agonists include nausea, daytime somnolence, confusion, hallucinations, leg edema, orthostatic hypotension, and erythromelalgia (ergot derivatives). The advantages and disadvantages of the various orally active DA should be compared in clinical practice. All available DA, with the exception of apomorphine, share the same efficacy profile (global class effect). However, the level of evidence available for the different drugs tends to vary because the effects of some older DA have never been thoroughly assessed. The best levels of evidence are, consequently, associated with newer nonergot derivatives, despite a lack of empirical evidence that older agonists are less effective that more recent ones. Safety is another critical aspect. Indeed, since fibrotic type B reactions appear to be much more frequent on ergot than on nonergot derivatives, ergot DA are no longer considered as the first-line drug therapy when treatment with this class of drugs is initiated.

It has frequently been reported that impulse control disorders (ICDs), defined as a failure to resist an impulse or temptation that is harmful to oneself or others, may develop in PD as a consequence of dopaminergic therapy. The prevalence of ICDs in some studies is as high as 14%, while the most commonly reported ICDs are pathological gambling, hypersexuality, compulsive shopping, and compulsive eating. Although some authors have claimed that ICDs are associated above all with treatment using nonergot compounds, these adverse events appear to represent a class effect of dopaminergic drugs that is not strictly specific to any compound. Though levodopa has also been reported to induce ICDs, it does so to a far lesser extent than DA.

Apomorphine has a limited but important role in cases with severe motor fluctuations; this compound when given subcutaneously, either by multiple injections or (better) continuous infusion with a portable pump, consistently reverses levodopa-resistant "off" periods. Studies based on this approach have revealed a significant reduction in "off" time and good drug tolerability. Parenteral apomorphine has been also used in PD to replace levodopa after major surgery or to treat the malignant syndrome induced by sudden levodopa withdrawal. The main side effect has been the occurrence of nodular skin lesions at the site of injection, particularly when continuous infusions are used.

Monoamine Oxidase-B (MAO-B) Enzyme Inhibitors These drugs, initially developed as antidepressants, are potent, irreversible, selective inhibitors of MAO-B that reduce the catabolism of dopamine and, in turn, increase the availability of this neurotransmitter at the synaptic level. The two compounds available on the market are selegiline and rasagiline, both of which have a moderate symptomatic benefit on PD cardinal symptoms, as well as on fatigue and mood, when used in early PD. They have also a marginal role, as an adjunct therapy to levodopa, in advanced PD. Their possible neuroprotective, or disease-modifying, role on dopamine cell loss is as yet unclear. Rasagiline is given at a dose of 1 mg once daily and selegiline at 5–10 mg once daily; titration is not required. Infrequent side effects are insomnia, nausea, dizziness and orthostatic hypotension. There are no direct comparative trials between selegiline and rasagiline. Drug interactions leading to a serotonin syndrome type may occur on rare occasions when MAO-B inhibitors are combined with some selective serotonin reuptake inhibitors (SSRIs) or with meperidine.

Catechol-*O*-methyltransferase (COMT) Enzyme Inhibitors Many patients with advanced disease experience a reduction in the bioavailability of levodopa, which causes motor fluctuations that are initially of the wearing-off type and then become less predictable. Add-on COMT inhibiting drugs may be used to extend the effects of levodopa and reduce these phenomena. These compounds, named tolcapone and entacapone, delay the enzymatic degradation of levodopa and dopamine; they are always administrated together with levodopa. Tolcapone, which exerts its effects at both the central peripheral levels, increases the release of dopamine in the central nervous system and is more powerful and longer-acting than entacapone. The side effects of tolcapone include urine dyscoloration, diarrhea and, in rare cases, serious hepatotoxicity. Since a small number of cases of sudden hepatic failure have been reported, tolcapone is now regarded as a second-choice drug. Informed consent is required and liver function tests must be monitored every 2 weeks for the first year of administration, every 4 weeks for the subsequent 6 months, and every 8 weeks thereafter.

Entacapone exerts its effects exclusively at the peripheral level and has a milder effect than tolcapone but is safer than the latter (side effects include increase of dyskinesia, urine discoloration, diarrhea). The dosage given with each dose of levodopa (three times daily or more frequently) is 200 mg and no liver function monitoring is required. The results of a recent study suggest that initiating levodopa therapy with entacapone in early PD is not recommended, limiting the indication for this compound to patients already experiencing fluctuations. In order to increase patients' compliance, a combination medication that contains levodopa, carbidopa, and entacapone has been marketed in the last decade (Stalevo˚).

Amantadine Amantadine is an old antiviral compound that may be used for initial symptomatic PD therapy. Although its mechanisms of action have yet to be fully understood, they are known to include not only dopaminergic action, but also antiglutamatergic and anticholinergic properties. Amantadine in PD patients helps to reduce parkinsonian signs, particularly tremor, at any stage of the disease, whereas in advanced PD it can be used to reduce dyskinesia, with a mild-to-moderate efficacy being attained in approximately half of the cases. The usual dosage is 100 mg two or three times a day. Side effects include insomnia, constipation, xerostomia, blurred vision, hallucinations, erythromelalgia, and livedo reticularis.

Anticholinergics Anticholinergics (*antimuscarinics)* are old drugs that may be still used in young patients with early PD and severe tremor. Owing to their common neuropsychiatric (memory loss, confusion) and autonomic (constipation, urinary retention, dry mouth) side effects and their limited clinical efficacy, these drugs are not recommended in elderly patients. The main compounds of anticholinergics are trihexyphenidyl and biperidene (2 mg three times daily).

Neuroprotective Agents Neuroprotection refers to a treatment that modifies the natural history of PD, reducing dopaminergic cell loss and disease progression. There is not as yet sufficient evidence to unequivocally demonstrate that substances such as antioxidant vitamins, coenzyme Q 10, creatine, dopamine agonists and inhibitors of MAO-B exert a neuroprotective effect in PD.

Pharmacological Treatment

The treatment of the main motor disorders of PD should take into account several crucial factors such as age at onset, disease duration, occupation, comorbidities, and patients' expectations. In Figures 28.1 through 28.4 are reported flow charts with the current recommendations for early (untreated), advanced, and dyskinetic (peak-dose and dyphasic) PD patients.

For delayed on status or complete dose failure, in the advanced stages of the disease, the gold standard is to optimize levodopa treatment (see flow charts 2–4). In addition, it could be useful to chew the tablets instead of swallowing them and to take medication on an empty stomach, to achieve a quicker onset of action of each dose. To get a more stable response to levodopa therapy, with caution (avoid malnutrition), dietary protein restriction has shown some results. When severe recurrent off periods appear in advanced PD (wearing off), levodopa may need to be administered up every 2 hours during the waking day (occasionally with additional doses during the night) and the total daily requirement of the drug may reach 1500 mg or more (see flow chart 2). In this situation, however, dopamine-related side effects may become severe, often forcing to reduce the total dose of levodopa.

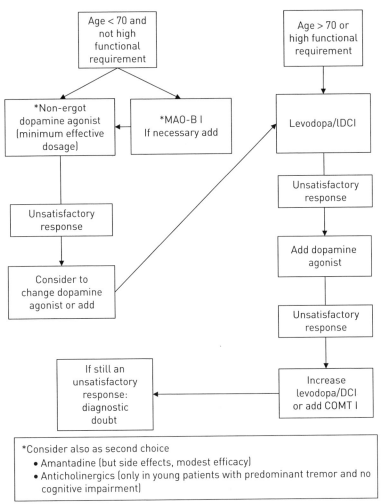

FIGURE 28.1

Management of Early PD.

MAO-B I: monoamineoxidase B inhibitors; COMT I: Cathecol-O-methyltransferase inhibitors; DCI: Dopadecarboxylase inhibitors.

Waking-day subcutaneous apomorphine or intraduodenal soluble levodopa remain an option, when the above mentioned measures are ineffective. They can be proposed before functional neurosurgery, or when this is contraindicated.

Nonpharmacological Treatment

Physical Therapy Most studies of physical therapy, speech therapy, and rehabilitation programs as an adjunctive therapy in PD report improvement in at least one outcome measure. However, it is difficult to interpret the clinical value of these improvements, and particularly its long-term cost-effectiveness. For the often disabling symptom of freezing of gait the use of alternative motor strategies (e.g., starting to walk with a military step, marching on the spot before beginning walking, making oscillatory trunk movements), or the addition of auditory or visual stimuli (walking in time to

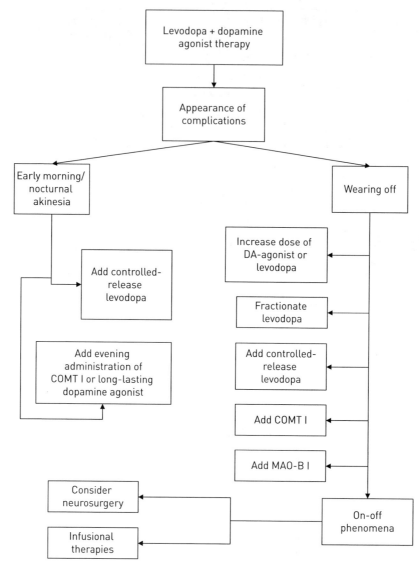

FIGURE 28.2
Management of advanced PD.

a metronome, following the lines of the paving stones, attempting to reach a target placed on the floor) may be useful.

Surgical Therapy The surgical interventions performed in PD, which were first proposed in the mid 1940s, are targeted lesions and deep brain stimulation (DBS) in basal ganglia areas. Thalamotomy and pallidotomy (more often unilateral), which was initially the intervention of choice, improve mainly tremor and dyskinesia on the contralateral side of the body in approximately 80% of cases. Several side effects are linked to this type of surgery: symptomatic infarction is documented in 3.9% of patients (with a mortality rate about 1.2%), while speech problems, facial paresis, and depression are even more

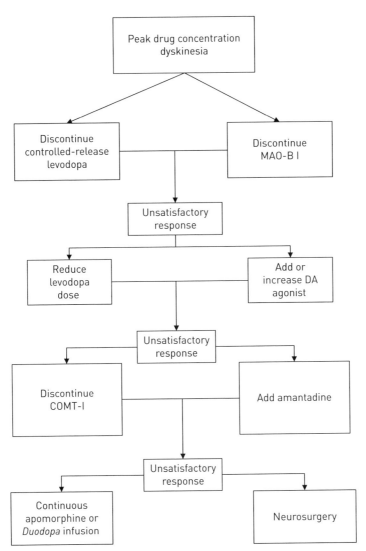

FIGURE 28.3
Management of PD with peak-dose dyskinesia.

frequent. DBS is a more modern technique, consisting in the stimulation through electrodes of the subthalamic nucleus (STN) or the internal pallidum. Both lead to a significant improvement in dyskinesia, a decrease in the severity and frequency of motor blocks; STN-DBS also leads to a reduction of up to 60% in levodopa intake. STN-DBS is now considered more effective than pallidal DBS by most authors. There are two types of adverse effects: those related to surgery (ischemic stroke, hemorrhage, seizures, mental confusion), and those related to electrode dysfunction (infections, fibrosis, need for repositioning of stimulator). Cognitive deficit and severely depressed mood are exclusion criteria because they may be exacerbated by DBS. Weight gain, dysphagia, apathy, and oculomotor disturbances have also been described following DBS.

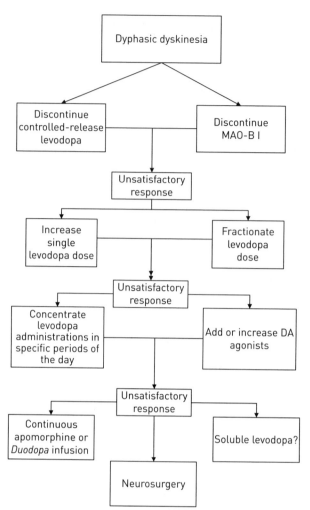

FIGURE 28.4
Management of PD with dyphasic dyskinesia.

Non–Motor Symptoms Treatment

Non–motor symptoms (NMS) occur across all stages of PD, are still underreported, and are a key determinant of quality of life of the patients; NMS are gaining increasing relevance in the management of patients with PD, and the use of dedicated questionnaires and scales may facilitate their clinical recognition and assessment. Several studies have now shown that almost all PD patients complained of one or more NMS (cognitive, behavioral, sleep, cardiovascular, gastrointestinal, genitourinary), all emphasizing their clinical relevance for both patients and care-givers. NMS may show a variable response to antiparkinsonian medications (Table 28.2), suggesting that NMS impairment is variably driven by dopaminergic denervation, whereas other drugs may be helpful for specific symptoms.

NMS Treatment Approach

Dementia The prevalence of dementia in idiopathic PD ranges from 20% to 40% according to different studies. The most frequent clinical pictures are mental slowness, frontal behavior, and psychotic features. In cases of dementia, drugs such as

Table 28.2 PD Symptoms Poorly Responsive to Dopaminergic Drugs

Postural instability

Freezing

Trunk postural abnormalities

Dysarthria

Dementia

REM sleep behaviour disorder

Orthostatic hypotension

Constipation

Bladder hyperreflexia

Sweating abnormalities

Sensory phenomena

Modified from Jankovic and Marsden. Therapeutic strategies in Parkinson's disease, in *Parkinson's Disease & Movement Disorders*, Tolosa E & Jankovic J (eds), Williams & Wilkins; 3rd edition, 1998.

central-acting anticholinergics, tricyclic antidepressants, tolterodine, oxybutynin, and benzodiazepines must be discontinued, if they are being used. A second step is to add acetylcholinesterase (AChE) inhibitors, such as rivastigmine, donepezil, and galantamine. It should be borne in mind, however, that the cognitive improvement achieved by adding AChE inhibitors may be relatively modest in such patients, and that tremor may be worsened. Other possible reasons for discontinuing AChE inhibitors are side effects such as nausea, vomiting and cardiac arrhythmias.

Psychosis All antiparkinsonian medications may cause delirium or transient psychosis, which are among the most disabling nonmotor complications of PD. Since infections and metabolic disorders can trigger psychosis, this potential underlying cause should be investigated in such cases (Table 28.3). The following step is to withdraw anticholinergic drugs, dopamine agonists and MAO-B inhibitors. As a rule, an antiparkinsonian polypharmacy is not recommended; indeed, patients should receive a single-drug therapy with carbidopa/levodopa at the lowest dose possible. Atypical

Table 28.3 Management of Psychotic Symptoms in PD: Sequential Approach

Remove trigger factors (dehydration, infections)

Stop unnecessary drugs

Stop antiparkinsonian drugs

    Anticholinergics

    Amantadine

    MAO-B inhibitors

    Dopamine agonists

    COMT-inhibitors

    Levodopa (dose reduction only)

Introduce atypical antipsychotics

    Clozapine

    Quetiapine

Consider cholinesterase inhibitors

antipsychotics, such as clozapine (12.5–75 mg at bedtime) are first-line drug therapy, according to current evidence. Leukopenia and agranulocytosis, despite being very rare, do occur as adverse events of clozapine use, so patients must be monitored by means of complete weekly blood counts for the first 18–24 weeks of treatment. Quetiapine (25–100 mg at bedtime) is a valid substitute and does not require blood counts. Olanzapine, risperidone, and typical (classical) antipsychotics should not be used because they clinically exacerbate parkinsonism. Evidence has recently emerged that AChE inhibitors may improve psychosis in PD.

Depression Depression affects about 40% of PD patients. It may occur at any stage of the disease, or even before the onset of motor symptoms. In PD patients who do not have optimal control of the motor disorder, it is important to optimize antiparkinsonian therapy (e.g., by introducing DA, which could have a secondary antidepressant effect as shown by recent reports). Specific therapeutic options are tricyclic antidepressants and SSRIs. Tricyclic drugs are those with the best evidence of efficacy. Conversely, SSRIs are less likely to produce cardiovascular or gastrointestinal side effects in PD patients than tricyclics, but when added to dopaminergic therapy they may induce a "serotonin syndrome." Other mixed action antidepressants such as reboxetine and venlafaxine are reported to be useful in PD-associated depression.

Sleep Disturbances Sleep disorders are common in PD (~65% prevalence), being even more frequent in patients with cognitive deficits. As some patients do not sleep comfortably because of their rigidity, they may require more dopaminergic medications. Patients who experience nocturnal insomnia may be treated with antidepressants or sedatives. Daytime somnolence is typical in patients treated with DA. Stimulant drugs such as modafinil (100–200 mg), methylphenidate (5–10 mg), and caffeine have been proposed as a means of reducing excessive daytime sleepiness. REM sleep behavior disorder (RBD) is a frequent and clinically relevant nocturnal disturbance for all stages of PD. It increases with age and disease duration and may contribute to the nocturnal problems of patients with PD and their bed partners. Clonazepam has been the drug of choice in those without significant cognitive impairment nor obstructive sleep apnea, and is usually effective at 0.25–0.5 mg/night, but doses above 1 mg nightly are necessary in some patients. Recent experience with melatonin shows that doses ranging from 3 to 12 mg/night can be effective either as sole therapy, or in conjunction with clonazepam.

Orthostatic Hypotension Cardiovascular autonomic dysfunction leading to orthostatic hypotension is common in PD (up to 50% of the cases). It sometimes represents a side effect of symptomatic medical therapy of PD: levodopa, DA, selegiline, and amantadine may all induce or increase orthostatic hypotension. General measures include safety measures, such as avoiding exposure to warm environments, alcohol and antihypertensive drugs. Increasing salt intake and wearing elastic stockings may also help to avoid orthostatic hypotension. In patients in whom orthostatic hypotension only occurs postprandially, the size of individual meals should be reduced. Specific symptomatic therapies may consist of adrenergic drugs, such as midodrine (2.5–5 mg three times daily), and/or mineralocorticoids (fludrocortisone 0.1–0.3 mg daily). The side effects of the frequent use of corticosteroids are hypertension, hypokalemia, and ankle edema.

Erectile Dysfunction Phosphodiesterase inhibitors, such as sildenafil or tadalafil, can be used to effectively treat erectile dysfunction in PD. Side effects include flushing, headache, visual blurring, priapism, and, in rare cases, severe hypotension and cardiac arrest. Adding DA such as apomorphine or pergolide may also improve erectile function.

Urinary Incontinence Detrusor hyperactivity with urge incontinence is frequent in PD. This bothersome symptom may be treated by adding anticholinergic compounds that act at the peripheral level, such as oxybutinin, tolterodine, and amitriptyline; oxybutinin is also available as a long-acting (3-day) patch. Other general measures include reducing the intake of water, or other drinks, before bedtime.

Gastrointestinal Problems Reduced gastric motility and constipation, which are frequent symptoms in PD, are often aggravated by antiparkinsonian medications. General measures need to be adopted to avoid constipation, such as a correct diet (with plenty of liquids and high-fiber foods); it may be eventually needed to reduce the dose, or eliminate, some of the antiparkinsonian drugs (particularly anticholinergics), and to use laxatives (macrogol). Domperidone (10–20 mg three times daily), a peripheral dopamine receptor blocker, reduces several dopamine-related gastrointestinal symptoms, such as nausea, anorexia, bloating, and constipation.

Sialorrhea This is frequent and bothersome symptom in advanced PD. Botulinum toxins type A and B, injected percutaneously in the salivary glands, are efficacious and with limited side-effects.

SUGGESTED READING

Berardelli A, Wenning GK, Antonini A, et al. EFNS/MDS-ES/ENS recommendations for the diagnosis of Parkinson's disease. Eur J Neurol 2013;20:16–34.

Chaudhuri KR, Schapira AH. Non-motor symptoms of Parkinson's disease: Dopaminergic pathophysiology and treatment. Lancet Neurol 2009;8:464–474.

Fox SH, Katzenschlager R, Lim SY, et al. The Movement Disorder Society Evidence-Based Medicine Review Update: Treatments for the motor symptoms of Parkinson's disease. Mov Disord 2011;26(Suppl 3):S2–S41.

Goetz CG, Poewe W, Rascol O, et al. Evidence-based medical review update: Pharmacological and surgical treatments of Parkinson's disease: 2001 to 2004. Mov Disord 2005;20:523–539.

Horstink M, Tolosa E, Bonuccelli U, et al. European Federation of Neurological Societies; Movement Disorder Society-European Section. Review of the therapeutic management of Parkinson's disease. Report of a joint task force of the European Federation of Neurological Societies (EFNS) and the Movement Disorder Society-European Section (MDS-ES). Part II: Late (complicated) Parkinson's disease. Eur J Neurol 2006;13:1186–1202.

Horstink M, Tolosa E, Bonuccelli U, et al. European Federation of Neurological Societies; Movement Disorder Society-European Section. Review of the therapeutic management of Parkinson's disease. Report of a joint task force of the European Federation of Neurological Societies and the Movement Disorder Society-European Section. Part I: Early (uncomplicated) Parkinson's disease. Eur J Neurol 2006;13:1170–1185.

Miyasaki JM, Martin W, Suchowersky O, et al. Practice parameter: initiation of treatment for Parkinson's disease: An evidence-based review: Report of the Quality Standards Subcommittee of the American Academy of Neurology. Neurology 2002;58:11–17.

Rascol O, Goetz C, Koller W, et al. Treatment interventions for Parkinson's disease: an evidence based assessment. Lancet 2002;359:1589–1598.

29 Atypical and Secondary Parkinsonism

Luca Marsili and Carlo Colosimo

ATYPICAL PARKINSONISM

Atypical parkinsonism (AP) consists in a heterogeneous group of neurodegenerative pathologies that include both α-synucleinopathies (multiple system atrophy [MSA] and dementia with Lewy bodies [DLB]) and tauopathies (progressive supranuclear palsy [PSP] and corticobasal degeneration [CBD]) (see Table 29.1). In all these disorders, parkinsonian signs are accompanied by signs of other neuronal systems dysfunction, such as ataxia, autonomic dysfunction, pyramidal involvement, and dementia. In addition, all these conditions are characterized by a general poor response to levodopa and a faster disease progression compared with Parkinson disease (PD). We review here the symptomatic therapy of these diseases, including DLB, which, because of the constant association of cognitive and behavioral features with the motor disorder, is also discussed in the section on dementia (chapter 32).

MSA

This is a relatively rare presenile degenerative disorder, in which parkinsonian features are usually combined with dysautonomia and cerebellar ataxia. To date, there is no real effective treatment for the cerebellar features of the disease and medical treatment is mainly focused on the parkinsonian signs and dysautonomia.

Treatment of Parkinsonism

Levodopa response in MSA is variably seen 30–70% of the patients, and it should be tested by giving at least for 2 months increasing doses of this compound, beginning with 100 mg (with a decarboxylase inhibitor) three times daily up to 1000 mg per day. The response typically declines after a few years of treatment. Peak-dose dyskinesia emerges in half of the patients treated with levodopa and they are commonly dystonic and mainly affecting the orofacial region. For doses and formulations of levodopa in MSA and other forms of AP, see the section on PD (chapter 28).

Dopamine agonists (see also the section on PD) are no more effective than levodopa and usually poorly tolerated by many patients. To date, literature about the use of these compounds in MSA is scarce and only small trials with bromocriptine and lisuride are available, showing only minor clinical effects. Therefore, they are not routinely

Table 29.1 Classification of Parkinsonism

Primary parkinsonism
Idiopathic Parkinson's disease
Juvenile hereditary parkinsonism
Dopa-responsive dystonia
Secondary parkinsonism
Drugs
    Neuroleptics, calcium channel blockers, antiemethics, litium, SSRI
Vascular
Infectious
    Encephalitis letargica, AIDS, syphilis, fungal, CJD
Metabolic
    Basal ganglia calcification/parathyroid abnormalities
    Acquired hepatolenticular degeneration
Hydrocephalus
Neoplastic
Psychogenic parkinsonism
Toxins
    MPTP, carbon monoxide, manganese, ethanol
Traumatic
Atypical parkinsonism
Multiple system atrophy
    Cerebellar type
    Parkinsonian type
Dementia syndromes
    Dementia with Lewy bodies, Alzheimer's disease,
Progressive supranuclear palsy
    Richardson's syndrome
    PSP-parkinsonism
    Pure akinesia with gait freezing
Corticobasal degeneration
Progressive pallidal, pallidonigral, and pallidoluysionigral degenerations
Heredodegenerative disorders
Wilson's disease
Huntington's disease
Neuroacanthocytosis
Frontotemporal dementia-parkinsonism linked to chromosome 17
Familial basal ganglia calcifications (Fahr's disease)
Neurodegeneration with brain iron accumulation
Pantotenate kinase–associated neurodegeneration
Fatty acid hydroxylase–associated neurodegeneration
Mitochondrial protein–associated neurodegeneration
Spinocerebellar ataxias

AIDS, acquired immune deficiency syndrome; CJD, Creutzfeldt–Jacob disease; MPTP, 1-methyl-4-phenyl-4-propionoxypiperidine; PSP, progressive supranuclear palsy; SSRI, selective serotonin reuptake inhibitor. Modified from Kompoliti and Goetz, 2005.

recommended in the treatment of the motor disorder of MSA. Amantadine is a drug with mixed pharmacological properties (including NMDA receptor antagonist), which has been occasionally reported to be beneficial in MSA; however, open trials and a small controlled study using also high doses (up to 600 mg per day) have not shown any significant antiparkinsonian benefit in MSA patients. Anticholinergics are usually used to treat hypersalivation (see later), since they are not particularly effective in improving motor symptoms.

Blepharospasm and limb dystonia are frequently observed in MSA patients and may respond well to local injections of botulinum toxin A, which is different from antecollis, in which the treatment does not lead to significant benefit and is often complicated by dysphagia.

Surgical strategies such as subthalamic deep brain stimulation (DBS) or pallidotomy have been used in selected cases to treat parkinsonian signs and dystonic postures with only partial benefits, but they are not routinely recommended for this condition.

To date, clinical trials exploring disease-modifying therapies in MSA have failed to show any change in the natural history of this severe disease.

Treatment of Autonomic Dysfunction

Cardiovascular Symptoms
Orthostatic hypotension can be alleviated avoiding trigger factors (e.g., abundant meals, drugs, alcohol). Elastic stockings, increased dietary salt, head-up tilt of the bed, and, when indicated, cardiac pacing may be used as other nonpharmacological support. When needed, several drugs can be employed: midodrine (α1-agonist) is the first line treatment for orthostatic hypotension (standard dosage: 2.5–10 mg three times daily). Alternatives are fludrocortisone and desmopressin, which reduce natriuresis and expand plasma volume, clonidine and yohimbine, which induce release of noradrenaline, and ergot derivatives which act on α-2 receptors with a vasoconstrictor effect. Droxidopa (L-threo-DOPS), a precursor of noradrenaline, has been investigated in phase 3 trials for neurogenic orthostatic hypotension also in MSA but the results are not univocal. Over time, clinostatic hypertension could usually associate with orthostatic hypotension and it has to be treated if systolic blood pressure exceeds 180–200 mm Hg. Evening time short-acting calcium-antagonists or ACE inhibitors are the standard treatment for clinostatic hypertension.

Sialorrhea should be treated, as we mentioned above, with oral anticholinergics or with botulinum toxin type A or B injections in the salivary glands (20–50 onabotulinumtoxin A U per side).

Genitourinary Symptoms
Anticholinergics with peripheral action (e.g., oxybutynin 2.5–5 mg twice daily or three times daily) may be used for detrusor hyperreflexia, but not infrequently they cause urinary retention. Sometimes desmopressin given at night may reverse nocturia; when incomplete bladder emptying appears, intermittent or permanent catheterization is required. Recent data show that bladder hyperreflexia or associated prostatic hyperplasia can be treated using botulinum toxin A injections.

Male impotence, almost universal in MSA, can be treated using different molecules as sildenafil or tadalafil but with the risk of inducing or aggravating orthostatic hypotension. Other therapeutic choices are prostaglandins, intracavernosal papaverine, or, eventually, penile implants.

Respiratory Symptoms

Continuous positive airway pressure may be helpful in selected cases with sleep apnea or when laryngeal stridor become prominent. Tracheostomy could be necessary in some cases in the advanced phase of the disease, but its feasibility should be always well-discussed in advance with the patient and the caregivers.

DLB

DLB is the second most common form of degenerative dementia, in which cognitive dysfunction is variably associated with behavioral and sleep disorders, parkinsonism and autonomic dysfunction. Response to levodopa therapy is reduced in DLB patients compared to PD patients, and may precipitate psychosis. In the course of DLB, psychotic features can be treated with low-dose clozapine (but 6 months of continuous weekly followed by 6 months of continuous biweekly white blood cell count is required). Randomized controlled trials indicate that quetiapine is less effective than clozapine to treat psychotic symptoms. Cholinesterase inhibitors, especially rivastigmine, are a therapeutic alternative for treating both psychotic and cognitive symptoms. Anticholinergics often induce delirium in demented patients, so it is important to avoid this kind of drugs. The same problem is associated with the use of dopamine agonists and amantadine. The following therapeutic algorithm for drug treatment is suggested: at first is important to stop anticholinergics and other second-line antiparkinsonian medications and if necessary to reduce levodopa. Cholinesterase inhibitors should be used until the maximum tolerated dose. If there is no adequate response, quetiapine is recommended and if is not effective, it could be switched to clozapine.

Recent RCTs tested the efficacy of the NMDA receptor antagonist memantine in patients with DLB, showing significant improvement of clinical global impression of change and behavioral symptoms in these patients. These studies demonstrated that memantine could be a valid therapeutic option for treatment of DLB patients.

PSP

This is a progressive and severe degenerative disease severe, which in its classic form, redenominated Richardson's syndrome (RS), is characterized by early impairment of vertical eye movements and of balance (leading to repeated falls). Axial rigidity, pseudobulbar signs and fronto-limbic dementia are other common features of RS. Symptomatic therapy with levodopa has poor efficacy in RS, while a better response is often reported in another and less common clinical variant, denominated PSP-parkinsonism (PSP-P) which may be initially confused with PD.

Evidence with symptomatic therapy of PSP is very scarce. Levodopa response should be always tested with modalities similar those described for MSA. Amantadine has several modes of action that may help patients with PSP. Despite less than 10% of PSP patients reporting significant benefit in gait freezing, speech or swallowing, amantadine should be probably tried (100 mg twice to t.i.d. daily) in all patients with PSP, except those with severe constipation or dementia. If no benefit is observed after one month it should be then tapered and discontinued. In a small double blind trial amitriptyline improved rigidity muscle pain, hypophonia, and dysphagia in three of four PSP patients. Amitriptyline is usually started at a dosage of 10 mg/day at bedtime, up to the maximum dosage of 20 to 25 mg twice daily. Some patients report worsening of postural instability. Botulinum toxin A is indicated for blepharospasm (and eyelid opening apraxia) and in some cases for severe retrocollis and arm dystonia. The main adverse effects to avoid in PSP patients when treating neck muscles are dysphagia and "floppy" neck. Other important strategies in management of PSP patients include SSRIs for depression and pseudobulbar symptoms, with very little evidence to guide this choice; benzodiazepines and related drugs (zolpidem) are used for primary insomnia and frequent awakenings, and—according to a few reports—zolpidem could also improve motor features of PSP. In addition, consideration should be given to early addition of vitamin D and calcium supplements to promote bone mineralization and minimize fracture risk. A hip protector should also be considered in those at high risk of falls.

To date, no disease-modifying agents are currently indicated for PSP. However, in a small pilot trial coenzyme Q10, a compound that has an antioxidant effect and could improve mitochondrial dysfunction in PSP, was compared with placebo and was able to improve cerebral metabolism, and some clinical features of the disease. The long-term effect of coenzyme Q10 administration (doses are up to 1200 mg per day) on disease progression in PSP is still under investigation and large controlled trials are needed.

CBD

The classic clinical phenotype of CBD (asymmetric akinetic-rigid syndrome, dystonia of affected hand, alien limb, myoclonus, abnormal eye movements, dysarthria, and gait disorders) has been widely described since the late 1960s. However, in recent years it has become clear that similar clinical pictures (corticobasal syndrome) may be caused by different pathological conditions, and probably PSP is the commonest cause of this misdiagnosis.

Levodopa and other dopaminergic medications are largely ineffective in CBD as in all tauopathies. Clonazepam should be used to suppress myoclonus if present, and local botulinum toxin may be helpful for treating CBD-associated limb dystonia. Early speech, physical, and occupational therapy may improve functioning and reduce complications such as aspiration pneumonia and falls. With time, however, most patients lose their independence and mobility. Throughout the course of this rare illness (particularly when it is advanced), caring for the caregiver becomes as important as caring for the patient.

Other Palliative Strategies

These measures remain a very important aspect in the management of all patients with AP in the advanced stages. Exercise programs that focus on the coordination of muscle activity while maintaining posture and movement can facilitate performance of skills and activities such as grasping, rolling over in bed, or preserving balance. Additionally, the changes in posture can be corrected by applying verbal or visual feedback; for example, using a mirror. Assist devices such as a rolling walker may help initially in patients with gait disorders; the wheelchair becomes then mandatory for postural instability and gait ataxia but not for akinesia and rigidity directly.

At the same time, speech therapy can improve speech and swallowing and provide communication aids. Dysphagia requires thickeners for thin fluids and, in the advanced phases of the disease, feeding through a nasogastric tube or even percutaneous endoscopic gastrostomy often become necessary.

For gaze paresis in PSP, rarely prisms for the downgaze palsy are successful, while single-lens prism may help the dysconjugate gaze that is frequently observed in the advanced phase of this disorder. Practical measures to compensate for gaze paresis include elevating reading material and to bring food to a level horizontal with the eyes. Despite often neglected, occupational therapy helps to limit the handicap resulting from the patient's disabilities and should include a home visit. Support groups can be helpful for patients and their caregivers. Published caregivers' information booklets provide helpful advice for home care and confidence to nonprofessional carers. Psychological support for both patients and partners needs also has great importance.

SECONDARY PARKINSONISM

The occurrence of secondary (or symptomatic) parkinsonism is not a rare event. In a large post-mortem cohort study of 620 total cases with parkinsonian syndrome, secondary parkinsonism accounted for 10.8% of all cases. For a detailed classification of secondary parkinsonism, see Table 29.1.

Among secondary parkinsonism, drug-induced parkinsonism (DIP) is one of the most frequent causes, and it should not be missed since it is potentially reversible. The classical causative drugs are typical antipsychotic, but many other drugs, usually biochemically related to neuroleptics (e.g., calcium channel blockers) may be responsible for DIP. The risk associated with antipsychotics is often dose dependent and related to dopamine D2 striatal occupancy. The risk is less, but not negligible, for the second-generation atypical antipsychotics. Regression of symptom will be observed in most cases after a mean delay of 3 months after cessation of treatment. However, in one-tenth of cases, symptoms persist after drug withdrawal leading to the diagnosis of underlying idiopathic PD. The diagnosis is clinical (helpful features are the presence of acute or subacute onset, bilateral and symmetric picture, and association with akathisia and orobuccolingual dyskinesia). In selected cases, cerebral dopamine transporter tomoscintigraphy (DaTSCAN*) can represent a useful diagnostic aid, since the exam is normal in DIP. Usually, if clinical features are not so severe, it is recommended to stop the responsible drug and wait 6–8 months before starting any dopaminergic therapy. Patients with DIP usually show a good response to levodopa therapy.

SUGGESTED READING

Albanese A, Colosimo C, Bentivoglio A, et al. Multiple system atrophy presenting as parkinsonism: clinical features and diagnostic criteria. J Neurol Neurosurg Psychiatry 1995;59:144–151.
Bhatia KP, Lee MS, Rinne JO, et al. Corticobasal de generation look-alikes. Adv Neurol 2000;82:169–182.
Boesch SM, Wenning GK, Ransmayr G, Poewe W. Dystonia in multiple system atrophy. J Neurol Neurosurg Psychiatry 2002;72:300–303.

Bower JH, Maraganore DM, McDonnell SK, Rocca WA. Incidence and distribution of parkinsonism in Olmsted County, Minnesota, 1976 to 1990. Neurology 1999;52:1214–1220.

Colosimo C, Albanese A, Hughes A. Some specific clinical features differentiate multiple system atrophy (striatonigral variety) from Parkinson's disease. Arch Neurol 1995;52:294–298.

Colosimo C, Riley DE, Wenning GK. Handbook of atypical parkinsonism. Cambridge, UK: Cambridge University Press; 2011.

Colosimo C, Bak TH, Bologna M, Berardelli A. Fifty years of progressive supranuclear palsy. J Neurol Neurosurg Psychiatry 2014;85:938–944.

Kompoliti K, Goetz G. Approach to the patient presenting with parkinsonism. In M Flint Beal, A E. Lang, A Ludolph, editors. Neurodegenerative diseases. Cambridge, UK: Cambridge University Press; 2005:552.

Kompoliti K, Goetz CG, Boeve BF, et al. Clinical presentation and pharmacological therapy in corticobasal degeneration. Arch Neurol 1988;55:957–961.

Newmann GC. Treating of PSP with tryciclic antidepressants. Neurology 1985;35:1189–1193.

Quinn N. Multiple system atrophy. In CD Marsden, S Fahn, editors. Movement disorders, ed 3. London, UK: Butterworth-Heinemann; 1994:262–281.

Stamelou M, de Silva R, Arias-Carrion O, et al. Rational therapeutic approaches to progressive supranuclear palsy. Brain 2010;133:1578–1590.

Wenning GK, Krismer F, Poewe W. New insights into atypical parkinsonism. Curr Opin Neurol 2011;24:331–338.

30 Hyperkinetic Movement Disorders

Carlo Colosimo, Maria Cristina
Martinez-Torrens, and Luca Marsili

INTRODUCTION

There are several neurological diseases characterized by involuntary movements (called hyperkinetic movement disorders, or hyperkinesia, or dyskinesia). Based on the phenomenology, hyperkinetic movement disorders are usually characterized into five main categories: tremor, dystonia, chorea/ballism, myoclonus, and tics. The pathophysiology of hyperkinetic movement disorders is, in the vast majority of the cases, linked to basal ganglia dysfunction due to variable causes. Discerning the underlying condition can be difficult given the range and variability of symptoms. Notwithstanding, recognizing the phenomenology and understanding the etiopathogenesis are essential to ensure appropriate treatment. For this reason, each category of involuntary movements will be described separately, underlying its specific clinical features, the commonest causes and the relative treatment. The last part of this chapter is devoted to a common clinical condition, restless legs syndrome, which is not an hyperkinetic movement disorder from the strictly clinical point of view, but because of its pathophysiology and treatment deserves to be described here.

Tremor

Introduction

Tremor is an involuntary oscillating movement on a joint axis with a relatively symmetric movement in both directions. Tremor is usually due to rhythmic alternating contraction of agonist and antagonist muscles. Its oscillatory nature (movement around an axis) is critical and helps distinguish tremor from other rhythmic movements. Tremor is labeled as a "rest tremor," "postural tremor," or "kinetic tremor" according to the condition under which it occurs. Frequencies of different tremors are quite variable, but except for some rare causes of tremor, frequency is usually not helpful in the differential diagnosis among the most common causes of this disorder.

There are many causes of tremor, which are listed in Table 30.1. Some of these are potentially reversible (e.g., drug-induced, metabolic) and need to be promptly recognized by the treating physician. Asymptomatic fine tremor may be present in the outstretched limbs of normal subjects.

Table 30.1 Causes of Tremor

Common
- Enhanced physiological (e.g., hyperthyroidism)
- Essential tremor (familial or sporadic)
- Parkinsonian tremor
- Dystonic tremor syndromes
- Cerebellar tremor (e.g., multiple sclerosis)
- Drug induced or drug withdrawal states

Uncommon
- Psychogenic
- Post-traumatic tremor

Rare
- Primary orthostatic tremor
- Holmes' (rubral) tremor
- Neuropathic tremor (IgM paraproteinaemia)

Some of these causes are discussed in other parts of this volume (e.g., tremor in Parkinson's disease, tremor in multiple sclerosis), and we will concentrate here on the most common cause of pathological tremor, essential tremor (ET).

Definition and Epidemiology

ET is a monosymptomatic, predominant postural and kinetic tremor that is usually slowly progressive over time. ET is the most common movement disorder with a widely estimated prevalence of 0.4–3.9%, higher among people over 65 years of age (4.6%).

Clinical Features

This is a disorder characterized by a 6- to 12-Hz postural and kinetic tremor involving the arms and less commonly the head, lower limbs and voice, accompanied by a family history of a similar tremor in 50% of the cases. Impaired balance (tandem walking) and upper-extremity rest tremor can be seen in advanced stages. ET is considered benign in term of its lack of effect on life expectancy.

Diagnosis

Diagnosis of ET is still based solely on neurological history and clinical examination (Figure 30.1), as specific biological markers or diagnostic tests are not available. The response to ethanol intake is an important supportive criterion. The most widely used diagnostic criteria are those developed by a consensus committee of the Movement Disorder Society (Table 30.2).

Treatment

Patients with minor, nondisabling tremor can be left untreated if the involuntary movements are not bothersome, or if the patient prefers not to pursue active treatment. The

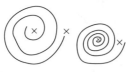 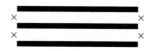

FIGURE 30.1

Archimedes spiral and handwritten lines represent a standard component of the neurological exam to detect tremor.

main drugs used to symptomatically treat ET are reported in Table 30.3. Functional neurosurgery may be considered only in severe cases that are not responding adequately to drugs (Table 30.4).

DYSTONIA

Introduction

Dystonia is an hyperkinetic movement disorder, characterized by sustained agonist/ antagonist muscle co-contractions that generate twisting movements and abnormal postures. As for other movement disorders (such as tremor), the term *dystonia* has historically been used at the same time to refer to the clinical phenomenology and to the numerous dystonia syndromes.

Table 30.2 ET: Movement Disorder Society Consensus Criteria

Inclusion criteria	Exclusion criteria
Bilateral, largely symmetrical postural or kinetic tremor involving hands and forearms that is visible and persistent	Other abnormal neurological signs; particularly dystonia
Additional or isolated tremor of the head might occur but in absence of abnormal posturing	Presence of known causes of enhanced physiological tremor, including current or recent exposure to tremorogenic drugs or presence of a drug withdrawal state
	Historical or clinical evidence of psychogenic tremor
	Convincing evidence of sudden onset or evidence of stepwise deterioration
	Primary orthostatic tremor
	Isolated voice tremor
	Isolated position-specific or task-specific tremors, including occupational tremors and primary writing tremor
	Isolated leg tremor
	Isolated tongue or chin tremor

Table 30.3 Pharmacological Treatment of ET

Treatment	Dosage	Evidence level	Side effects	Contraindications
Beta-blockers Propranolol (PRP) Other beta-blockers	PRP 120–240 mg divided in three daily doses or PRP–long acting (LA) to achieve better compliance	Strong recommendation low quality of evidence, 1C Strong recommendation very low quality of evidence, 1D. Weak quality of evidence (2D) were attributed to the others	Hypotension, bradycardia, body coldness, depression, apathy, dizziness, sleepiness, fatigue and dryness of mouth. Majority of side effects were observed during long-term PRP-LA therapy. Cases of severe bradycardia, syncope and discontinuation due to a severe skin eruption were observed with PRP-LA.	Asthma, heart congestive failure, manifest bradycardia, 2° and 3° grade heart blocks, arterial peripheral circulation problems, Prinzmetal angina, not treated pheocromocitoma, Hypoglicemia, metabolic acydosis.
Anticonvulsants Topiramate, primidone, levetiracetam, zonisamide, other anticonvulsants	25–400 mg daily in two administrations 250–750 mg daily in 1–3 administrations Levetiracetam 1000 mg/day and zonisamide 160–250 mg/day	Strong recommendation moderate quality of evidence, 1B strong recommendation very low quality of evidence, 1D Weak recommendation and low quality of evidence (2C) weak recommendation and very low quality of evidence (2D)	Adverse effects usually described in these pharmacological classes like confusion, sedation, somnolence, and dizziness	

Table 30.3 Continued

Treatment	Dosage	Evidence level	Side effects	Contraindications
Neuroleptics				
Clozapine Olanzapine Quetiapine	Clozapine 12.5–100 mg/day Olanzapine 10–20 mg/day Quetiapine 25–50 mg/day	Weak recommendation, due to the safety profile, the low number of studies and their low quality of evidence, 2C very low quality of evidence (2D)	Risk of agranulocytosis, arrhythmias, weight increase, hyperglicemia and diabetes, parkinsonism	
Other Amantadine	100–200 mg/day	Not recommended in ET treatment (strong recommendation very low quality of evidence, 1D).		
Botulinum toxin type A (BTX-A)	Doses: 60–150 U (onabotulinumtoxin A) in neck muscles	Strong recommendation and low quality of evidence (1C) were attributed to BTX-A in patients with defined limb or head ET. There is too low quality of evidence to support or exclude efficacy of BTX-A in voice ET.	Side effects are limited and temporary and include muscle weakness, pain at the injection site, dysphagia (when injected for head or voice tremor), and a breathy vocal quality (when injected for voice tremor). Muscle weakness is observed in 30–70% of treated patients, but the exact impact of this adverse effect on global functioning following treatment-induced tremor attenuation needs further investigation.	Myastenia, pregnancy

Table 30.4 Nonpharmacological Treatment of ET

Thalamotomy	Unilateral VIM-thalamotomy could be useful in the treatment of limb ET	Weak recommendation, moderate quality of evidence, 2B	Surgical risks include brain hemorrhage and infection.
Deep brain stimulation (DBS)	Unilateral thalamic-DBS is effective for treating contralateral limb tremor	Strong recommendation, moderate quality of evidence, 1B	Surgical risks include brain hemorrhage and infection. Side effects of the stimulation include Paresthesias, paresis, imbalance, dysarthria, and, in rare cases, dysphagia.
	There are no sufficient data regarding the superiority of bilateral stimulation on reducing tremor.	Level of evidence for bilateral thalamic-DBS is low (weak recommendation, 2C).	Not indicated in voice tremor and in very advanced age
	STN-DBS could be a target for long-term treatment of ET; for patients below the age of 70 years old, however, the VIM seems to be a preferable target	weak recommendation, moderate quality of evidence, 2B)	Oral anticoagulants, main contraindications to surgical procedures

Epidemiology

Dystonia is one of the most frequent movement disorders, although underdiagnosed. The exact incidence is not precisely known, because of the variability of design on the studies that have been performed. Recent studies report a prevalence range between 2 and 50/1,000,000 for early-onset dystonia and between 30 and 7320/1,000,000 for late-onset dystonia.

Clinical Features

Other characteristic features of dystonia are represented by the presence of:

I.   *Geste antagoniste*; sometimes dystonia decreases intensity by touching a body part, like grabbing the neck in cervical dystonia
II. Motor overflow, dystonic contraction diffusion, co-contractions
III. Mirror movements: dystonia could be activated by a specific task, performed by the opposite normal body part

Diagnosis

Although the dystonic agonist/antagonist muscle co-contractions could be demonstrated by electromyography (EMG), the diagnosis of this disorder is mainly clinical. In Table 30.5 are reported the European Federation of Neurological Societies (EFNS) guidelines on diagnosis of dystonia.

Treatment

Pharmacological: Treatment options include anticholinergics (effective in generalized dystonia), benzodiazepines (useful in mild cases of dystonia), baclofen (useful in oromandibular and generalized dystonia) and botulinum toxin local injections, which represent the first-line treatment for most cases of focal and segmental dystonia (Table 30.6). Only in the rare genetic forms of DOPA-responsive dystonia, low doses of levodopa (50–600 mg/day) almost abolish clinical symptoms.

Nonpharmacological: GPi-DBS is currently used in selected cases of dystonia, with positive results mainly in the primary dystonia group (generalized forms or focal forms not responding to BTX-A or BTX-B treatments). In secondary dystonia, the results are not promising yet.

Chorea

Introduction

Chorea is an hyperkinetic movement disorder characterized by involuntary movements that are brief and abrupt, resulting from a continuous flow of random muscle contractions. When choreic movements are proximal and more severe, they are called ballism. When ballism is unilateral (hemiballism) is often due to a vascular brain lesion, and in most of these cases the clinical picture is spontaneously reversible after some time from the onset. Chorea can affect any muscular group and it can be suppressed

Etiological:

Primary or idiopathic

Primary pure dystonia: just manifests with dystonia (tremor may be also present)
E.g.: DYT1 dystonia

Primary plus dystonia: dystonia is associated to other features as myoclonus, chorea, parkinsonism. e.g.: DYT5 dystonia

Primary paroxysmal dystonia: occurs by brief periods of time, as patient moves (kinesigenic) or patient stands still (non kinesigenic).

Heredodegenerative dystonia

Secondary dystonia: symptom of a specific neurological condition (cerebrovascular disease, drug-induced, neurodegenerative disease)

Anatomical:

Focal: single body region

Segmental: contiguous body regions

Multifocal: noncontiguous body regions

Generalized: both legs and at least one other body region (usually one or both arms)

Age of onset:

<26 year old: early onset, probably will progress to generalized: e.g.: DYT1 dystonia

>26 year old: late onset, most probably will remain focal. e.g.: cervical dystonia

Genetical:

Primary torsion dystonia (PTD), where dystonia is the only clinical sign (except for tremor) (DYT1, 2, 4, 6, 7, 13, 17, and 21)

Dystonia plus loci, where other phenotypes in addition to dystonia, including parkinsonism or myoclonus, are present (DYT3, 5/14, 11, 12, 15, and 16)

Paroxysmal forms of dystonia/dyskinesia (DYT8, 9, 10, 18, 19, and 20)

---

only for a short time. It often gets better during sleep and it can be seen in a wide range of disorders (Table 30.7). The prototype of a choreic disorder is Huntington's disease (HD), and in most of the other causes of chorea a similar approach to symptomatic treatment may be used.

Epidemiology

HD is an autosomal dominant disorder representing the most frequent cause of genetic chorea, with reported prevalence rates in North America and Europe ranging from 3 to 7 per 100,000.

Clinical Features

Typical age at onset is between the third and the fifth decade. Its time course and the body parts distribution depend mainly on its cause. In HD, the choreic movements are often associated with other involuntary movements such as dystonia and tics, typically associated to signs of motor impersistency. In later stages, parkinsonian features often appear, whereas hyperkinetic features become much less evident.

Table 30.6 Pharmacological Treatment of Dystonia

Drug	Dosage	Adverse effects
Anticholinergics (trihexyphenidyl)	6–120 mg/day (tid)	Constipation, hallucinations, cognitive impairment, nausea, vomiting, glaucoma
Benzodiazepines (clonazepam and diazepam)	Diazepam 2–40 mg/day (tid) Clonazepam 0.5–6 mg/day (tid)	Somnolence, asthenia, confusion, amnesia
Baclofen	Oral 75–100 mg/day (tid) Intrathecal (injectable solution) 800–1500 mg/day	Confusion, ataxia, psychosis, syncope, hypertonia, bradycardia, dyspnea, venous thrombosis
Botulinum toxin type A (BTX-A) onabotulinumtoxin A (*) Or abobotulinumtoxin A (#)	Expressed in U Per region (*): cervical dystonia (CD) 100–190, blepharospasm (BP) 20–50, focal hand dystonia 20–70, oromandibular dystonia 70–100 Per region (#): CD 500–1000, BP 100–200	Side effects are limited and transient and include, pain at the injection site and muscle weakness in the injected region (e.g., ptosis, strabismus, diplopia, dysphagia, dysphonia, dry mouth)
Botulinum toxin type B (BTX-B)	CD 5000/10,000 (in nonresponders to BTX-A)	

Diagnosis

This is initially clinical, with later support from laboratory tests such as genetic testing, neuroimaging studies, and blood analyses.

Treatment

Pharmacological: Symptomatic drug treatment should only be considered when choreic movements become severe, interfering with the patient's activities of daily living. Antidopaminergic drugs (phenotiazines and butyrophenones) have long been the principal pharmacological treatment of chorea, regardless of its cause (Table 30.8). Long-term clinical experience indicates that drugs such as atypical neuroleptics (olanzapine, quetiapine, and clozapine), despite some theoretical advantages in term of lessened side effects, have limited roles in the treatment of chorea. A compound that is now considered as the gold standard to counteract chorea is tetrabenazine. The precise mechanism by which tetrabenazine exerts its antidyskinetic effects is unknown, but it is believed to be mainly related to its effect as a reversible depletor of monoamines from nerve terminals, inhibiting the vesicular monoamine transporter 2 (VMAT2).

Table 30.7 Causes of Chorea

GENETIC	ACQUIRED
Huntington's disease	Immunological (Sydenham chorea and variants [chorea gravidarum and contraceptive-induced chorea], systemic lupus erythematosus, antiphospholipid antibody syndrome, paraneoplastic syndromes)
Huntington's disease–like illnesses	
Neuroacanthocytosis	
McLeod's syndrome	
Wilson's disease	
Benign hereditary chorea	
Spinocerebellar atrophy type 2, 3, 17	Drug-related (amantadine, amphetamine, anticonvulsants, carbon monoxide, central nervous system stimulants [methylphenidate, pemoline, cyproheptadine], cocaine, dopamine agonists, levodopa, dopamine-receptor blockers, ethanol, lithium, tricyclic antidepressants)
Dentatorubropallidoluysian degeneration	
Ataxia-teleangectasia	
Ataxia associated with oculomotor apraxia	
Neuroferritinopathy	
Pantothenate kinase associated neurodegeneration	
Leigh disease and other mitochondrial disorders	Endocrine-metabolic dysfunction (hyper/hypocalcemia, hyper/hypoglycemia, liver failure, others)
Lesch–Nyhan disease	Vascular (post-pump chorea, stroke, subdural hematoma)
	Infections (bacteria, protozoa, parasites, AIDS related)
	Miscellaneous (anoxic encephalopathy, cerebral palsy, kernicterus, multiple sclerosis)

Table 30.8 Pharmacological Treatment of Chorea

Drug	Dosage	Adverse effects
Tetrabenazine	37.5–150 mg/day (tid, start with low doses)	Sedation, akathisia, parkinsonism depression (reversible with a decrease in dosage), leukopenia Dysphagia and neuroleptic malignant syndrome (rare)
Haloperidol, pimozide, fluphenazine, thioridazine, sulpiride, and tiapride (typical neuroleptics)	Haloperidol 2–15 mg/day, Pimozide: 1–10 mg/day, Sulpiride 50–100 mg/day (increase slowly, 1 mg/week)	parkinsonism, akathisia, acute dystonia, and tardive dyskinesia
Olanzapine	5–20 mg/day	Parkinsonism
Risperidone	1–3 mg/day	Parkinsonism
Clozapine	25–100 mg/day	Severe leukopenia (rare)

Nonpharmacological: DBS of the GPi has been described as an effective short-term treatment in some patients with severe chorea due to HD. It is difficult to predict the long-term impact of this procedure and to determine the optimal stimulation parameters, because of the difficulty in predicting disease course in HD. To date long-term clinical data on DBS are not available.

Myoclonus

Introduction

Myoclonus is an hyperkinetic movement disorder, characterized by sudden, brief, shock-like muscular contractions (positive myoclonus), or interruptions of it (negative myoclonus or asterixis)

Epidemiology

Pathological and persistent myoclonus, has a lifetime prevalence of 8.6/100,000, and it may reach the 0.5% prevalence in older subjects living in nursing homes.

Clinical Features

Because of its sudden onset and brief duration, myoclonus can be distinguished from other hyperkinetic movement; in addition, this is also nonsuppressible, not preceded by an urge to move, generally arrhythmic, and not influenced by a *geste antagoniste*. Myoclonus can be synchronous and stimulus-sensitive, rarely incorporated in voluntary actions, and does not show entrainment. However, myoclonic jerks regularly occur in patients with other movement disorders, and electrophysiological studies might be needed for a correct diagnosis. Electroencephalography can help in differentiating the cortical and subcortical types, while EMG is useful in diagnosing the peripheral forms.

Classification

There are three main different classifications of myoclonus: clinical, etiological, and anatomical (Table 30.9). These classifications are interrelated and are crucial for both diagnosis and treatment.

Treatment

Therapy should focus on the cure of the underlying disorder; however, symptomatic treatment is often needed when treatment of an underlying cause is impossible or ineffective. Because of a generally low level of evidence, therapeutic options are mainly based on small observational studies or case reports (Table 30.10).

Table 30.9 Classification of Myoclonus

a. Clinical features

Distribution	Focal, segmental, axial, generalised
Temporal pattern	Usually irregular (arrhythmic) or oscillatory
Synchrony	Synchronised jerks or asynchronous.
Relation to movement	At rest or associated to voluntary movement
Muscular activity	Positive or negative (*asterixis*)
Sensitive stimulus response (tactile, auditive)	Positive/negative

b. Etiology

Type or cause	*Characteristics*
Physiological	Not pathological. Common in healthy individuals (e.g., sleep jerks and hiccups)
Symptomatic	Most common, approximately 70% of cases. Manifestation of an underlying disorder; as post-hypoxic syndrome, Alzheimer's disease, drug-induced myoclonus, and toxic–metabolic myoclonus.
Epileptic myoclonus	Second most common. Myoclonus might be the only symptom, can be a component of a seizure, or one of the seizure types
Essential myoclonus	Usually hereditary. Currently described as myoclonus-dystonia
Psychogenic	Should be considered when organic causes have been excluded

c. **Anatomical origin:** *mainly based on electrophysiological characteristics and can additionally be guided by clinical signs and etiological classification.*

Type	*Example*	*Characteristics*
Cortical	Myoclonic seizures as those of progressive myoclonic epilepsy syndromes, Posthypoxic cortical reflex myoclonus and myoclonus in neurodegenerative syndromes	The natural history and prognosis follows that of the cause (it can be severe in progressive myoclonic epilepsy)
Subcortical	Myoclonus-dystonia, Opsoclonus-myoclonus syndrome Palatal myoclonus,	Inherited autosomal-dominant with reduced penetrance disorder (mutations in the epsilon-sarcoglycan gene, *DYT11*, among others)

(*continued*)

Table 30.9 Continued

	Orthostatic myoclonus	Onset in early childhood with benign course
		Alcohol responsiveness
		Psychiatric symptoms associated.
		Rare entity characterized by irritability, chaotic ocular movements with vertical, horizontal, rotatory components (opsoclonus) along with myoclonus and ataxia.
		Symptomatic palatal myoclonus (also known as palatal tremor) is caused by a lesion in the triangle of Guillain and Mollaret and is associated with hypertrophic olivary degeneration that has multiple causes.
		Essential palatal tremor has no currently demonstrable cause and no accompanying physical or radiological signs
		Stand-up myoclonus
Spinal	Segmental and propriospinal myoclonus	Uncommon disorder
Peripheral	Hemifacial spasm (HFS) and others	HFS is very common, in most cases determining only minor disability

Tics

Introduction

This type of hyperkinetic movement disorder represents the core feature of Gilles de la Tourette's syndrome (GTS), but it can also present transiently during childhood or be classified as chronic motor or vocal tic disorder without the variety of psychiatric and behavioral disorders seen in GTS. Other conditions that can be accompanied by tics are drug intoxication or withdrawal (including cocaine and amphetamine), HD and Wilson's disease, tardive syndrome due to neuroleptics, cerebrovascular disease, and cerebral palsy.

Epidemiology

Epidemiological studies indicate a prevalence of GTS of 0.5–1% in school-aged children.

Clinical Features

Tics may be motor or phonic and simple or complex. They tend to occur in clusters or bouts, and they are divided in myoclonic or dystonic, according to their main phenomenology. Tics are often preceded by a premonitory sensation—tight feeling around the

Table 30.10 Pharmacological Treatment of Myoclonus

Type	First line treatment
Cortical	Levetiracetam (up to 3000 mg/day)
	Piracetam (2·4–21·6 g/day)
	Clonazepam (up to 15 mg/day)
	Valproic acid (1200–2000 mg/day)
Subcortical	Clonazepam (up to 6 mg/day),
Myoclonus-dystonia	Trihexyphenidyl (up to 6 mg/day)
Opsoclonus-myoclonus	Rituximab, ACTH, intravenous
Hyperekplexia	immunoglobulin therapy, clonazepam
Palatal myoclonus (palatal tremor)	Clonazepam (up to 6 mg/day)
Orthostatic myoclonus	Clonazepam, carbamazepine, phenytoin,
	barbiturates, valproic acid, baclofen,
	anticholinergics, tetrabenazine,
	lamotrigine, sumatriptan, piracetam, BTX-A,
	tinnitus masking device
Spinal	Clonazepam (up to 6 mg/day)
Segmental	
Propriospinal	
Peripheral	BTX-A (25 U of onabotulinumtoxin A is the
Hemifacial spasm	usual dosage to initiate treatment)

area of the tic, or a mental feeling. Tics can be suppressed for a short while, but with an increase of internal tension, while the tic itself often brings relief from the tension.

Diagnosis

Clinical symptoms should start before the age of 18 and be present for at least 1 year.

Treatment

Haloperidol (2–15 mg daily) and pimozide (2–18 mg daily) are the only drugs approved and usually used to treat these involuntary movements, while there is insufficient evidence-based data on new generation antipsychotics, except risperidone (1–6 mg daily). The associated symptoms of affective psychosis may be treated with antidepressants, while in severe cases DBS (pallidal, subthalamic, or thalamic) has been also proposed.

Restless Legs Syndrome

Introduction

Restless legs syndrome (RLS) is described as an idiopathic disorder, or a secondary syndrome often due to iron deficiency (<50 μg/L ferritine) or terminal renal disease.

About half of idiopathic cases has an hereditary origin, with an autosomal dominant pattern, and high penetrance level.

Clinical Features

RLS is characterized by the urgency to move the legs, sometimes associated by different uni- or bilateral sensitive symptoms, unpleasant sensations like tingling or leg pain mainly when the patient is laying down. This improves when the motor activity begins, such as during walking. When illness progresses, these symptoms can involve the arms, in a great percent of the patients.

Epidemiology

A prevalence of 3–10% in the general population has been reported. In 2004, a very large RLS epidemiologic study (N = 23,052) reported a 9.6% of subjects who fulfilled the criteria for this disorder. The age of its presentation has a very wide range, from the childhood until the ninth decade.

Diagnostic Criteria

The diagnosis is mainly clinical. The RLS criteria were identified in 1995 by the RLS study group and were revised in 2002 (Table 30.11).The polysomnographic evaluation is reserved to cases with a diagnostic doubt, probable leg periodic movement syndrome, or other clinical suspect. The clinical history and physical examination are enough in the majority of cases

Treatment

Nonpharmacological: Sleep hygiene, avoid trigger drugs, diagnose and treat a secondary cause of RLS, and start moderate exercise.

Pharmacological: The two most frequently used group of drugs are dopaminergics (at low dosage) and opioids (in refractory cases). Other alternatives have been

Table 30.11 Diagnostic Criteria for RLS

Essential Diagnostic Criteria*
Leg moving urge, associated to unpleasent sensation of discomfort
Leg moving urge that get worse in rest
Leg moving urge that get worse in rest that gets better during activity
Get worse by night
Supportive Criteria
Good treatment response
Periodic leg movement
Family history of RLS

*All four essential criteria must be present for the diagnosis.

Table 30.12 Pharmacological Treatment of RLS

Drug	Dosage (mg/daily)
Dopaminergic	
Levodopa + decarboxylase inhibitor (DCI)	100–200 + DCI
Pramipexole	0.125–1.5
Ropirinole	0.25–6
Opioids	
Tramadol	50–400
Oxycodone	5–20
Hydrocodone	5–20
Methadone	5–40
Benzodiazepines	
Clonazepam	0.5–4
Anticonvulsants	
Gabapentin	300–2400

reported without the same efficacy. The doses of the main compounds used to treat RLS are reported in Table 30.12.

SUGGESTED READING

Albanese A, Asmus F, Bhatia KP, et al. EFNS guidelines on diagnosis and treatment of primary dystonias. Eur J Neurol 2011;18:5–18.

Albanese A, Jankovic J, editors. Hyperkinetic movement disorders: Differential diagnosis and treatment. Hoboken, NJ: Wiley; 2012.

Deuschl G, Bain P, Brin M. Consensus statement of the Movement Disorder Society on Tremor. Ad Hoc Scientific Committee. Mov Disord 1998;13(Suppl 3):2–23.

Dijk JM, Tijssen MA. Management of patients with myoclonus: available therapies and the need for an evidence-based approach. Lancet Neurol 2010;9:1028–1036.

Fabbrini G, Defazio G, Colosimo C, et al. Cranial movement disorders: clinical features, pathophysiology, differential diagnosis and treatment. Nat Clin Pract Neurol 2009;5:93–105.

Martino D, Leckman JF, editors. Tourette syndrome. New York, NY: Oxford University Press; 2013.

Novak MJ, Tabrizi SJ. Huntington's disease: Clinical presentation and treatment. International Rev Neurobiol 2011;98:297–323.

Postuma RB, Lang AE. Hemiballism: revisiting a classic disorder. Lancet Neurol 2003;2:661–668.

Trenkwalder C, Högl B, Winkelmann J. Recent advances in the diagnosis, genetics and treatment of restless legs syndrome. J Neurol 2009;256:539–553.

Zappia M, Albanese A, Bruno E, et al; Italian Movement Disorders Association (DISMOV-SIN) Essential Tremor Committee. Treatment of essential tremor: A systematic review of evidence and recommendations from the Italian Movement Disorders Association. J Neurol 2013;260:74.

31 Cerebellar Ataxia

Luca Marsili and Carlo Colosimo

INTRODUCTION

The term *cerebellar ataxia* is commonly used to designate specific diseases of the nervous system in which progressive ataxia due to cerebellar involvement is the prominent clinical manifestation. Classification of ataxia could be based on neuropathological, etiological, or genetical criteria. In the early 1980s, Harding proposed a new classification that was mainly based on clinical and genetic criteria that gained wide acceptance. This classification distinguishes between congenital, hereditary, and nonhereditary ataxia (Table 31.1). Hereditary ataxia are divided into autosomical recessive (such as Friedreich's ataxia [FRDA], ataxia-teleangectasia [AT]) and autosomical dominant or spinocerebellar (SCA) ataxia. The number of genes responsible of SCA has been increasing progressively during the past 20 years. The nonhereditary ataxia include idiopathic neurodegenerative diseases and symptomatic ataxia in which the etiology is well known.

To date, although many advances in the diagnostic work-up of ataxia have been made, specific therapeutic approaches are not available for most of ataxic diseases.

We will describe specific treatment of single causes of ataxia (where available) in the following section, but unfortunately only supportive treatment is available in most cases. In these cases, focused physiotherapy and speech therapy are crucial. The main aim of these supportive therapies is to maintain the patient's autonomy as long as possible and to prevent secondary complications.

The treatment of other medical and neurological symptoms associated with cerebellar ataxia should not be neglected, such as cardiomyopathy and diabetes in FRDA and autonomic failure or parkinsonism in multiple system atrophy (MSA; see Chapter 29). Most important, it should not be missed the possibility of curative therapies: examples are the withdrawal of toxic compounds in ataxia due to toxic agents, vitamin supplementation (B1, E) in the alcoholic and vitamin deficiency variants, thyroid hormone supplementation in ataxia linked to hypothyroidism, administration of statins in cerebrotendineous xanthomatosis (CTX), and, finally, the use of intravenous immunoglobulins in the Miller-Fisher syndrome–related ataxia.

ETIOLOGICAL THERAPY

Etiological treatment approaches are available only for some rare forms of ataxia with known biochemical deficits, such as FRDA, AT, ataxia due to isolated vitamin E deficiency (AVED), abetalipoproteinemia (ABL), Refsum's disease (RD), and CTX.

Table 31.1 Classification of Ataxia

331

Cerebellar Ataxia

Hereditary Ataxia

Autosomal Recessive Ataxia

Friedereich ataxia

Ataxia Teleangectasia

Abetalipoproteinemia

Ataxia with oculomotor apraxia (type 1)

Ataxia with vitamin E deficiency

Refsum disease

Autosomal Dominant Cerebellar Ataxia

Spinocerebellar ataxia (SCA)

Episodic ataxia

Inborn errors of metabolism

Adrenoleukodystrophy

Wilson's disease

Mitochondrial disorders

MELAS

MERRF

NARP

Acquired Ataxia

Degenerative

Multiple system atrophy, cerebellar type

Sporadic adult onset ataxia of unknown origin

Symptomatic ataxia

Toxic (alcohol, drugs, other)

Vascular (ischemic or hemorragic stroke)

Paraneoplastic, neoplastic, metastatic

Inflammatory demyelination (MS, ADEM)

Infectious (HIV, viral cerebellitis, Miller-Fisher syndrome)

Prion (CJD)

Ataxia due to acquired vitamin deficiency or metabolic disorders (B1, E deficiency; celiac disease)

Structural (Arnold-Chiari malformation)

Endocrine (decreased T4)

Abbreviations: MELAS, mitochondrial encephalophathy with lactic acidosis and stroke-like episodes; MERRF, myoclonic epilepsy with ragged red fibers; NARP, neuropathy, ataxia, retinitis pigmentosa; MS, multiple sclerosis, ADEM, acute demyelinating encephalomyelitis; HIV, human immunodeficiency virus; CJD, Creutzfeldt-Jakob disease.

Friedreich's Ataxia

Given that the mitochondrial iron imbalance and the oxidative stress are involved in the pathogenesis of FRDA, iron chelators such as desferioxamine have been widely used to treat this cerebellar disease. The limits of desferioxamine are its several side effects and the lack of specific targeting on mitochondrial iron deposit. For this reason, 2-pyridylcarboxaldehyde isonicotinoyl hydrazone (PCIH), an agent that removes mitochondrial iron deposits, has been introduced, but to date studies about its real efficacy are lacking. Alternatively, based on the same rationale, it has been proposed an antioxidant therapy with idebenone (analogue of coenzyme Q10). However, idebenone has been found more effective than placebo in the treatment of cardiomyopathy associated with FRDA, but it seems unable to improve the neurological symptoms of this disease. Other trials using coenzyme Q10 and vitamin E resulted in a significant improvement of cardiac function, with a slowing of the progression of certain clinical features.

Ataxia-Teleangectasia

Despite the great advances in understanding molecular genetics of AT, we still do not have effective etiopathogenetical therapies. AT treatment is mainly focused on the supportive care, the management of associated infections, tumors, and immunodeficiency, and finally on the rehabilitative approach (including intervention on swallowing and nutrition). Single case reports have shown some benefit using amantadine, buspirone, and fluoxetine. Cerebellar tremor could be treated using anticonvulsivants as clonazepam or gabapentin. Recent small-sample trials showed an improvement of cerebellar functions in AT patients treated with betamethasone (0.1 mg/kg/day) for a 10 days, possibly related to antioxidative mechanisms. These data showed that the clinical amelioration was inversely correlated with the level of cerebellar atrophy, as revealed by magnetic resonance imaging.

Ataxia Due to Isolated Vitamin E Deficiency

In this rare condition, lifelong high-dose oral vitamin E supplementation is necessary to bring plasma vitamin E concentrations into the high-normal range; if supplementation is started early in the course of the disease, this results in cessation of progression of neurological symptoms and mental deterioration and, in some cases, even in the amelioration of established neurological abnormalities. α-Tocopherol given at 800 mg twice daily, associated with meals containing fat, raises the serum level of vitamin E to the desired range. Prevention of primary manifestation with vitamin E administration in presymptomatic children carriers of homozygous α-tocopherol transfer protein (TTPA) mutations prevents symptoms development, whereas heterozygous children for TTPA mutation do not need vitamin supplementation. Moreover, individuals with AVED needs to avoid smoking because it further lowers plasma vitamin E concentrations.

Abetalipoproteinemia

Reduction of dietary lipids to prevent steatorrhea and administration of vitamin E to prevent progression of neurological and retinal degeneration is the gold standard therapy.

Refsum's Disease

The clinical biochemical feature of RD is represented by the increased plasmatic levels of phytanic acid. This acid, in humans, is exclusively of nutritional origin, and beef and fish are the most common sources. Phytanic acid–free diet is warranted by green vegetables, pork, and poultry, which do not contain this element. Usually, ataxia, neuropathy, ichthyosis, and cardiac arrhythmia respond to the lowering of plasmatic levels of phytanic acid, whereas other symptoms (retinitis pigmentosa and ocular signs in general, bony abnormalities) are irreversible. Plasmapheresis and lipapheresis could be used to rapidly achieve a clinical response in most severe cases.

Cerebrotendineous Xanthomatosis

Daily treatment with chenodeoxycholic acid (CDCA) up to 1000 mg and statins (usually simvastatin or lovastatin) at dosage of 10 mg daily is usually the gold standard. In the follow-up, it is important to constantly monitor the serum cholestanol levels. The effect of long-term administration of CDCA on polyneuropathy associated with CTX is still debated, even if recent reports suggest that CDCA treatment daily promotes myelin synthesis in nerve fibers with residual unaffected axons.

SYMPTOMATIC THERAPY

Although the exact mechanism of action is unclear, it has been repeatedly described that buspirone, a 5-HT1$_A$ agonist and D2 dopamine antagonist/agonist, has some transient beneficial effects in both younger and older individuals with ataxia, at a dosage of 1 mg/kg/day (60 mg/day maximum). In FRDA, and sporadic late-onset cerebellar atrophy some evidence supports that 5-hydroxytryptophan is more effective than placebo improving neurological symptoms. Some other centrally acting drugs, such thyrotropin-releasing hormone, and D-cycloserine (a partial NMDA allosteric agonist), have a minor antiataxic action and improve cerebellar ataxia (in particular, in some forms of SCA). However, these observations are controversial, since they relie on single case-reports or studies in small case series The effect of sulfamethoxazole-trimethoprim antibiotic therapy in SCA3/Machado-Joseph disease (MJD) has been reported, although this therapy seems to improve spasticity and rigidity but not ataxia. Its effect could be due to an increase in biopterin and homovanillic acid levels, which are decreased in the cerebrospinal fluid of SCA3/MJD patients However, initial data based on small series were not confirmed in a subsequent double-blind crossover study on the same disease.

A specific therapy for the deficient cholinergic system using choline or choline derivatives has been experimented in FRDA and other cerebellar ataxia, but the result are not definitive and need further investigations. Based on a similar rationale, a positive effect mainly on axial cerebellar symptoms has been recently reported with varenicline, a partial agonist at nicotinic cholinergic receptors, which is already marketed for smoking cessation. Twenty patients with SCA3/MJD were studied in a 2-month controlled trial. These interesting results need now confirmation in larger, independent trials.

Finally, in selected cases, deep brain stimulation of the ventral intermediate nucleus of the thalamus is an adequate operative intervention that can help in patients with a severe disabling kinetic limb tremor without prominent associated ataxia.

SUGGESTED READING

Ginanneschi F, Mignarri A, Mondelli M, et al. Polyneuropathy in cerebrotendinous xanthomatosis and response to treatment with chenodeoxycholic acid. J Neurol 2013;260:268–274.

Klockgether T. Approach to the patient with ataxia. In M Flint Beal, AE Lang, and A Ludolph, editors. Neurodegenerative diseases. New York, NY: Cambridge University Press: 2005.

Kohlschutter A. Abetalipoproteinemia. In T Klockgether, editor. Handbook of ataxia disorders. Vol. 50. New York, NY: Dekker: 2000:205–221.

Meiner V, Leitersdorf E. Cerebrotendinous xanthomatosis. In T Klockgether, editor. Handbook of ataxia disorders. Vol. 50. New York, NY: Dekker: 2000:257–269.

Ogawa M. Pharmacological treatments of cerebellar ataxia. Cerebellum 2004; 3:107–111.

Sakai T, Matsuishi T, Yamada S, et al. Sulfamethoxazole-trimethoprim double-blind, placebo-controlled, crossover trial in Machado-Joseph disease: sulfamethoxazole-trimethoprim increases cerebrospinal fluid level of biopterin. J Neural Transm Gen Sect 1995;102:159–172.

Trujillo-Martin MM, Serrano-Aguilar P, Monton-Alvarez F, et al. Effectiveness and safety of treatments for degenerative ataxias: a systematic review. Mov Disord 2009;24:1111–1124.

32 Dementia

Alessandro Padovani and Barbara Borroni

INTRODUCTION

The change in global age demographics and the predicted rise in the incidence of age-related diseases, including dementia, are of major public health concern. Dementia affects 5.4% of people over 65 years of age, and its prevalence further increases with age. The number of people living with dementia worldwide is currently estimated at 35.6 million; Western Europe is the region with the highest number of people with dementia (7.0 million), closely followed by East Asia with 5.5 million, South Asia with 4.5 million, and North America with 4.4 million. These numbers will double by 2030 and more than triple by 2050 according to the World Health Organization. The total number of new cases of dementia each year worldwide is nearly 7.7 million, implying that one new case occurs every 4 seconds. Despite the fact that there is significant evidence for the benefits of early diagnosis, treatment, and social support, the rate of diagnosis and treatment in people with dementia varies considerably, even in Western countries. Primary care physicians play a major role in the identification, diagnosis, and management of patients with dementia, while the involvement of specialists, especially neurologists, geriatricians, and psychiatrists, is mandatory for advanced diagnostic techniques and management of the complex needs of patients and caregivers during the course of the dementia disease.

Physicians often define dementia based on the criteria given in the *Diagnostic and Statistical Manual of Mental Disorders, Fourth Edition (DSM-IV)*. To meet *DSM-IV* criteria for dementia, symptoms must include decline in memory *and* in at least one another cognitive abilities (ability to generate coherent speech or understand spoken or written language, and/or ability to recognize or identify objects, assuming intact sensory function, and/or ability to execute motor activities, assuming intact motor abilities and sensory function and comprehension of the required task, and/or ability to think abstractly, make sound judgments and plan and carry out complex tasks) and the decline in cognitive abilities must be severe enough to interfere with daily life.

To establish a diagnosis of dementia, a physician must determine the cause of the dementia-like symptoms ruling out all those conditions that mimic dementia but that, unlike dementia, can be reversed with treatment. These treatable conditions include depression, delirium, side effects from medications, thyroid problems, certain vitamin deficiencies, and excessive use of alcohol. In contrast, most dementias are caused by irreversible damage to brain cells. Different types of dementia are associated with distinct symptom patterns and brain abnormalities, as described in Table 32.1.

However, increasing evidence from long-term observational and autopsy studies indicates that demented patients, especially elderly individuals, have brain abnormalities associated with more than one type of dementia. Thus, estimates of the

Table 32.1 Common Types of Dementia

Type of Dementia	Clinical Picture
Alzheimer's disease (AD)	Most common type of dementia; accounts for an estimated 60 to 80% of cases. Difficulty remembering names and recent events is often an early clinical symptom; apathy and depression are also often early symptoms. Later symptoms include impaired judgment, disorientation, confusion, behavior changes and difficulty speaking, swallowing and walking. New criteria and guidelines for diagnosing AD were proposed and published in 2011. They recommend that AD be considered a disease that begins well before the development of symptoms. Hallmark abnormalities are deposits of the protein fragment beta-amyloid (plaques) and twisted strands of the protein tau (tangles) as well as evidence of nerve cell damage and death in the brain.
Vascular dementia (VaD)	Impaired judgment or ability to make plans is more likely to be the initial symptom, as opposed to the memory loss often associated with the initial symptoms of AD. Occurs because of brain injuries such as microscopic bleeding and blood vessel blockage. The location of the brain injury determines how the individual's thinking and physical functioning are affected.
Dementia with Lewy bodies (DLB)	Patients with DLB usually have initial or early symptoms such as sleep disturbances, well-formed visual hallucinations, and parkinsonism. Lewy bodies are abnormal aggregations of the protein alpha-synuclein. When they develop in the cerebral cortex, dementia can result. Alpha-synuclein also aggregates in the brains of people with Parkinson's disease, but the aggregates may appear in a pattern that is different from DLB. The brain changes of DLB alone can cause dementia, or they can be present at the same time as the brain changes of Alzheimer's disease and/or vascular dementia, with each entity contributing to the development of dementia. When this happens, the individual is said to have "mixed dementia."
Parkinson's disease dementia	As Parkinson's disease progresses, it often results in a severe dementia similar to DLB or AD. Problems with movement are a common symptom early in the disease. Alpha-synuclein aggregates are likely to begin in the substantia nigra, causing degeneration of the nerve cells that produce dopamine.
Frontotemporal dementia (FTD)	Typical symptoms include changes in personality and behavior and difficulty with language. No distinguishing microscopic abnormality is linked to all cases, and either Tau-inclusions or TDP43 inclusions are the most common neuropathological hallmarks. Mutations in a number of genes causing autosomal dominant inherited disorder have been identified.

proportion of dementia cases attributable to each of these must be interpreted with caution since these are clinical diagnoses based on typical patterns of onset and course. Neuroimaging biomarkers are routinely available for cerebrovascular disease, but imaging of amyloid plaques as well as cerebrospinal fluid and plasma biomarkers has only recently become available not only as research techniques but possibly as diagnostic tools. Evidence from neuropathological studies challenges the notion of discrete subtypes. Mixed pathologies are much more common than "pure" ones—particularly for Alzheimer's disease (AD) and vascular dementia (VaD), and AD and dementia with Lewy bodies (DLB). In one case series of over 1000 post-mortem examinations, while 86% of all those with dementia had pathology related to AD, only 43% had pure AD, 26% had mixed AD and cerebrovascular pathology, and 10% had AD with cortical Lewy bodies. Findings were similar for those who had been given a clinical diagnosis of AD: "pure" VaD was comparatively rare (7.3%), and uncommon subtypes of dementia, including frontotemporal dementia (FTD), tended to be misdiagnosed in life as AD. Furthermore, the relationship between AD neuropathology and dementia syndrome is less clear-cut than previously thought. Some individuals with advanced pathology do not develop dementia, and cerebrovascular disease may be an important co-factor determining dementia onset. Therefore, estimates of the proportion of cases accounted for by AD, VaD, mixed dementia, DLB, FTD, and other dementias represent, at best, the relative prominence of these different pathologies.

MANAGEMENT OF ALZHEIMER'S DISEASE

The management of a patient with AD is a complex and evolving task because the natural history of AD is one of progressive decline; patients' cognitive, physical, and social functions gradually deteriorate. One of the key aspects of optimal management of dementia is realistic expectations for therapeutic benefits, including treatment effects and potential outcomes; it is, therefore, mandatory that physicians are aware of these issues and discusses them with both the patient and caregiver. To be effective, interventions for patients with dementia ideally will improve functional status to a level that is detectable by caregivers or health care providers.

AD is associated with the presence of beta-amyloid (Abeta) in plaques, intracellular aggregates of tau protein, forming neurofibrillary tangles, and progressive neuronal loss. Abeta plays a primary role in AD pathophysiology. Oligomer species of aggregated Abeta exert toxic effects on synaptic and cellular functions, finally leading to neurodegeneration and cognitive impairment, as well as behavioral and psychological symptoms (BPSD). Although many neurotransmitter systems are affected in AD, degeneration in the cholinergic system occurs earlier and more consistently than in other systems, and these changes are closely correlated with the presence of neuropathological hallmarks. Acetylcholine (ACh) plays a key role in learning and memory, and the predictable degeneration of cholinergic neurons of the hyppocampi, the enthorinal cortex, and the neocortex observed in patients with AD contributes significantly to the first presenting symptoms of the disease. In this view, the replacement of cholinergic deficit has been the main target of AD treatment, and cholinesterase inhibitors (ChEIs) have been the cornerstone of treatment for the past decade.

As AD progresses, deterioration of multiple domains over than memory is observed, including cognition, behavior, and function (see Table 32.2). Specific symptoms

Table 32.2 Main Clinical Characteristics Across Severity Stages of Alzheimer Disease

Early Stage	Middle Stage	Late Stage
The early stage is often overlooked. The onset of the disease is insidious.	In this stage, limitations become clearer and more restricting.	The last stage is characterised by nearly total dependence and inactivity.
• Become forgetful, especially regarding things that just happened • Difficulty in finding words • Getting lost • Lose track of the time, including time of day, month, year, season • Have difficulty carrying out complex tasks • Mood and behavior: – may become less active and motivated and lose interest in activities and hobbies – may have behavioral changes, including depression or anxiety	• Forgetfulness and lose track of the time • Have increasing difficulty with communication • Need help with personal care and with activities of daily living • Need supervision and support • Mood and behavior: wandering, disinhibition, aggression, disturbed sleeping, hallucinations	• Usually unaware of time and place • Have difficulty understanding what is happening around them • Unable to recognize relatives, friends and familiar objects, to eat without assistance, may have difficulty in swallowing • Bladder and bowel incontinence • Behavior changes, may escalate and include aggression towards carer, nonverbal agitation

vary between patients and between stages, and treatment targets should be revised accordingly.

PHARMACOLOGICAL INTERVENTIONS

There are currently no means of reversing the pathological processes of AD. Currently available medications do not halt the underlying degenerative process but can slow disease progression and therefore delay symptomatic decline. The specific goals of therapy are to preserve cognitive and functional ability and minimize behavioral disturbances, with maintenance of patients' and caregivers' quality of life. Nevertheless, realistic expectations of treatment outcomes are needed because the impact for most patients is likely to be modest and temporary, with not every patient responding to treatment. The main benefit of pharmacotherapy is an attenuation of decline over time along with a modest improvement in cognitive or behavioral symptoms. It is important to discuss this point with patients and their families, who may expect improvement rather than relative stability.

Four drugs are commonly used for treating AD: three ChEIs approved for mild to moderate disease, one of which also is approved for severe AD, and a glutamate N-methyl-D-aspartate (NMDA) antagonist approved for moderate to severe disease.

Moreover, along with specific pharmacological management, there is evidence that antihypertensives, nonsteroidal anti-inflammatory agents, statins, and hormone replacement therapy; high education; diet; physical activity; and engagement in social and intellectual activities are protective preventive factors in AD. However, whether modifying these factors reduces risk of dementia is not yet known and, currently, no clear recommendations about dementia prevention can be made.

Furthermore, no treatments have demonstrated clear efficacy for preventing or delaying development of AD in subjects with mild cognitive impairment, while evidence exists that ChEIs, vitamin E, Gingko biloba, and anti-inflammatory drugs are not substantively helpful.

Cholinesterase Inhibitors

Donepezil, rivastigmine, and galantamine are the only approved ChEIs for the treatment of AD. This class of drugs has shown sustained clinically benefit on cognitive function, behavior, global outcome, and activities of daily living. There have been few direct comparisons between ChEIs and those that have been undertaken have been small in size and not produced consistent evidence of better efficacy of one drug over another. On the other hand, large-scale trials with the three ChEIs have shown efficacy in patients with mild to moderate AD, usually defined as a Mini-Mental State Examination (MMSE) between 16 and 26. Further, it has been demonstrated that ChEIs decreased the risk of institutionalization and caregiver burden. Clinical trials of ChEIs in more severe AD (MMSE < 10) have also shown positive results, and a Cochrane review concluded that trials supported evidence of benefit in mild, moderate, and severe AD. In light of current evidence, limiting the prescribing of ChEIs to only mild to moderate AD subjects does not seem justified. Although a point will be reached in severe AD when ChEIs are unlikely to continue to have benefit, it is currently unclear at what point in the disease process ChEIs should be withdrawn.

A disease-modifying effect of ChEIs has been proposed and has some basic scientific support, but no strong clinical data, either from trials of clinical end points or of those using biomarkers, have been forthcoming to support these claims. Effects on BPSD have also been shown, though, as with cognition effect sizes, they are modest. There remains uncertainty as to which particular noncognitive symptoms may respond best, although effects on psychosis, apathy, wandering, and sleep have been consistently described.

Starting dosages, titrated ratio, and target dosages are described in Table 32.3. These drugs should be avoided in presence of breathing problems (such as asthma, chronic obstructive pulmonary disease), fainting, heart disease (such as sick sinus syndrome, other heart conduction disorders), seizures, stomach/intestinal disease (such as ulcers, bleeding), and trouble urinating (such as enlarged prostate). ChEIs are generally well tolerated, although common gastrointestinal adverse effects such as nausea, diarrhea, and vomiting may lead to discontinuation of treatment in some patients. Tolerance to these side effects often develops after a few weeks of treatment. It is important to remember that the three CHEIs have different metabolism, elimination, and protein binding, thus asking for caution when treating patients with somatic comorbidities and polipharmacology (see Table 32.4).

If side effects occur, the drug should be administered at the lowest tolerated dosage. There is some evidence from open-label studies that patients who do not tolerate or do not seem to benefit from one ChEI may tolerate or draw benefit from the other.

Table 32.3 ChEIs Currently Used in the Treatment of AD.

Drug	Route	Action	Metabolism and Elimination*	Starting dosage	Titration	Target dosage
Donepezil	Oral	AChE	CYP2D6 and CYP3A4 *Hepatic	5 mg once daily	increase after 4 weeks to 10 mg	10 mg one daily
Rivastigmine	Oral	AChE and BuChE	Plasma, ACHE hydrolysis *Renal	1.5 mg twice daily	increase after 4 weeks each dose by 1.5 mg	6 mg twice daily
Rivastigmine	transdermal	AChE and BuChE	Plasma, ACHE hydrolysis *Renal	4.6 mg/ 24 h	increase after 4 weeks to 9.5 mg	13.3 mg/24 h
Galantamine	oral	AChE and nicotinic receptor	CYP2D6 and CYP3A4 *Hepatic	4 mg twice daily	increase after 4 weeks each dose by 4 mg	12 mg twice daily

AChE: Acetylcholinesterase; BuChE: Butyrrilcholiesterase

One of the ChEIs, rivastigmine, is now available in a transdermal (patch) formulation that appears to have lower incidence of side effects and better compliance than oral administration but equal efficacy.

Periodic monitoring and assessment of global cognitive impairment by standardized assessment tools (MMSE, Alzheimer's Disease Assessment Scale, Clinical Dementia Rating) and of functional abilities (Activities of Daily Living) are highly recommended.

Memantine

Memantine is a low- to moderate-affinity, non-competitive (channel blocking), NMDA-receptor antagonist that seems to block pathologic neural toxicity associated with prolonged glutamate release. Blockade of NMDA receptors by memantine could confer disease-modifying activity in AD by inhibiting the "weak" NMDA receptor–dependent excitotoxicity that contributes to the neuronal loss underlying the progression of dementia. Studies in moderate to severe AD have been more consistently positive than those in mild to moderate AD; previous reviews of the literature have concluded that there is a significant effect in cognition at all severities, whereas effects on global outcome, activities of daily living, and behavior were only apparent in the moderate to severe studies. Modest effects on behavior were also found in a pooled

Table 32.4 Drug-Drug Interaction of CHEIs

341

Dementia

Donepezil	1. Highly protein bound, may displace other protein bound drugs such as digoxin or warfarin.
	2. CYP 2D6 inhibitors such as fluoxetine, cimeditine can raise level of donepezil.
	3. CYP 3A4 inhibitors such as grapefruit juice, amiodarone, ketoconzaole can raise level of donepezil.
	4. May increase the risk of antipsychotic-related extrapyramidal symptoms.
	5. Excessive cholinergic stimulation with other cholinergic agents.
	6. Concurrent use with beta-blockers may cause bradycardia
Rivastigmine	1. Anticholinergics: effects may be reduced with rivastigmine
	2. May increase the risk of antipsychotic-related extrapyramidal symptoms.
	3. Cigarette use increases the clearance of rivastigmine by 23%
	4. Depolarizing neuromuscular blocking agents effects may be increased
	5. Patients may be at increased risk for peptic ulcers or GI bleeding with concomitant NSAIDS use.
Galantamine	1. Drugs that are inhibitors of CYP2D6 and CYP3A4 such as paroxetine, cimeditine, ketoconazole, and erythromycin can increase galantamine level.
	2. Concurrent use with beta-blockers, calcium blockers, amiodarone may lead to bradycardia.
	3. Synergistic effects with cholinergic agents, leading to worsening of cholinergic side effects.
	4. Concurrent use with NSAIDS may lead to gastric ulcers.
	5. May increase the risk of antipsychotic-related extrapyramidal symptoms.

analysis of six studies that included all those with MMSE <20, with delusions, agitation/aggression, and irritability being the most responsive symptoms, though studies of subjects primarily selected for the presence of these behavioral features have not yet been reported. Once-daily dosing has been shown to be as effective as the original recommendation of administration twice daily. Memantine is generally well tolerated, and adverse effects include fatigue, pain, hypertension, headache, constipation, vomiting, back pain, somnolence, and dizziness. Combination therapy of a ChEI and memantine is rational from a pharmacologial perspective because the agents have different mechanisms of action. Further studies are needed before clear recommendations can be made about the benefits of combining memantine to ChEIs.

In Figure 32.1, pharmachological management of AD is reported. There are several ongoing clinical studies aimed at modifying the underlying disease process, including international trials of passive and active amyloid immunisation. However, recommendations about the usefulness of these and other agents must await definitive results from rigorous Phase III studies.

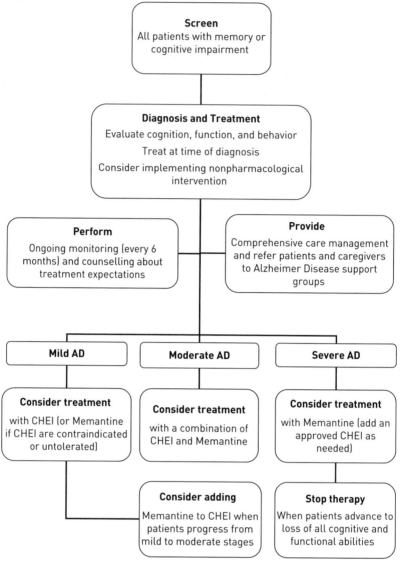

FIGURE 32.1

Treatment and management of Alzheimer disease.

MANAGEMENT OF NONALZHEIMER DEMENTIAS

With few exceptions, there are no established pharmacological treatments approved by the regulatory agencies for non-Alzheimer dementias. However, as the underlying proteinopathies in the individual neurodegenerative entities are being elucidated, the targeting of pathological protein misfolding has become an attractive goal for future mechanism-based treatments.

Frontotemporal Dementia

There is no approved treatment for any of the FTDs. One study demonstrated that despite the lack of evidence from randomized, placebo-controlled clinical trials, off-label use of established ChEIs and memantine is common in behavioral variant FTD (bvFTD). There are three notable open-label studies with each of the ChEIs and three open-label studies with memantine in FTD: all failed to provide robust evidence for efficacy. A recent systematic review stated that antidepressant treatment significantly improves behavioral symptoms in FTD, but most studies were small and uncontrolled; serotonergic treatments with SSRIs appeared to provide inconsistent improvement in the behavioral but not cognitive symptoms of FTD. In a small, randomized controlled trial with trazodone, the cognitive measure MMSE remained unchanged, while there was a significant improvement in behavioral symptoms. Dopaminergic replacement in FTD may ameliorate only the motor symptoms with no evident effect on cognition and on behavior.

Dementia with Lewy Bodies and Parkinson's Disease Dementia

There is evidence that patients with DLB respond to ChEIs with improvement in cognitive and psychiatric symptoms. The Cochrane Library review on ChEI treatment in DLB and Parkinson's disease dementia (PDD) concluded that there was evidence that rivastigmine had a moderate effect on cognition. Patients with DLB show a propensity to have exaggerated adverse reactions to neuroleptic drugs, with a significantly increased morbidity and mortality.

Vascular Dementia

The main goal of treatment in VaD is to prevent further cerebrovascular disease by optimal control of major risk factors in people with a history of stroke. However, there is still no good evidence that aspirin is effective in treating patients with VaD. However, it is still useful as secondary prevention of cerebrovascular disease. Risk factor modification to reduce the risk of stroke should also be started, including physical activity, dietary modification, cholesterol lowering, blood pressure control, and diabetes/glucose control. There have been a few trials of antihypertensive drugs in the treatment or prevention of dementia or cognitive decline. The results of two trials suggested an effect of angiotensin-converting enzyme (ACE) inhibitors (i.e., perindopril in the PROGRESS study) and calcium-channel blockers (i.e., nitrendipine in the SYST-EUR study) in the prevention of both AD and VaD. Systematic reviews have found benefit with nimodipine, another calcium-channel blocker, and also ACE inhibitors and diuretics. However, the results of other large trials of blood pressure lowering were negative for prevention of cognitive decline. Antihypertensive treatment for the prevention of cerebrovascular disease is demonstrated and hence should be used for this purpose, an indirect effect of which may be the prevention of stroke-related cognitive decline.

Increasing evidence supports the involvement of the cholinergic system in VaD, similar to that seen in AD. However, no ChEIs have been approved to date for the treatment of VaD, despite positive results in clinical trials with this medication. However, it is necessary to ensure that the patient does not have a coexistent AD that may warrant such treatment. Mixed dementia with coexisting AD and VaD is thought to occur in up to 50% of dementia cases.

TREATING BEHAVIORAL SYMPTOMS IN NEURODEGENERATIVE DEMENTIAS

Traditionally, cognitive function has been the main focus of interest in treatment and research of people with dementia. It is becoming increasingly recognized, however, that noncognitive symptoms are those that are most disturbing to families and caregivers and may seriously impact not only the patient's well-being, but also the family's, caregivers', and providers' approaches to managing the patient. The most common symptoms are agitation, aggression, mood disorders/behavioral disturbance, apathy, depression, psychosis and hallucinations, with sexual disinhibition, elation/euphoria, appetite and eating disturbances, and abnormal vocalizations occurring less frequently. These may vary according to dementia diagnosis and clinical stage. These have been grouped together under the umbrella term *behavioral and psychological symptoms of dementia* (BPSD) by the International Psychogeriatric Association.

Management of BPSD should focus to careful search for trigger and/or exacerbating factors including environmental cues, physical problems (infections, constipation), medication, and depression or psychosis.

Both conventional and atypical antipsychotics reduce BPSD, with particular effects demonstrated for agitation/aggression and psychosis (see Table 32.5). However, antipsychotics have important and potentially serious side effects, most especially increased stroke risk, increased mortality, parkinsonism, and cognitive impairment. They should be used with caution, at low dose, and for the shortest period needed

Table 32.5 Most Common Antipsychotic Drugs Used in Treating Dementia

Atypical antipsychotics	Dose	Comment
Risperidone	Initial dosage: 0.25 mg/day at bedtime; maximum dosage: 2–3 mg/day, usually twice daily in divided doses	Current research supports use of low dosages; extrapyramidal symptoms may occur at 2 mg/day
Olanzapine	Initial dosage: 2.5 mg/ day at bedtime; maximum dosage: 10 mg/day, usually twice daily in divided doses	Generally well tolerated
Quetiapine	Initial dosage: 12.5 mg twice daily; maximum dosage: 200 mg twice daily	More sedating; beware of transient orthostasis
Typical antipsychotics		
Haloperidol	Initial dosage: 0.5 mg three times/day; maximum dosage: 2-3 mg three times/daily	Anticipated extrapyramidal symptoms; if these symptoms occur, decrease dosage or switch to another agent; avoid use of benztropine or trihexyphenidyl
Clozapine	Initial dosage: 25 mg once daily; maximum dosage: 100 mg three times/day	Agent with "in-between" side-effect profile. Effective in Dementia with Lewy Bodies

only for those with moderate to severe symptoms causing distress and after careful assessment of risk and benefit and after discussion with caregiver and, where possible, patient. There is no evidence that conventional agents are any safer in regard to risk of stroke or mortality than atypical agents, and they have a less-established evidence base and greater side effects. Low doses of antipsychotics should be used with careful monitoring and drugs prescribed for the minimum period required. Atypical antipsychotics have diminished risk of developing parkinsonism compared to conventional agents.

When BPSD have settled, antipsychotics can be withdrawn in most cases without reemergence of BPSD, unless behavioral disturbance is still present.

Different drugs have been used for the spectrum of BPSD in dementia. Mood stabilizers have been used in cases of control of agitation, repetitive, and combative behaviors (see Table 32.6 for drugs and dosages). For depression in dementia, although there is little placebo-controlled evidence to guide practice, clinical experience indicates that

Table 32.6 Pharmacological Approaches to BPSD in Dementia

Mood-stabilizing drugs	Dose	Comments
Trazodone	Initial dosage: 25 mg/day; maximum dosage: 200 to 400 mg/day in divided doses	Use with caution in patients with premature ventricular contractions
Carbamazepine	Initial dosage: 100 mg twice daily; titrate to therapeutic blood level (4–8 µg/mL)	Monitor complete blood cell count and liver enzyme levels regularly; carbamazepine has problematic side effects
Divalproex sodium	Initial dosage: 125 mg twice daily; titrate to therapeutic blood level (40–90 µg/mL)	Generally better tolerated than other mood stabilizers; monitor liver enzyme levels; monitor platelets, prothrombin time, and partial thromboplastin time as indicated.
SSRIs		
Fluoxetine	Initial dosage: 10 mg every other morning; maximum dosage: 20 mg every morning	Activating, very long half-life
Citalopram	Initial dosage: 10 mg/day; maximum dosage: 40 mg/day	Generally well tolerated
Sertraline	Initial dosage: 25–50 mg/day; maximum dosage: 200 mg/day (morning or evening)	Well tolerated; compared to other SSRIs, it has less effect on metabolism of other medications
Paroxetine	Initial dosage: 10 mg/day; maximum dosage: 40 mg/day (morning or evening)	Less activating but more anticholinergic than other SSRIs
Fluvoxamine	50 mg twice daily; maximum dosage: 150 mg twice daily	Exercise caution when using fluvoxamine with alprazolam or triazolam

selective serotonin reuptake inhibitors (SSRIs) are safe and effective in treating mood disorders in dementia and do not have the adverse anticholinergic effects of tricyclics. SSRIs may prolong half-life of other drugs by inhibiting various cytochrome P450 isoenzymes, and typical side effects include sweating, tremors, nervousness, insomnia or somnolence, dizziness, and various gastrointestinal and sexual disturbances (see Table 32.6). For anxiety, benzodiazepines are considered the elective treatment, but regular use can lead to tolerance, addiction, depression, and cognitive impairment; paradoxic agitations occur in about 10% of patients treated with benzodiazepines. Cholinesterase inhibitors improve the apathetic syndrome in AD and may decrease or prevent psychotic symptoms, particularly hallucinations, in AD and DLB.

SUGGESTED READING

Caltagirone C, Bianchetti A, Di Luca M, et al; Italian Association of Psychogeriatrics. Guidelines for the treatment of Alzheimer's disease from the Italian Association of Psychogeriatrics. Drugs Aging 2005;22(Suppl 1):1–26.

Gauthier S, Patterson C, Chertkow H, et al; CCCDTD4 participants. 4th Canadian Consensus Conference on the Diagnosis and Treatment of Dementia. Can J Neurol Sci 2012;39(6 Suppl 5):S1–S8.

Qaseem A, Snow V, Cross JT Jr, et al; American College of Physicians/American Academy of Family Physicians Panel on Dementia. Current pharmacologic treatment of dementia: a clinical practice guideline from the American College of Physicians and the American Academy of Family Physicians. Ann Intern Med 2008;148:370–378.

Sorbi S, Hort J, Erkinjuntti T, et al; EFNS Scientist Panel on Dementia and Cognitive Neurology. EFNS-ENS Guidelines on the diagnosis and management of disorders associated with dementia. Eur J Neurol 2012;19:1159–1179.

SECTION TEN
CENTRAL NERVOUS SYSTEM TUMORS

33 Low-Grade Gliomas

Paola Gaviani, Andrea Salmaggi,
and Antonio Silvani

INTRODUCTION AND EPIDEMIOLOGY

Low-grade gliomas (LGGs) are a heterogeneous group of relatively slow-growing primary brain tumors. The World Health Organization (WHO) classified these tumors as grade I and grade II.

Grade I gliomas include pilocytic astrocytoma (PA), dysembryoplastic neuroepithelial tumor (DNET), and ganglioglioma. It is important to distinguish grade I glioma from other LGGs because of their benign prognosis.

Grade II gliomas are subdivided based on the microscopic appearance of the tumor. The more common subtypes are diffuse astrocytomas, oligodendrogliomas; pleomorphic xanthoastrocytoma (PXA) is less common. Diffuse astrocytomas include fibrillary, protoplasmic, and gemistocytic variants; the mitotic activity in WHO grade II astrocytomas is very low, but the gemistocytic variant is more prone to malignant progression. Mixed gliomas consist of mixtures of various tumor subtypes (such as diffuse astrocytoma and oligodendroglioma). These tend to behave similarly to diffuse astrocytomas. Low-grade diffuse fibrillary astrocytomas have a well-known tendency to become histologically and clinically more severe over time, progressing toward anaplastic astrocytomas and finally glioblastoma multiforme.

Low-grade tumors make up approximately 10–20% of glial tumors in adults and 25% in children. The median age of patients diagnosed with a low-grade astrocytoma, approximately 35 years, is younger than that of patients with more malignant gliomas. In randomized studies, the 5-year overall (OS) and progression-free survival (PFS) rates range from 58–72% and 37–55%, respectively. Several factors can influence survival, such as the histopathology of the tumor (oligodendrogliomas have a better prognosis than astrocytomas, whereas oligoastrocytomas have an intermediate outcome) or the type of therapy received. Younger age (<40 years) and better performance status at the time of diagnosis, as well as the absence of preoperative neurological deficits also have a positive influence on long-term survival.

Finally, molecular features can correlate with prognosis: for example, combined loss of 1p/19q is a favorable marker in oligodendroglioma or oligoastrocytoma; also, *IDH1* mutation has been recently suggested as an independent favorable prognostic factor.

CLINICAL PRESENTATION AND RADIOLOGICAL FEATURES

Most patients with LGG present between the second and fourth decades of life. The symptoms of LGG can vary greatly depending on the size and location of the tumor and whether it has infiltrated into other areas of the brain or spine.

A seizure is the first symptom of an LGG in 72–89% of patients, and often seizures can be resistant to drug therapy. Mental status changes or signs of increased intracranial pressure, such as headache and nausea, are both possible symptoms, as well as focal neurological deficits, present in 2–30% of patients. However, it is important to note that patients may have normal neurological examinations.

Conventionally, these lesions have been diagnosed and investigated using computed tomography (CT) and magnetic resonance Imaging (MRI). CT demonstrates an area of hypodensity, but tumors may be difficult to detect or substantially larger than visualized, often being near isodense. Calcification may be seen in 20% of diffuse astrocytomas and 40% of oligodendrogliomas The typical MRI features of low-grade astrocytomas include a relatively well-defined usually homogeneous mass that displays little or no mass effect, with minimal or no vasogenic edema and little or no enhancement after contrast administration (Figure 33.1).

However, conventional MRI alone may not always be reliable for predicting the histopathologic grading of a given brain astrocytomas, and therefore new MRI techniques can be helpful. In particular because of their low cellularity, LGGs have a higher apparent diffusion coefficient (ADC) on diffusion-weighted MRI and perfusion can

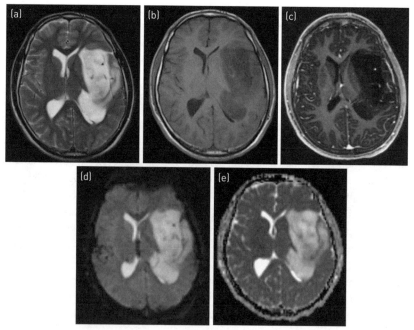

FIGURE 33.1

Radiological features in low-grade glioma that appears hyperintense on T2-weighted images (a), hypointense in T1-weighted images (b) without contrast enhancement (c). Perfusion (d), and diffusion (e) sequences show slow activity.

show low regional blood flow (rCBV). Metabolism and proliferation (assessed by MR spectroscopy or PET) are usually normal or lower than normal brain in LGGs.

After diagnosis, MRI is very important to follow patients with an LGG, as these tumors show either gradual enlargement of the nonenhancing mass or anaplastic progression from low-grade tumor to high-grade tumor; moreover, each new MRI study should be compared with previous studies over as long a period as possible to detect the presence of gradual interval growth.

Sometimes, the findings on the brain CT or MRI are sufficiently clear and the diagnosis of an LGG is fairly certain. In such cases, a histological assessment may not be necessary. However, in most cases, a histological assessment biopsy is recommended to establish the type of tumor.

PROGNOSTIC FACTORS

Clinical factors such tumor size or location, patient age, and performance status have been recognized as prognostic markers in the management of patients with LGGs. Molecular biomarkers are increasingly evolving as additional factors that facilitate diagnostics and therapeutic process.

Isocitrate dehydrogenase (IDH) mutations, 1p deletion, or 1p/19q codeletion have the strongest prognostic impact on survival of treated patients with LGGs, however, so far, no known biomarker is of any relevance for the postoperative course of disease in the absence of an adjuvant treatment. In particular, loss of heterozygosity (LOH) 1p/19q, strongly associated with oligodendroglial brain tumors, was first recognized as a good marker for chemosensitivity; however, it appears to lose its prognostic impact when LGG patients after tumor resection do not receive any further treatment with radiotherapy or chemotherapy.

Moreover, although *IDH1/IDH2* mutations are widely recognized in gliomas (*IDH1/IDH2* mutations have been confirmed as early mutations in LGGs and are associated with a younger age) their prognostic significance remains controversial.

In this settings the study of prognostic biomarkers could be very important affecting possible therapeutic decisions of patients with LGGs, for examples to support the possibility of a primary watch-and-wait strategy in younger patients (<40 years) with few symptoms and clinically stable disease.

TREATMENT

The optimal treatment of LGG (particularly the timing of treatment) is controversial, and treatment decisions must balance the benefits of therapy against the potential for treatment-related complications.

Surgery

Surgery (biopsy or resection) is necessary to provide a histological diagnosis and to assess the molecular status of tumors. The effect of the extent of surgery on OS and PFS is still uncertain, because there are no randomized trials that have specifically addressed this question. However, most clinical series have shown that patients who undergo gross total resection have the longest survival durations. Moreover, total resection improves seizure control, particularly in patients with a short epileptic history and insular tumors. Even subtotal resection is of benefit if the tumor can be removed safely. The timing of surgery is particularly controversial in patients who are young, present with an isolated seizure (medically well controlled), and present with small tumors. In those cases, some clinicians favor a "wait-and-see" approach. However, the risk of deferring surgery includes managing at a later time point a larger tumor, which may have undergone anaplastic transformation. Most reports suggest that removing as much tumor as possible is beneficial even if all neoplastic cells cannot be removed owing to the infiltrating nature of gliomas.

In this setting, intraoperative neurophysiological monitoring has been used increasingly in the last few years. This technique is important to localize anatomical structures, which helps guide the surgeon during intervention mainly in lesions involving functionally important regions of the brain. For example, intraoperative cortical mapping can help to achieve a greater extent of resection and is often used in combination with awake craniotomy.

RADIOTHERAPY

Radiotherapy after surgery of LGGs is still a topic of debate. Long-term toxicity and side effects must also be taken into consideration in LGGs compared with malignant gliomas because patients have an overall longer survival. Some controversies in the use of radiotherapy for LGGs concern the optimal timing of RT and the optimal radiation dose; however, a standardized dose and timing of radiotherapy are relatively established.

As the timing of RT is concerned, phase III randomized trials (Figure 33.2) show that although improved PFS was demonstrated for patients treated with immediate RT, this did not translate into improved OS. This lack of survival benefit with immediate adjuvant radiotherapy has been used as a justification to postpone radiation until disease progression, trying to postpone or avoid potential radiation damages. As the right dose of RT is concerned, randomized trials showed no advantage for higher versus lower doses, with an increased toxicity when higher doses are used. Moreover, patients treated with whole-brain RT seem to have a higher incidence of leukoencephalopathy and cognitive deficits in comparison with patients treated with focal RT. In an EORTC study with 343 patients with LGGs, doses between 45 Gy over 5 weeks and 59.4 Gy yielded no significant difference in overall or progression-free survival between these two regimens. Another phase 3, prospective, randomized trial on 203 patients comparing low-dose 50.4Gy over 28 fractions versus high-dose 64.8 Gy found a higher incidence of radiation necrosis in the high-dose radiotherapy arm.

Chemotherapy

Unfortunately, a large number of LGGs with a diffuse growth pattern cannot be removed without substantial compromise of healthy brain tissue. In this group of patients, the use of chemotherapy can be considered. Results from observational studies indicate that chemotherapy may be effective in patients with oligodendroglial tumors, but the role of chemotherapy in diffuse low-grade astrocytomas is less clear. PCV (procarbazine, CCNU, and vincristine) and TMZ seem to show similar objective

Study	Number of Patients	Treatment	5-Years pfs %	5-Years os %
EORTC 22845	311	Surgery vs surgery + RT	37% (surgery group) vs 44% (surgery + RT) p = 0.02	66% (surgery group) vs 63% (surgery + RT) p = ns
RTOG 94.02	251	Surgery + Rt vs surgery + RT + CT (PCV	46% (Surgery + RT) vs 63% (surgery + RT + CT), p = 0.005	63% (Surgery + RT) vs 72% (surgery + RT + CT), p = ns
EORTC 22844	343	Surgery + Rt 45Gy vs Surgery + Rt 59.4 Gy	47% (Surgery + RT 45Gy) vs 50% (Surgery + Rt 59.4 Gy) p = ns	58% (Surgery + RT 45Gy) vs 59% (Surgery + Rt 59.4 Gy) p = ns
NCCTG	203	Surgery + Rt 50.4 Gy vs Surgery + Rt 64.8 Gy	55% (Surgery + RT)50.4 Gy vs 52% (Surgery + Rt 64.8 Gy) p = ns	72% (Surgery + RT 50.4 G) vs 64% (Surgery + RT 64.8 Gy) p = ns

Legend: RT (radiotherapy), CT (chemotherapy), PCV (procarbazine, vincristine and CCNU), na (not available), ns (not significant)

FIGURE 33.2

Phase III Trials on Adjuvant Treatment in Low Grade Glioma.

radiological response rates (45–62%) and duration of response (10–24 months), especially in patients with 1p/19q deletion and methylated MGMT promoter. TMZ seems to have a better toxicity profile. In fact, TMZ has been shown in multiple studies to be a well-tolerated alkylating agent that can improve radiographic response, symptom benefit, and progression-free survival. Due to its favorable toxicity profile, TMZ has been proposed as a therapeutic alternative to radiotherapy in the first-line treatment, especially when patients are young or tumor growth would require a too extensive field of radiation.

At the moment, there are numerous clinical trials in LGG patients that investigate different dosing schedules, combination therapies, and safety profiles of new therapies. Moreover, the study of prognostic biomarkers could be very important in possible therapeutic decisions of this group of patients; as a matter of fact, newer agents, such as angiogenesis inhibitors or monoclonal antibodies, signal transduction inhibitors, as well as new approaches to drug delivery, such as drug-impregnated sustained-release polymers and convection-enhanced delivery, remain to be investigated in this group of tumors.

SYMPTOM MANAGEMENT

Seizures, cerebral edema (swelling in the brain around the tumor), and obstructive hydrocephalus (increased pressure within the brain due to blockage of the flow of cerebrospinal fluid within the brain) can all result in serious symptoms. Each of these requires a different therapeutic approach.

Seizures occur as a presenting symptom in more than 50% of LGG cases and have a cumulative frequency of 80%. Furthermore, patients with WHO grade II diffuse astrocytomas often experience neuropsychological and psychological problems that are aggravated by epilepsy and its treatment. The same medications used to treat epilepsy are usually useful in controlling seizures associated with brain tumors. However, seizures may be more difficult to control in brain tumor patients, particularly in LGGs.

Cerebral edema usually can be treated successfully with steroids; the most commonly used steroid is dexamethasone that may be particularly useful in the late phases.

TAKE-HOME MESSAGES ON TREATMENT

- Surgery represents the first treatment option, with the goal to maximal resection of the tumor whenever possible, minimizing the postoperative problems (for example, with the identification of eloquent cerebral areas), and when surgery is not feasible with an indication of a biopsy (either stereotactic or open) that should be performed to obtain a histological diagnosis.
- Radiation therapy and chemotherapy are generally used in the settings of incomplete resection and recurrent disease, and these strategies are being investigated in prospective clinical trials.
- For patients with unfavorable prognostic factors an adjuvant treatment is indicated at any time, and this is more commonly RT, with a standard total RT dose of 50–54 Gy.
- Chemotherapy is an option as initial treatment for patients with large residual tumors after surgery or unresectable tumors or it is an option for patients with recurrence after surgery and radiation therapy.
- Since LGGs represent a heterogeneous group of tumors with variable natural histories, the risks and benefits of therapies must be carefully balanced with the data available from limited prospective studies.

SUGGESTED READING

Hafeez S, Cavaliere R. Recent innovations in the management of low-grade gliomas. Curr Treat Options Neurol 2012;14:369–380.

Jakola AS, Myrmel KS, Kloster R, et al. Comparison of a strategy favoring early surgical resection vs a strategy favoring watchful waiting in low-grade gliomas. JAMA 2012;308:1881–1888.

Lang FF, Gilbert MR. Diffusely infiltrative low-grade gliomas in adults. J Clin Oncol 2006;24:1236–1245.

Shaw EG, Tatter SB, Lesser GJ, et al. Current controversies in the radiotherapeutic management of adult low-grade glioma. Semin Oncol 2004; 31:653.

Soffietti R, Baumert BG, Bello L, et al. Guidelines on management of low-grade gliomas: report of an EFNS-EANO Task Force. Eur J Neurol 2010;17:1124–1133.

Weller M, Wick W. Molecular predictors of outcome in low-grade glioma. Curr Opin Neurol 2012;25:767–773.

34 High-Grade Gliomas

Andrea Salmaggi, Anna Fiumani,
and Antonio Silvani

INTRODUCTION

High-grade gliomas (HGGs) are tumors arising in the central nervous system from cells of the glial lineage, that is, astrocytes, oligodendrocytes, and ependymal cells.

According to the WHO 2007 classification, they include grade IV gliomas (glioblastoma and gliosarcoma) and grade III gliomas (anaplastic astrocytoma, anaplastic oligodendroglioma, anaplastic oligoastrocytoma, and anaplastic ependymoma).

Their prevalence is of approximately 6 or 7 cases/100.000/yr, with a higher frequency in males. The most frequent subtype is represented by glioblastoma, which accounts by itself for 50% of HGGs. Median age at onset is around 60 years in glioblastomas, while it is lower in grade III gliomas. Tumor location is generally in the white matter of cerebral hemispheres, although deep-seated tumors are also encountered such as those in the basal ganglia. Cerebellar, brainstem, and spinal location are rare in adults. As far as ependymomas (grade III) are concerned, they may arise at the spinal, infratentorial, and supratentorial levels.

Glioblastomas may either arise de novo or be the end-stage of a previous lower-grade glioma at progression. These two varieties of glioblastoma differ from a molecular biology standpoint, with primary glioblastoma showing amplification of the epidermal growth factor receptos variant III (EGFRvIII), and also clinically, with a higher frequency of seizures in secondary glioblastoma. Clinical features include localizing signs and symptoms and/or signs of generalized brain dysfunction or the syndrome of intracranial hypertension.

In a prospective study in 349 glioblastoma patients, symptoms or signs at disease onset included seizures in 29%, headache in 24%, language disorder in 22%, cognitive/behavioral abnormalities in 22%, paresis in 22%, and other symptoms and signs in 8%. Brain CT and MRI show the typical features of HGG, with areas of hypointensity in T1- and hyperintensity in T2-weighted images, mass effect with effacement of sulci, and an irregular enhancement ring with often a nodular portion surrounding a central necrotic area. Calcifications may be present in secondary glioblastomas arising, especially from oligodendrogliomas. Digitate vasogenic edema is present in most cases. Hydrocephalus may complicate tumors obstructing cerebrospinal fluid (CSF) flow or reabsorption.

A minority of HGGs do not display contrast enhancement but their CT/MRI features are suggestive of highly cellular malignancies.

In cases in which doubts arise on the possible diagnosis, other tools such as diffusion~perfusion MRI, spectroscopic MRI, FDG, and methionine PET may help in discriminating HGG from other tumor or nontumor conditions such as giant multiple sclerosis plaques and brain abscess.

However, sensitivity and specificity of these techniques do not attain 100%. Definite diagnosis requires histological assessment, which is obtained either by stereotactic biopsy in those cases not deemed to be amenable to surgical resection or by tumor resection in those cases in which total-subtotal removal is a reasonable option with low risk of neurological deficit.

THE ROLE OF SURGERY

No large scale randomized phase III trial has ever been conducted to assess the role of surgery and its impact on survival in HGGs.

Accumulating evidence suggests that—apart from the palliative role of surgery—a substantial cytoreductive intervention, the minimal extent of which is debated, may positively impact on survival. The extent of tumor resection above which this effect is detected may be as low as 78% according to recent data. In controversial cases, such as those at risk for postoperative deficits, or those with very poor performance status or with significant medical comorbidities, a multidisciplinary evaluation is suggested involving radiotherapist, neuro-oncologist, and palliative care physician.

When surgery is planned, presurgical MRI with tractography may help clarify the relationships between tumor and long fibers. Also, awake anesthesia is helpful in preventing neurological deficits, as well as intraoperative monitoring of cortical and subcortical activity. Intraoperative use of 5aminolevulinic acid (5Ala) helps the surgeon in achieving as maximal a resection as possible.

The surgeon should provide information on the risks of surgery or biopsy, including the risk of nondiagnostic histology when stereotactic biopsy is considered. Life expectancy in glioblastoma varies according to well-known prognostic factors (i.e., age, performance status, extent of tumor resection, methylated MGMT promoter), with longer survival in younger, fitter, MGMT promoter methylated patients undergoing gross total resection. Median ST is 14 months after surgery, RT, and chemotherapy with temozolomide.

POSTSURGICAL TREATMENTS

Glioblastoma

A standard of care exists for patients with glioblastoma aged 18 to 70 and with a WHO PS of 2 or less, since the 2005 EORTC trial. This includes focal radiotherapy for a total of 60 Gy over 6 weeks, concomitant with temozolomide 75 mg/per square meter/day and followed by temozolomide 150–200 mg per square meter per day for 5 days every 28 days up to six cycles. Phase IV experience shows that only 70–80% of patients are able to complete the chemotherapy treatment, due to either tumor progression or side effects. Controversy exists regarding the attitude in patients in whom good general conditions and neurological conditions, no side effects, and no evidence of tumor regrowth are seen at the end of the six cycles of temozolomide. No standard of care exists for fit patients over 70 and for any patient with PS higher than 3.

Recent trials suggest that either radiation therapy alone at standard or reduced *45 Gy dose or temozolomide alone at 150/200 mg/sq^2/day for 5 days every 28 days for

6 to 12 cycles may be of some benefit in fit elderly patients. In elderly patients with poor PS, chemotherapy alone or schedules of hypofractionated radiotherapy may be a worthwhile option.

The ongoing EORTC trial will clarify whether addition of concomitant and adjuvant temozolomide is worthwhile in combination with radiotherapy for 45 Gy in elderly and fit HGG patients. An alternative therapeutic standard to the Stupp regimen includes positioning of carmustine-loaded polymers in the postsurgical cavity at the end of surgery, followed by standard radiotherapy. This option may be chosen in selected patients in whom total tumor resection without opening of the ventricles has taken place. Side effects may include brain abscess, seizures, and brain edema.

No phase III trials have been conducted comparing the Stupp approach to the Gliadel approach.

Only phase II trials have assessed the safety, toxicity, and preliminary efficacy of combining the Stupp regimen with Gliadel. Note that the mean increase of overall survival provided by either systemic or locoregional chemotherapy is of approximately 2 months. The patients with methylated MGMT promoter may benefit more from the Stupp schedule in terms of increased survival. The percentage of survivors at 2 years is of nearly 50% with the Stupp schedule and of nearly 10% at 5 years, suggesting that a subset of patients may become long-term survivors. In the few patients displaying either allergic reactions to temozolomide or difficulties in swallowing, intravenous treatment with nitrosureas such as BCNU may be an option, which has been proved of some efficacy at a meta-analysis level.

The addition of intravenous bevacizumab to the Stupp schedule in first diagnosis glioblastoma has been shown by two large randomized trials to improve progression free survival without inducing any prolongation in overall survival when compared with the standard Stupp regimen.

Radiotherapy

Radiotherapy in HGG should start for GBM within 6 weeks from surgery and be targeted to the tumor bed as detected by CT or MRI plus a 2.5-cm margin to reduce the rate of local relapse. Single daily fractions of 2 Gy are delivered by LINAC over 6 weeks. During radiotherapy, monitor the patient for early side effects, including brain edema.

Also assess possible side effects in patients receiving chemotherapy and antiepileptic medication, including myelosuppression, infections, and allergic reactions. In elderly people with good PS, a trial by Keime Guibert et al has shown superiority of a shortened and lower-dose radiotherapy versus best supportive treatment.

POSTSURGICAL CARE IN GRADE III GLIOMAS

Grade III gliomas include anaplastic astrocytoma, anaplastic oligoastrocytoma, and anaplastic oligodendroglioma.

Prognostic factors in these tumors include age, extent of resection, and presence or absence of LOH at 1p and 19q chromosomes.

Median survival is shorter in purely astrocytic grade III neoplasms, which display a median survival time (MST) of approximately 3 years. Survival is longer in anaplastic oligodendrogliomas, with intermediate values in mixed-grade III gliomas.

The strongest predictive factor on survival appears to be the genetic profile with codeleted patients displaying survival times of many years. Surgery in these tumors has the aim of resecting the neoplasm totally or subtotally. Radiation therapy after surgery is standard.

Concerning anaplastic oligoastrocytoma and anaplastic oligodendroglioma, long-term results of two large trials have been published in 2012, both showing that early chemotherapy with PCV after surgery improves both progression free and overall survival, at the expense of a higher frequency of side effects.

Both the effect on progression free survival and that on overall survival are substantially restricted to patients positive for LOH 1p/19q codeletions.

In grade III oligodendrogliomas and oligoastrocytomas with positive LOH at 1p and 19q, seriously consider addition of chemotherapy after surgery and prior to or after radiation therapy.

Concerning purely anaplastic astrocytoma, postsurgical radiotherapy is standard, with nitrosurea-based chemotherapy having been shown to be effective only at meta-analytic level. Widespread prescription of both adjuvant temozolomide and Stupp schedule is observed but not based on level A evidence.

Anaplastic ependymoma management includes surgery followed by radiation therapy on the operated field. No solid data are available for the putative effect of chemotherapy in addition to radiotherapy on clinical outcome.

Always remember that craniospinal contrast-enhanced MRI should be part of the presurgical staging in the suspicion of ependymoma, or follow surgery.

MANAGEMENT OF TUMOR-RELATED SEIZURES

Seizures occur at presentation in 20–40% of HGGs, but their frequency increases during the course of the disease. They may be either simple partial or complex partial or secondarily generalized.

Seizures associated with HGGs are produced by a number of pathophysiological mechanisms involving both the tumor and, more importantly, the tumor infiltration area surrounding the main tumor mass. Among these mechanisms, microbleeding, ionic imbalances, and amino acid shifts play a role. Recent evidence suggests that glutamate produced by the tumor may enhance neuronal hyperexcitability, leading to seizures.

Expression of drug resistance molecule in the context of the tumor and surrounding area may partly explain the difficulties in achieving a satisfactory seizure control.

There is no need to start prophylactic antiepileptic treatment in patients not having displayed previous seizures. Perioperative prophylaxis may be performed, but it should be tapered down in a few weeks after surgery.

In patients with seizures, treatment must be started after the first episode and it is advisable to continue at least until the end of radiation therapy. Most cases will have to go on indefinitely, perhaps with the exception of grade III oligodendroglioma with total resection and favorable prognosis.

It is preferable to consider non–enzyme-inducing antiepileptic drugs, which show less interference with metabolism of chemotherapeutic agents. Consider either oxcarbazepine or levetiracetam or lamotrigine or valproic acid, with the last being an enzyme suppressor.

The frequency of partial complex seizures is probably underestimated in HGGs.

Brain edema associated with brain tumors often produces clinical signs and symptoms so severe to affect severely both performance status and quality of life of patients.

In clinical practice, brain edema associated with brain tumor is commonly treated by steroid administration. Steroid treatment in patients with mass-effect secondary to brain edema frequently gives a marked improvement of clinical conditions.

Low doses of dexamethasone (4 mg) may actually be enough to get such clinical improvement. A clinical trial on patients with brain edema associated to brain metastases has showed that 16 mg of dexamethasone did not further the improvement of the performance status obtained with 4 mg. On the other hand, in severe edematous reactions, doses even higher than 16 mg are sometimes required.

The guidelines recommend to stop steroid administration when symptoms are over, but actually, in clinical practice, stopping or even just reducing steroid administration meets with lots of obstacles, including persisting mass effect. Side effects might be relevant and drug-dependence patterns often occur. The current abuse of steroids in neuro-oncology is then detrimental, as the comorbidity induced by the side effects is able to worsen significantly both performance status and quality of life, even to threat of survival. Diabetes, water retention with gaining of body weight, hypertension, osteoporosis with vertebral collapses, immunosuppression with opportunistic infections, insomnia, mental changes, and myopathy are the most common complications.

As an alternative to steroids, which presumably give BBB stabilization, the available notions on brain edema pathophysiology suggest the use of other drugs, such as VEGF antagonists (bevacizumab), which induce a marked brain edema reduction in HGG relapses, with relevant clinical improvement, even if general survival seems to be not significantly increased.

Recently, a controlled clinical trial has confirmed the putative role of boswellic acid (H15) in brain edema treatment of neuro-oncological patients after radiotherapy. H15 is administered per os and its use might let reduce steroids doses (steroids sparing) or even stop their administration.

Osmotic agents may be used to manage acute brain edema. Mannitol 100 mL i.v. every 4 to 6 hours for a few days is effective but should not be used for longer time.

MANAGEMENT OF HIGH-GRADE GLIOMA AT RELAPSE

No phase 3 trials have been performed in HGGs at relapse, except for the trial comparing repeat surgery plus gliadel to repeat surgery alone. That trial showed a statistically significant improvement in survival in patients with glioblastoma treated with repeat surgery and gliadel at relapse.

The FDA has authorized, on the basis of a phase II randomized non comparative trial, the use of bevacizumab; however, this view has not been shared by the European regulatory authorities.

If time elapsed from first surgery is not exceedingly short, repeat surgery may be a worthwhile option in fit patients.

Also, second-line chemotherapy with dose-dense temozolomide or with fotemustine or with PVC may be proposed, keeping in mind that no phase III trials are available.

The FDA has also authorized electric field–based therapy in recurrent HGG.

Focal radiosurgery with a cyber knife may be proposed for lesions not larger than 3.5 cm.

Note that treatment in the context of HGG relapse is not standard. Whenever possible, patients should be referred to clinical trials; when this is not feasible, an individualized approach with a focus on side effects and patient preferences should be entertained, since survival is likely not to be longer than 10 months in this setting, whatever the treatment chosen.

PALLIATIVE CARE IN HIGH-GRADE GLIOMA

Due to the poor outlook in the short term in many HGG patients, palliative care and end of life issues are relevant points in the clinical management.

Empathic communication by the medical and nursing staff, psychological support when needed, assessment of the needs of patients and their supportive group are important issues.

In the end stage of the disease, when patients are bedridden and with swallowing difficulties, shift to i.m. antiepileptic therapy has to be planned.

SUGGESTED READING

Buckingham SC, Campbell SL, Haas BR, et al. Glutamate release by primary brain tumors induces epileptic activity. Nat Med 2011;17:1269–1274.

Cairncross JG, Wang M, Shaw EG, et al. Chemotherapy plus radiotherapy versus RT alone for patients with anaplastic oligodendroglioma. Long term results of the RTOG 9402 phase III study. Abstract of 2012 ASCO annual meeting.

Chinot O.L., Wick W., Mason W., et al. Bevacizumab plus radiotherapy-temozolomide for newly diagnosed glioblastoma. N Eng J Med 2014;370:709–722.

Friedman HS, Prados MD, Wen PY, et al. Bevacizumab alone and in combination with irinotecan in recurrent glioblastoma. J Clin Oncol 2009;27:4733–4740.

Gallego Perez-Larraya J, Ducray F, Chinot O, et al. Temozolomide in elderly patients with newly diagnosed glioblastoma and poor performance status. An ANOCEF phase II trial. J Clin Oncol 2011;29:3050–3055.

Gilbert M.R., Dignam J.J., Armstrong T.S., et al. A randomized trial of bevacizumab for newly diagnosed glioblastoma. N Eng J Med 2014;370:699–708.

Keime-Guibert F, Chinot O, Taillandier L, et al. Radiotherapy for glioblastoma in the elderly. N Engl J Med 2007;356:1527–1535.

Kirste S, Treier M, Wehrle SJ, et al. Boswellia serrata acts on cerebral edema in patients irradiated for brain tumors: a prospective, randomized, placebo-controlled, double-blind pilot trial. Cancer 2011;117:3788–3795.

Laperriere N, Weller M, Stupp R, et al. Optimal management of elderly patients with glioblastoma. Cancer Treatment Rev 2012;1:1–8.

Roth P, Wick W, Weller M. Steroids in neurooncology: actions, indications, side-effects. Curr Opin Neurol 2010;6:597–602.

Rudà R, Trevisan E, Soffietti R. Epilepsy and brain tumors. Curr Opin Oncol 2010;6:611–620.

Salmaggi A., Silvani A., Merli R. et al. Multicentre prospective collection of newly diagnosed glioblastoma patients. Update on the Lombardia experience. Neurol Sci 2008;29:77–83.

Sanai N., Berger M.S. Glioma extent of resection and its impact on patient outcome. Neurosurgery 2008;62:753–766.

Stupp, R., Mason W.P., van den Bent M.J., et al. Radiotherapy plus concomitant and adjuvant temozolomide for glioblastoma. N Engl J Med 2005;352:987–996.

Van den Bent M.J., Hoang-Xuan K., Brandes A.A. et al. Long term follow-up results of EORTC 26951. A randomized phase III study on adjuvant PCV chemotherapy in anaplastic oligodendroglial tumors. Abstract of 2012 ASCO annual meeting.

Westphal M., Hilt D.C., Bortey E., et al. A phase 3 trial of local chemotherapy with biodegradable carmustine (BCNU) wafers (Gliadel wafers) in patients with primary malignant glioma. Neurooncology 2003;5:79–88.

Wick W, Platten M, Meisner C, et al. Temozolomide chemotherapy alone versus radiotherapy alone for malignant astrocytoma in the elderly. The NOA-08 randomized, phase 3 trial. Lancet Oncol 2012;13:707–715.

35 Gliomatosis Cerebri

Paola Gaviani, Andrea Salmaggi, and Antonio Silvani

INTRODUCTION AND PATHOLOGICAL FEATURES

Diffuse cerebral gliomas are a rare form of infiltrating tumor, in which invasion by glial neoplastic cells involves more than two lobes (bilaterally in nearly half the cases and sometimes the major part of the brain), occasionally extending to infratentorial structures or the spine, with the preservation of anatomical architecture and a sparing of neurons. It is not uncommon to have the frontal and temporal lobes involved with the basal ganglia and thalami. Brainstem involvement is not unusual, with the midbrain and pons being affected more commonly than the medulla. An interesting observation consists in the fact that gliomatosis has a predilection for the right side of the brain, which in most people is the nondominant, less active hemisphere. Compared with active regions, in fact, less active regions show a lower metabolism and blood circulation and therefore a possibly lower immune surveillance.

Diffuse cerebral gliomas were termed gliomatosis cerebri (GC) by Nevin in 1938, and this condition has been included in the World Health Organization (WHO) classification of brain tumors. From a pathogenic point of view, it is not clear if GC represents a diffuse neoplastic transformation with multicentric origin of transformed glial cells or a direct spread from one or more localized neoplastic foci, and this point raises a question as to whether GC represents a separate entity or a highly infiltrative subtype of common glial neoplasm. In this setting, according to the 2007 WHO classification, GC is listed as a subtype of diffuse glioma, considering GC as a growth pattern of astrocytomas (most commonly), oligodendrogliomas, and oligoastrocytomas.

To date, it is difficult to find specific genetic alterations that distinguish GC from other gliomas; molecular genetic and immunohistochemical alterations found in GC are the same as in other low-grade astrocytic tumors, especially genetic alterations of *TP53* or chromosome 1p deletion in GC with oligodendroglial differentiation, although no significant alterations that frequently occur primarily in high-grade gliomas have been reported. The role of MGMT promoter methylation status is unknown at the moment. It has been reported that some cell adhesion factors, such as L1, are expressed more abundantly in GC than in other gliomas; since L1 could play an important role in the migration process, it might be significantly involved in the invasive potential of GC. Moreover, the frequency of *IDH1* in GC is relatively high in secondary GC, caused by the progression of diffuse astrocytomas, whereas no *IDH1* mutation was observed in primary GC. GC is usually an aggressive neoplasm corresponding to WHO grade III in a majority of cases; although GC often demonstrates histological and molecular findings of WHO grade II gliomas, the formation of secondary malignant foci may occur, including, in this case, GC, in WHO grade III gliomas.

CLINICAL FEATURES AND DIAGNOSIS

Clinically, GC shows the same age and sex distribution of other gliomas; it can occur at any age but is usually found in 40- to 50-year-olds and presents a slight male prevalence.

Gliomatosis can produce nonspecific symptoms as a result of increased cerebral pressure, as well as symptoms as result of specific tumor location. The duration of symptoms varies from a slow, insidious onset to more rapid presentations. Clinical manifestations are variable and not specific and include seizures, intracranial hypertension, changes in mental status or focal neurological deficits. For this reason clinical changes are not really helpful to establish the diagnosis. Laboratory findings are mostly normal and not specific and regarding cerebrospinal fluid findings, there are discrepancies in the literature.

Therefore neuroimaging is an important tool in the diagnosis of GC The radiologic findings of gliomatosis cerebri reflect the diffuse infiltrative nature of this tumor. CT can appear normal because lesions are often isodense to normal brain parenchyma. There is relative lack of mass effect and distortion. There may be an asymmetry or subtle hypoattenuation to the involved brain parenchyma. The imaging study of choice is MRI (Figure 35.1) and radiologic-pathologic correlation indicates that tumor delineation should be based mainly on T2-weighted MRI.

The T2-weighted images demonstrate the tumor involvement through the white matter in multiple lobes of the brain with diffuse increased signal intensity and loss of distinction between grey and white matter. The increase in signal intensity is usually mild to moderate on T2-weighted images, whereas some areas of the lesion may show higher signal intensity, possibly representing anaplastic components. The T1-weighted sequences may show mild decrease in signal intensity. Contrast enhancement is not usually evident or minimal, and if a focal area of enhancement is seen degeneration into a more malignant glioma should be suspected (Figure 35.2).

Differential diagnosis involves a number of other diseases. GC could be misinterpreted as ischemic or infectious disease (for example, leukoencephalopathy); a challenging differential diagnosis could be demyelinating disease; however, in GC, neurons and axons are usually better preserved and the large plaques in multiple sclerosis are usually more circumscribed than the changes in GC. Gliomatosis could be differentiated from multifocal gliomas by its continuity of cellular infiltration and lack of clear distinction from adjacent normal brain tissue.

The definite diagnosis of GC was formerly made only at autopsy. However, recent improvements in imaging and biopsy now allow for ante-mortem diagnosis. Because the diagnosis of GC requires radiopathological correlation, brain biopsy and histopathological examination are mandatory. However, it is important to know that the biopsy sample may not be representative of the entire lesion, because some parts of the tumor can show no mitotic activity or little anaplasia, and other parts could be the expression of diffusely infiltrating form of high-grade glioma. To date, brain biopsy based on MRI is the method recommended to establish the diagnosis; however, there could be limits due to possible misinterpretation of imaging findings for the localization of ideal biopsy as well as the sampling error. When possible, the center of diffuse

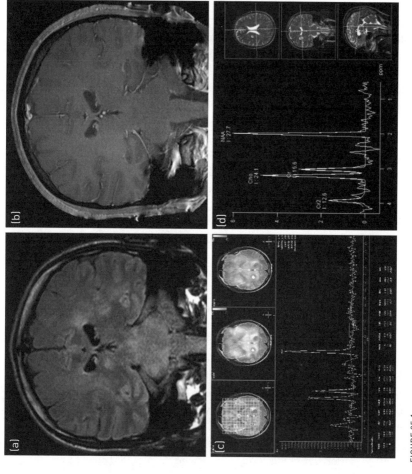

FIGURE 35.1

Gliomatosis cerebri on MRI. FLAIR images (a) show tumor involvement through the white matter in multiple lobes, T1-weighted images, (b) show the absence of enhancement and spectroscopy, and (c and d) indicate a low cell turnover.

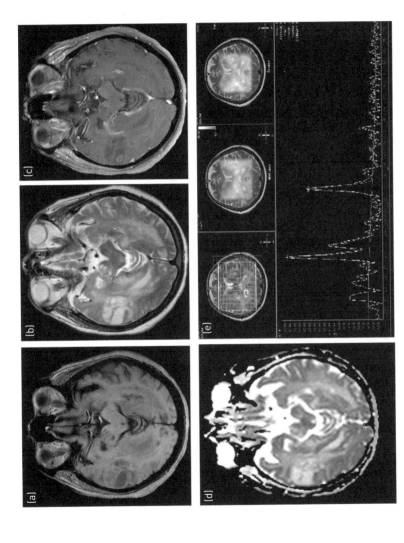

FIGURE 35.2

MRI axial T1-weighted (a), T2-weighted (b), T1-weighted post contrast (c), ADC (d), and MRS (e) images of a progressive high-grade gliomatosis.

infiltrative lesion (in cases without contrast enhancement on MRI) or the center of enhanced area (in cases with contrast enhancement on MRI), should be selected by neurosurgeons during stereotactic biopsy to point the most representative lesion.

PROGNOSIS AND TREATMENT

Generally, prognosis of patients with GC is poor probably due to the highly infiltrative activity of glioma cells. The 1-, 2-, and 3-year reported survival rates are 48%, 37%, and 27%, respectively, not very different from those in glioblastoma. However, survival for patients who did not receive treatment is highly variable and can range from weeks to years.

Age and performance status at diagnosis, as well as histological features, seem to be the most important prognostic factors. Early detection by MRI, active management of increased intracranial pressure, and radiation therapy with optimal dose and field may account of cases with a better outcome.

The optimal treatment for gliomatosis cerebri is still controversial.

The main problem in studies on GC patients is the small number of patients due to the rarity of the disease, so often the studies are anecdotal or unrandomized and patient population is heterogeneous: this precludes meaningful statistical analysis of real factors affecting outcome. Moreover, another important limit in studying this group of patients consists in the fact that patients with GC are mainly excluded from clinical trials due to the fact that these tumors are unresectable and that the patients often present a poor performance status; therefore there are no guidelines for therapy in this group of tumors.

Surgery

Surgery, outside diagnostic purposes, is of little benefit given the extensive and diffuse spread of the disease in the brain. Craniotomy can be useful in some situations to decompress the brain in patients with significantly increased intracranial pressure and to relieve from local mass effect.

Radiotherapy

The literature contains a number of anecdotal reports of radiation therapy as treatment. Given the widespread nature of gliomatosis, radiation can involve areas of diffuse brain involvement, leading to consider this type of treatment potentially effective; on the other hand the diffuse involvement of brain puts a large volume of brain at risk for radiation damage, and this is particularly important in patients who have a low grade variant of GC with a better prognosis in terms of survival. In general radiation may improve or at least stabilize the clinical conditions in patients with GC, and it seems that the outcome for patients who receive radiotherapy is relatively better than the outcome of patients who do not receive any treatment. However, based on literature, the real impact of brain radiotherapy on survival remains still not completely definite.

After radiotherapy clinical and radiological stabilization or improvement is often reported in literature; in a large review by Taillibert and colleagues on 296 cases of patients with GC, of 41 patients treated with radiation a response rate of 58% of clinical improvement and a response rate of 31% of radiological response are reported; however the impact of radiotherapy on overall survival remains questionable, with a median OS of 14.5 months among the whole population of patients and a median OS of 11 months among the 105 patients who did not receive any treatment.

Chemotherapy

The precise role of chemotherapy alone or associated with radiotherapy in GC is not definitely proved, even if promising. Chemotherapy typically includes the use of nitroureas as single treatment or as a combination (for example, lomustine-CCNU, nimustin-ACNU, or procarbazine) and has been reported to lead to radiological response rates from 25% to 45%, with a median OS of 25 months in patients who responded to treatments. However, it should be noted that a relevant problem with nitrosureas and other alkylating agents consists in severe and cumulative hematologic

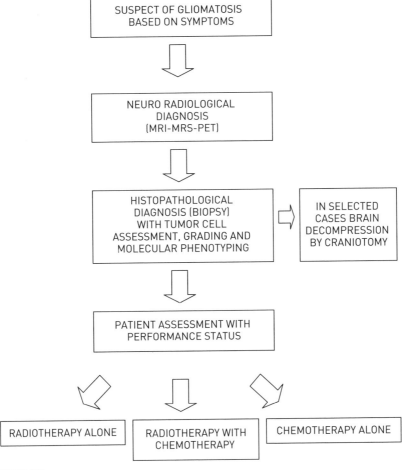

FIGURE 35.3
Possible algorythm for initial management of gliomatosis cerebri.

toxicity, especially increased during multidrug combination such as PCV scheme (procarbazine, lomustine, and vincristine). To date, it has been established that a significant proportion of patients might benefit from an initial chemotherapy with temozolomide, with objective responses in around half of patients treated, and good tolerability; in particular, significant neurological improvement can be observed in patients with either response or stable disease on MRI. Moreover, it is suggested that adjuvant chemotherapy with temozolomide following radiotherapy may be effective in prolonging survival and in delaying tumor progression. Experimental chemotherapy delivered concurrent or subsequent to radiation therapy is actively being investigated in the treatment of diffuse gliomatosis cerebri. For example, a combined low-dose chemotherapy with temozolomide and celecoxib (a cyclooxygenase-2 inhibitor) as antiangiogenic treatment following radiation therapy is reported to be a promising approach for treating these patients

In conclusion, the optimal treatment of GC is still unclear:

1. The role of surgery is limited to histological diagnosis.
2. Whole brain radiation therapy alone could affect positively clinical and radiological response rates but its role on overall survival is questionable.
3. Chemotherapy seems to be beneficial at least in some patients; in the future it is likely that treatment will be guided by molecular genetic findings that could direct a more individualized therapy (Figure 35.3).

SUGGESTED READING

Freund M, Hähnel S, Sommer C, et al. CT and MRI findings in gliomatosis cerebri: a neuroradiologic and neuropathologic review of diffuse infiltrating brain neoplasms. Eur Radiol 2001;11(2):309–316.

Glas M, Rasch K, Wiewrodt D, et al. Procarbazine and CCNU as initial treatment in gliomatosis cerebri. Oncology 2008;75(3–4):182–185.

Kim DG, Yang HJ, Park IA, et al. Gliomatosis cerebri: clinical features, treatment and prognosis. Acta Neurochir 1998;140:755–762.

Kong DS, Kim ST, Lee JI, et al. Impact of adjuvant chemotherapy for gliomatosis cerebri. BMC Cancer 2010;10:424.

Perkins GH, Schomer DF, Fuller GN. Gliomatosis cerebri: improved outcome with radiotherapy. Int J Radiat Oncol Biol Phys 2003;56(4):1137–1146.

Romeike BFM, Mawrin C. Gliomatosis cerebri: growing evidence for diffuse gliomas with wide invasion. Exp Rev Neurotherapeut 2008;8(4):587–597.

Sanson M, Cartalat-Carel S, Taillibert S, et al. Initial chemotherapy in gliomatosis cerebri. Neurology 2004;63(2):270–275.

Seiz M, Kohlof P, Brockmann MA, et al. First experiences with low dose anti angiogenic treatment in gliomatosis cerebri with sign of angiogenic activity. Anticancer Res 2009;29:3261–3267.

Taillibert S, Chodkiewicz C, Laigle-Donadey F, et al. Gliomatosis cerebri: a review of 296 cases from the ANOCEF database and the literature. J Neurooncol 2006;76:201–205.

36 Pituitary Adenomas

Andrea Saladino, Roberto Attanasio,
Francesco Di Meco, and Renato Cozzi

INTRODUCTION AND EPIDEMIOLOGY

Pituitary adenomas are the most common cause of sellar masses, accounting for up to 10% of all intracranial neoplasms. They are benign tumors of the anterior pituitary gland; sometimes they show aggressive course and local malignancy.

There are only few studies on the incidence and prevalence of pituitary adenomas: current reports show that the prevalence of pituitary adenomas is four fold higher than previous estimates. Lactotroph adenomas are the most frequent (58%), followed by clinically nonfunctioning adenomas (29%); somatotroph and corticotroph adenomas are rarer. Mutations in some genes may play a role in the development of these tumors: *MEN1, Gs-alpha, PTTG* (pituitary tumor transforming gene), *FGF receptor-4* (fibroblast growing factor-4), *AIP* (aryl hydrocarbon receptor interacting protein).

CLASSIFICATION

Adenomas are classified according to size, invasiveness of local structures and hormonal secretion. Lesions smaller than 10 mm are classified as microadenomas, lesions larger than 10 mm as macroadenomas. They may be completely intrasellar or grow outside the sella turcica with invasion of bone or surrounding structures (pituitary walls, sphenoid and/or cavernous sinus), or with suprasellar extension. Adenomas can yield an increased secretion of hormone by a cellular type and/or decreased secretion of other hormones due to tumoral compression of normal pituitary gland. Lactotroph adenomas usually cause hyperprolactinemia, leading to hypogonadism in both sexes (amenorrhea in women, sexual dysfunction in men) and galactorrhea. Gonadotroph adenomas usually present as clinically non functioning tumors. Somatotroph adenomas cause acromegaly due to increased growth hormone (GH) secretion. Corticotroph adenomas cause Cushing's disease due to increased secretion of adrenocorticotropin (ACTH). Thyrotroph adenomas may cause hyperthyroidism due to increased secretion of thyroid-stimulating hormone (TSH).

CLINICAL MANIFESTATIONS

Pituitary adenomas can present with visual impairment, neurological symptoms, signs and symptoms related to impaired secretion or hypersecretion of pituitary hormones. Nowadays they often present as incidental findings on neuroradiological investigations performed for other reasons.

Visual impairment. Impaired vision is the most common symptom. Very often it is the only complaint and, unless a visual field examination is performed, the diagnosis is missed. One or both eyes may be affected to variable degrees. The most typical sign is bilateral hemianopia. The onset of visual field defect is usually gradual.

Neurological symptoms. Headache is common, but not specific. In rare cases headache is dramatic and may be associated to abrupt visual loss, diplopia, diabetes insipidus and acute hypopituitarism: this clinical picture, called pituitary apoplexy, is induced by sudden hemorrhage and/or infarction into the adenoma. Sometimes apoplexy is the first manifestation of a previously unrecognized adenoma. Diplopia, caused by lateral compression on oculomotor nerves in the cavernous sinus by the adenoma, may be transient if it is due to partial apoplexy of adenoma.

Endocrine picture. Hypopituitarism with impaired secretion of one or all pituitary hormones has often a blunted clinical picture. The most common deficiencies in pituitary hormone involve gonadotropins, resulting in hypogonadism in both sexes; in young females the cause of amenorrhea may be diagnosed earlier, in males the impairment of sexual desire is frequently unappreciated or attributed to other causes. In the most advanced cases, mostly in men, phenotype is peculiar, with hypopituitaric aspect; symptoms are vague and aspecific, and asthenia is the leading complaint of these patients.

DIAGNOSIS

Clinical

Hyperprolactinemia causes typical symptoms in premenopausal women and in men, but not in postmenopausal women. In premenopausal women hyperprolactinemia causes hypogonadism (oligomenorrhea, or amenorrhea) and less often galactorrhea. In men hyperprolactinemia also causes hypogonadism, with decreased libido, impotence, infertility, gynecomastia, or rarely galactorrhea. The presence of Cushing's syndrome is suggested by a peculiar phenotype (troncular obesity, moon face, easy bruising and thinning of the skin, striae rubrae on the abdomen, proximal muscle atrophy and weakness), hypertension, diabetes mellitus, menstrual irregularity up to secondary amenorrhea, depression, osteoporosis up to vertebral fractures. The diagnosis of acromegaly is easy in the patient with a typical clinical picture: facial disfigurement, enlargement of hands and feet, macroglossia, voice deepening, headache, arthritis. Despite the prominence of these findings at the time of diagnosis, the rate of change is so slow that only few patients seek care because of change in their appearance or other symptoms related to acral enlargement. TSH-secreting adenoma presents as hyperthyroidism, goiter and inappropriately assessable TSH levels. Clinically non functioning pituitary adenomas present with symptoms and signs of local growth (hypopituitarism, visual impairment, headache).

Imaging

MRI is the single best imaging procedure. Micro- and macroadenomas usually enhance after gadolinium (Gd) administration to a lesser degree than the normal pituitary, allowing to differentiate normal from pathological tissue.

Hormonal hyposecretion has to be looked for carefully in each patient with a macroadenoma. The most common deficiencies involve gonadotropin, responsible of hypogonadism, and GH, causing growth failure in children and a typical metabolic derangement in adult patients. TSH and ACTH deficiency (with central hypothyroidism and hypoadrenalism, respectively) are rarer, usually caused by a long-standing huge mass. Hormonal diagnosis of hypopituitarism is reached indirectly measuring the hormones secreted by the peripheral glands controlled by the pituitary hormones, i.e. cortisol for ACTH, FT4 for TSH, testosterone in males and gonadotropins or estrogens in amenorrheic or postmenopausal females.

The demonstration of hormonal hypersecretion identifies the lesion as a pituitary adenoma and the subtype of the adenoma. A serum prolactin (PRL) greater than 100–150 ng/mL (i.e., 2500–3750 microU/mL) generally identifies a prolactinoma; lower levels could be measured in PRL-secreting microadenomas or macroadenomas non–PRL-secreting but causing hypothalamopituitary disconnection. In acromegaly the best single test is the serum insulin-like growth factor (IGF)-1 level measurement, which should be matched for age and coupled to GH levels after an oral glucose load. Elevated 24-hour urinary free cortisol (UFC) associated to normal–high ACTH levels usually indicates a corticotroph adenoma, whereas high FT3 and FT4 levels coupled to inappropriately normal/high TSH levels characterize TSH-secreting adenomas. In pituitary incidentalomas the type of evaluation is based on the size: if macro, it should be assessed as described above; if micro, PRL levels are the most cost effective measurement to perform.

TREATMENT

Generalities for Surgical Treatment

Transnasal transsphenoidal microscopic or endoscopic approach is the usual procedure when surgical removal of a pituitary tumor is indicated (see later). This procedure, either microscopic or endoscopic, provides direct access to the pituitary fossa through the nasal cavities without any external scar on the scalp or forehead deformity following a craniotomy. It is an extraarachnoid approach, which allows internal tumor resection or debulking with no need for brain or nerve manipulation. In recent years, the combined use of CT and MR image guidance has implemented the safety of the approach during the transnasal and transsphenoidal times, improved the extent of tumor resection in macroadenomas and facilitated tumor identification in microadenomas surgery.

Relative limitations of transsphenoidal surgery are a minimal enlargement of the sella with a large suprasellar mass causing chiasmal compression, a dumbbell-shaped tumor with an extremely narrow waist at the junction of the intrasellar and suprasellar portion when the tumor is growing through a narrow discontinuation of the diaphragm sellae, a large subfrontal or parasellar extension, especially if there is a middle or posterior fossa mass larger than the intrasellar mass, and, sometimes, an unusually fibrous tumor. In these cases a transcranial approach can be used to remove the intracranial portion of the tumor causing mass effect to the surrounding structures.

The most common postoperative complication, presenting in up to 20% of patients, is hormonal imbalance. Transient alterations in antidiuretic hormone (ADH) secretion causing diabetes insipidus (DI) is frequent in the first postoperative period and a strict fluid and electrolytes balance is required before discharge, using vasopressin preparations or fluid intake restriction if needed. DI lasting more than 3 months is uncommon. Cortisol deficiency and TSH deficiency can also occur postoperatively and hormonal replacement with steroids (hydrocortisone) and levothyroxine is usually started and continued until the adequacy of endogenous hormones is established. The incidence of cerebrospinal fluid rhinorrhea is 3.5–5%, higher when an extended approach is performed for very large masses. Significant postoperative complications of transsphenoidal surgery are not common (≤ 1%) but potentially severe, including death or stroke from carotid artery injury and visual loss from postoperative intracranial hematoma.

Clinically Nonfunctioning Pituitary Adenomas

Surgery is usually indicated for nonsecreting pituitary adenomas causing mass effect because of large size, as there is no effective medical therapy in this setting. The typical indication is visual field impairment. Some surgeons recommend surgery for large macroadenomas elevating the chiasm even in the absence of visual field deficiencies, especially in younger and middle-aged patients (<65 years), to prevent injuries to the optic apparatus. Surgical debulking of macroadenomas can also be performed in elderly patients with visual field defect in order to relieve chiasmal compression and provide a better target for radiation therapy, if needed. In patients with hormonal deficiencies and an absent or mild visual field deficit, surgery can be delayed and a replacement therapy is started.

If visual field impairment is progressively worsening in consecutive tests a more urgent surgical approach is required. If there is an acute visual loss or other neurological deterioration, ischemia of the chiasm, hemorrhage and infarction (pituitary apoplexy) or abscess of the tumor must be suspected and investigated with neuroradiological imaging. The major danger is blindness and often requires emergent decompression; acute hypopituitarism can be associated and replacement therapy should be started soon.

Radiation therapy can also be used in patients with nonfunctioning pituitary adenomas and controls tumor growth in more than 90% of patients. In elderly or clinically unstable patients this could be the only treatment option at diagnosis. Radiation therapy, including radiosurgery, should be considered as a valuable alternative to surgery for recurrent or growing residual tumor, especially if the cavernous sinus is involved and the optic apparatus is well decompressed.

PRL-Secreting Tumors

A dopamine agonist drug (DA) should be the first treatment for each patient with a prolactinoma (micro or macro) since these drugs decrease the size of the tumor and PRL secretion in most cases. Other approaches must be considered for the minority of patients resistant or intolerant to DAs.

Several DAs have been used. Bromocriptine (Br) was the first ergot derivative used: it is a short acting medication and induces side effects such as nausea, vomiting and postural hypotension even at low doses, thus limiting its use. Pergolide was voluntarily withdrawn from the market in March 2007, whereas quinagolide was used only in few patients. Cabergoline (Cab) is a powerful and long-lasting DA with only few side effects; it is the initial choice in most cases as it is the most effective DA in treating hyperprolactinemic patients and the least likely to cause side effects. The initial Cab dose is 1 mg weekly, and an increase of the dose usually is effective even in patients resistant to the starting dose.

DAs decrease PRL secretion and reduce the size of the lactotroph adenomas in more than 90% of patients. Often the first administration of DA induces a dramatic fall in PRL levels and an improvement of visual acuity and/or of the visual field defect. These effects are more apparent in patients with larger tumors and higher PRL levels. Cab is superior to Br in decreasing PRL levels: in a retrospective study Cab normalized PRL levels in 86% of patients, including 70% of those who were resistant to Br. Visual fields abnormalities resolved in 70% of the patients with some defect before the treatment and tumor size decreased in 64% of patients harboring a macroadenoma. In patients with macroadenoma the fall in PRL levels usually precedes tumor shrinkage; in few patients the decline in PRL levels is not followed by a tumor size reduction and in some other cases tumor size increases in spite of PRL levels normalization. In most patients PRL fall and tumor shrinkage are progressive up to the normalization of PRL and of the visual field defect, and tumor disappearance, thus allowing to downtitrate the drug and extend the time period between administrations.

The consequences of discontinuation of DA treatment have been extensively evaluated. Recurrence of hyperprolactinemia and increase in adenoma size have been variable. Most patients with remnant macroadenoma have tumor recurrence during follow-up. In addition giant adenomas (>3 cm) may behave more aggressively, with rapid substantial regrowth within weeks of discontinuation of DA treatment. The remission chances are higher the longer PRL level has been normal and no adenoma has been seen on MRI scan: however, if PRL increases above normal while decreasing DA treatment, DA should be reincreased.

It has been reported that the administration of high doses of Cab in patients affected by Parkinson's disease is associated with an increased risk of valvular heart disease, but this risk is very low at the lower doses usually administered to hyperprolactinemic patients.

After the normalization of PRL levels and the shrinkage or the tumor, pituitary function may improve as well: in women menses and fertility recover and in men testosterone secretion, sperm count, and erectile function improve. Hypothyroidism and/or hypoadrenalism may also revert to normal function.

Surgery is not the treatment of choice for most PRL-secreting adenomas. Transsphenoidal resection is indicated for macroprolactinomas not controlled medically, when levels and/or tumor size increase despite optimal medical therapy. Surgery may also be needed for those invasive tumors causing bone erosion of the sphenoid, clivus and anterior petrosal bones, which shrink on medical treatment causing fluid leakage and a subsequent potential risk of bacterial meningitis. In these particular cases, the goal of surgery is not further removal of the tumor, but, if feasible, identification of the fistula and its repair. In these patients more than one operation at different times may be needed.

Transnasal resection of the tumor can also be offered to the subset of female patients, harboring a microprolactinoma, who are intolerant to DAs or not willing to assume them chronically.

GH-Secreting Adenomas

The goal of therapy is

1. to lower IGF-1 levels to within the reference range for the patient's age
2. to lower GH concentration to at least < 1 ng/mL after a glucose load
3. to ameliorate symptoms
4. to control the size of the adenoma
5. to prevent hypopituitarism
6. to reverse comorbidities and increased mortality.

By normalizing IGF-1 levels, life expectancy of patients with acromegaly is similar to that of the general population.

Surgery is currently regarded as the best initial treatment for GH-secreting adenomas, as surgical removal is the most effective treatment to provide a rapid hormone reduction and to eliminate compression on neural structures around the tumor. In case of microadenomas (accounting for less than one third of cases), surgery is curative in most cases and the preservation of pituitary function is as high as 95% in the best series. On the other hand, large invasive macroadenomas usually require adjuvant treatments to normalize GH levels, but surgery still plays an important role in reducing the tumor volume and the mass effect on surrounding structures.

It is a matter of debate if all acromegalic patients should have somatostatin analog (SA) treatment before surgery for up to 3–4 months to improve general condition, partially reverse soft tissue changes about the tongue and throat and lessen cardiac risks of anesthesia. It is certainly useful in patients with a marked clinical involvement and/or clear acromegalic comorbidities (see below). It is still controversial if surgery should be performed in elderly patients with acromegaly but no other symptoms, since the operation may not alter life expectancy in this group.

Medical treatment of acromegaly has dramatically changed the therapeutic strategy of the disease, improving its outcome. Drugs acting by suppressing GH hypersecretion, such as DAs and somatostatine analogues (SAs), or at the peripheral level, by blocking IGF-1 synthesis, such as Pegvisomant (Peg), a GH receptor antagonist (GHRA), are available. They can be used as adjuvant therapy, in cases of active disease persistence after surgery, and also as primary treatment, mainly in patients who have inacceptable surgical risks, refuse surgery or have adenomas that are unlikely to be cured surgically, due to the size of the adenoma or to very high GH levels.

Cab normalizes IGF-1 levels in up to 25–35% of patients, mainly in those with lower GH and IGF-1 levels at baseline. PRL hypersecretion is not a prerequisite for Cab effectiveness. Tumor shrinkage is occasionally reported. Cab is an oral compound that can be easily administered on a daily schedule, at a progressively escalating dosage (starting from 0.25 mg once/twice weekly up to 0.25–0.5 mg/day). Mean doses are higher than in patients with prolactinoma. As reported above, the recent report of cardiac valve deterioration observed in patients with Parkinson's disease after prolonged

Cab treatment at high dosage (3 mg/day), raised some concern. However, the first observational studies in prolactinoma patients are reassuring.

Octreotide and lanreotide are the presently available SAs. They inhibit effectively hormonal hypersecretion achieving safe GH and normal IGF-1 levels in at least 50% of patients, and considerable decrease of GH and IGF-I secretion in another 40%. Final outcome can be reliably predicted by early (3–6 months) results obtained during chronic treatment. High GH levels and a huge adenoma volume are not negative predictors of SA effectiveness according to some but not all authors. Long-term treatment does not induce any tachyphylaxis. SAs obtain a progressive amelioration of hormonal control. Clinical amelioration parallels hormonal control: headache, swelling, hyperhydrosis, and snoring markedly improve or disappear, as well as systemic comorbidities (cardiac involvement, sleep apnea, diabetes mellitus). Adjuvant medical treatment improves patients' outcome after unsuccessful surgery. SAs are parenteral drugs to be injected i.m. (octreotide LAR) or sc (lanreotide Autogel) every 4 weeks, starting with the intermediate strength commercially available dosage (20 and 90 mg, respectively). After 3 injections, the dosage has to be individually tailored, according to biochemical results. The occurrence and degree of tumor shrinkage are more impressive when SAs are used as primary treatment (greater than 50% vs baseline in over half of patients) than as adjuvant therapy (20%). Tumor shrinkage occurs in the first months of treatment; it may be quick and progressive during the prolongation of treatment, up to an empty sella or disappearance of the tumor. Adverse effects to SAs are scanty. Gastroenteric side effects (diarrhea, abdominal pain, flatulence, steatorrhea) are usually transient and mild to moderate in severity and relieve after pancreatic extracts administration. The net effects on carbohydrate metabolism are widely variable, but seldom of clinical significance; in diabetic patients glucose metabolism improves in most cases. In previously euglycemic patients, glycated hemoglobin may increase or remain unchanged. Gallstones are a frequent occurrence in acromegalic patients treated with SAs (1 out of 3 altogether) and may occur at any time.

At present, Peg is the available GHRA effective in normalizing IGF-I levels in 76% of patients resistant/intolerant to SAs. The higher the pretreatment IGF-I levels and the greater the patients weight, the higher the Peg doses needed. In Europe, Peg can be employed only in SAs-resistant/intolerant patients after neurosurgical failure or awaiting the effects of radiotherapy. Even though tumor growth remains uncontrolled during Peg treatment, "true" tumor size increase was noticed only in few patients, mainly those with aggressive disease, whereas tumor volume reportedly increased in a few cases after the withdrawal of previous SA treatment which had caused tumor shrinkage. Peg is a parenteral drug to be injected sc daily, starting with a 10 mg dose, to be stepwise increased at monthly intervals up to IGF-I normalization. Injection site reactions have been reported in 7.4% (lipohypertrophy, that in some cases may be worrisome and impair drug absorption) and liver toxicity in 5.2% [transaminases x 3 upper limit of normal range (ULN)].

Drugs can be combined to take advantage of their different mechanism of action and possible synergies. The combined use of SA and Cab obtained hormonal targets in 20% of patients partially sensitive to SA. The combined use of SA and Peg is a promising therapeutic option, since it concomitantly controls tumor growth and hormonal hypersecretion, normalizes IGF-1 levels in virtually each patient and permits a Peg sparing, thus improving compliance and quality of life. This treatment should be envisaged in all patients with an aggressive disease, in whom tumor shrinkage is demonstrated on MRI scan but hormone targets are not achieved on SA treatment alone.

A number of factors should be taken into account to select the right strategy of treatment, with the awareness that it seldom will be definitely successful in one step. The decision making should be influenced by the presence of severe and progressive visual field defect and/or neurological involvement, patient's clinical conditions, risk factors (such as comorbidities and age), MRI features of the adenoma and GH levels, as well as personal preference. Neurosurgery is the only treatment that can induce quick remission of the disease. However, in the best neurosurgical series this goal is achieved only in near half of patients with a macroadenoma. On the other hand, medical treatment dramatically improve the outcome of the disease and several reports have shown that SA adjuvant treatment after unsuccessful surgery obtains GH/IGF-1 suppressive effects similar to primary treatment. Altogether, these findings have modified the therapeutic strategy in acromegaly and this is the reason why the approach to the acromegalic patient must be individually tailored.

First-line neurosurgery is recommended in patients with:

1. clinically significant deterioration of visual field and neurological involvement and/or emergency conditions such as endocranic hypertension and tumor apoplexy, even though surgical cure cannot be achieved;
2. not invasive adenoma regardless of its volume (i.e. both micro- and macroadenoma) and without active invalidating comorbidities, with a high probability to undergo a definitive remission of the disease.

First-line medical therapy is recommended in patients:

1. who are not amenable to the primary neurosurgical treatment due to poor clinical conditions associated to severe comorbidities (cardiomyopathy, sleep apnea, arrhythmias) or metabolic derangements;
2. with a predictable poor surgical result (invasive adenoma, high GH levels);
3. who refuse surgery.

The possibility to prolong first-line medical treatment indefinitely may be considered in patients who achieve a good disease control on ongoing treatment, especially if they are likely to have a poor surgical result, they are in poor clinical conditions or still refuse surgery. Depot preparations of SA are recommended as the first choice of pharmacotherapy. Primary treatment with Cab is suggested rarely, mainly in patients with mild hypersecretion or refusing injections.

The decision upon a first-line medical treatment never excludes a second-line surgical treatment. Second-line surgery has to be considered if SA therapy does not normalize IGF-1 or contraindications to the operation have been overcome and patients have a high probability to undergo a definitive remission of the disease. Adjuvant drug treatment in patients with persistence of disease activity after surgery is recommended.

Cushing's Disease

Transsphenoidal surgery is the treatment of choice for most ACTH-secreting adenomas, with cure rates around 90% in microadenomas. A selective adenomectomy can be performed when the tumor is clearly visible on preoperative MRI, whereas exploration of the pituitary gland can be planned when the tumor is difficult to localize on the scans (25–45% of cases). In these cases, a seemingly identifiable tumor is found intraoperatively in 94% of cases, with histological confirmation in 82% of cases. Even if there is still controversy on this approach, some surgeons suggest total hypophysectomy when resolution of the hypercortisolemic state is an absolute necessity.

ACTH-secreting macroadenomas (~10% of cases) are obviously easier to identify pre- and intraoperatively, but surgical failure rate is higher than in microadenomas, mainly in long-term disease control. This may reflect a lateral invasion of the cavernous sinus dura or of the cavernous sinus itself by the tumor, which is not amenable to complete surgical removal as entering the cavernous sinus may significantly alter surgical morbidity.

Stereotactic radiation, administered by linear accelerator or gamma knife, can be used as an adjuvant treatment after failed initial or repeat surgery or in those cases of residual tumor around the cavernous sinus. Clinical long-term remission is reported to occur in a percentage of patients as high as 90% in some series, with an average time from treatment to remission ranging between 3 and 63 months. The results of radiation treatment are better if it is used as a second line treatment than as stand-alone treatment. Hypopituitarism is more common after RT than transsphenoidal surgery.

The main indications for medical therapy of Cushing's syndrome include:

1. Management of hypercortisolism when surgery is contraindicated
2. Control of hypercortisolism in preparation to surgery
3. Persistence or recurrence of hypercortisolism after surgery
4. Control of hypercortisolism while waiting for the effects of pituitary radiation.

Several drugs acting at different levels are available with different mechanisms of action.

Among the several drugs directed at the pituitary level that have been investigated, only Cab and the new SA pasireotide have shown promising results and potential benefit.

The outcome of chronic treatment with Cab is available in small series only. Recent studies have shown that Cab therapy (at doses of 1–7 mg weekly) reduces the excretion in UFC to less than 125 %ULNR in 12 out of 24 patients with Cushing's disease. Normalization of UFC was obtained in 30% of patients with up to five years of follow up. In another report the addition of ketoconazole (200–400 mg/day) normalized UFC in 6 out of 9 patients.

Pasireotide is a new SA, with a unique receptor-binding profile that targets four of the five somatostatin receptors, with the highest affinity for subtype 5. In a recent large study conducted in 162 patients, pasireotide normalized UFC in 21 out of 80 (26%) patients receiving 900 μg bid sc and in 12 out of 82 (15%) given 600 μg bid sc. The median UFC level decreased by approximately 50% by month 2 and remained stable in both groups. A normal UFC level was achieved more frequently in patients with baseline levels not exceeding 5 folds the ULNR than in patients with higher baseline levels. Clinical signs and symptoms of Cushing's disease diminished. As UFC levels decreased, systolic–diastolic blood pressure, lipids, weight, and health-related quality of life score improved. As for adverse effects, hyperglycemia occurred in 118 of 162 patients (73%) and 74 patients required starting a glucose-lowering medication. Pasireotide has been recently approved by European Agency of Drug for patients presenting persistent or recurrent Cushing's disease after surgery or in whom surgery is contraindicated for medical reasons.

Ketoconazole (Kcz), metyrapone, and etomidate inhibit one or more enzymes involved in cortisol synthesis. Kcz, the most widely agent used in Europe, inhibits mainly the first step in cortisol biosynthesis. It decreases also testosterone production, leading to gynecomastia, decreased libido and impotence in men. Kcz may be hepatotoxic, thus requiring a tight follow up of liver enzymes during treatment. Daily doses range from 200 to 1200 mg.

Mitotane is an adrenolytic agent used primarily for the treatment of adrenal carcinoma. It can also be used in patients with Cushing's disease. Its effect persists long after the drug withdrawal and may require replacement therapy with adrenal steroids.

Mifepristone is a glucocorticoid-receptor antagonist with antiprogestational and abortifacient effect. At very high doses it acts as a glucocorticoid receptor antagonist. It is rapidly effective notably in cortisol-induced psychosis. The follow-up on this treatment is cumbersome, since no hormonal testing is reliable.

The association of pasireotide, Cab, and Kcz shows additive effect increasing the number of patients with normalization of UFC.

TSH-Secreting Adenomas

They are usually very aggressive and invasive, making complete surgical removal not possible in most cases. The goal of surgery should be tumor debulking, followed by medical treatment, sometimes associated to radiation therapy.

SAs are effective in nearly all patients. They obtain FT3 and FT4 normal levels in a very large percentage of patients within one year, TSH fall by more than 50% in 92% of patients and normal values in 79%, tumor shrinkage in more than 50%. These nice results suggest that SAs can be used not only as adjuvant therapy, but also as primary therapy to reduce hormonal hypersecretion, to improve clinical conditions and to shrink tumor size in macroadenoma, to get easier their removal by the neurosurgeon. Bromocriptine and Cab have also proven effective in occasional patients.

Aggressive Tumors and Carcinomas

Aggressive pituitary tumors and pituitary carcinomas are associated to a poor prognosis. Management should be aggressive.

Multiple surgical procedures remain the first-line option. Most aggressive tumors will regrow because complete surgical removal is often impossible.

Medical treatments with DAs or SAs are unlikely to improve symptoms. Temozolomide (Tmz), an oral alkylating agent used in the management of glioblastoma, has shown significant antitumoral activity in pituitary carcinomas. More than 40 patients presenting either with a locally aggressive pituitary adenoma or with a pituitary carcinoma treated with Tmz have been reported. The mean tumoral response rate was 33%, with seven of 21 patients showing tumor volume decrease. Five additional patients had stable tumor volume during treatment, suggesting tumor control in about 50% cases. As for antisecretory efficacy, 12 out of 18 patients with ACTH-secreting tumors had decreased ACTH secretion (67%), whereas a reduction in tumor volume was observed in 10 patients (56%). In the group of PRL-secreting tumors, hormone response was observed in 11/15 patients (73.3%) while tumor shrinkage was noted in 10 patients (66.6%). Only one of three patients with GH-PRL secreting tumors achieved hormonal and tumoral response. Methylguanine-DNA methyltransferase, a DNA repair enzyme that specifically removes the alkylating bond induced by Tmz, could be a predictor of response to Tmz in pituitary tumors, but there is no consensus on this report.

SUGGESTED READING

Attanasio R, Cozzi R, Lasio G, Barbò R. Diagnostic evaluation of the lesions of the sellar and parasellar region. In Explicative Cases of Controversial Issues in Neurosurgery, Dr. Francesco Signorelli (Ed.). http://www.intechopen.com/books/explicative-cases-of-controversial-issues-in-neurosurgery/the-diagnostic-evaluation-of-the-lesions-of-the-sellar-and-parasellar-region; pp 97–166.

Barker FG, Klibanski A, Swearingen B. Transsphenoidal surgery for pituitary tumors in the United States, 1996–2000: mortality, morbidity, and the effects of hospital and surgeon volume. J Clin Endocrinol Metab 2003;88:4709–4719.

Beck-Peccoz P, Persani L. Thyrotropin-secreting pituitary adenomas, Chapter 13a, in: Thyroid Disease. http://www.thyroidmanager.org/chapter/thyrotropin-secreting-pituitary-adenomas/

Biermasz NR, Pereira AM, Neelis KJ, et al. Role of radiotherapy in the management of acromegaly. Exp Rev Endocrinol Metab 2006;1:449–460.

Cozzi R, Attanasio R. Octreotide LAR for acromegaly. Expert Rev Clin Pharmacol 2012;5:125–143.

Cozzi R, Baldelli R, Colao A, et al. AME Position Statement on clinical management of acromegaly J Endocrinol Invest 2009;32(Suppl 6).

Estrada J, Boronat M, Mielgo M, et al. The long-term outcome of pituitary irradiation after unsuccessful transsphenoidal surgery in Cushing's disease. N Engl J Med 1997;336:172–177.

Freda PU, Beckers AM, Katznelson L, et al. Pituitary incidentaloma: an Endocrine Society clinical practice guideline. J Clin Endocrinol Metab 2011;96:894–904.

Hentschel SJ, McCutcheon IE. Stereotactic radiosurgery for Cushing disease. Neurosurg Focus 2004;16:E5.

Katznelson L, Atkinson JLD, Cook DM, et al. AACE Acromegaly guidelines. Endocr Pract 2011;17(Suppl 4):1–44.

Kong DS, Lee JI, Lim do H, et al. The efficacy of fractionated radiotherapy and stereotactic radiosurgery for pituitary adenomas: long-term results of 125 consecutive patients treated in a single institution. Cancer 2007;110:854–860.

Melmed S, Casanueva F, Hoffman AR, et al. Diagnosis and treatment of hyperprolactinemia: an Endocrine Society clinical practice guideline. J Clin Endocrinol Metab 2011;96:273–288.

Molitch ME, Clemmons DR, Malozowski S, et al. Evaluation and treatment of adult Growth Hormone deficiency: an Endocrine Society clinical practice guideline. J Clin Endocrinol Metab 2011;96:1587–1609.

Nieman LK, Biller BMK, Findling JW, et al. The Diagnosis of Cushing's Syndrome: An Endocrine Society Clinical Practice Guideline J Clin Endocrinol Metab 2008;93:1526–1540.

Nomikos P, Buchfelder M, Fahlbusch R. The outcome of surgery in 668 patients with acromegaly using current criteria of biochemical "cure." Eur J Endocrinol 2005;152:379–387.

Raverot G, et al. Temozolomide treatment in aggressive pituitary tumors and pituitary carcinomas: a French multicenter experience. JClin Endocrinol Metab 2010;95:4592–4599.

Sheehan JM, Vance ML, Sheehan JP, et al. Radiosurgery for Cushing's disease after failed transsphenoidal surgery. J Neurosurg 2000;93:738–742.

Starke RM, Reames DL, Chen CJ, et al. Endoscopic transsphenoidal surgery for Cushing disease: techniques, outcomes, and predictors of remission. Neurosurgery 2013;72:240–247.

Starke RM, Williams BJ, Jane JA Jr, Sheehan JP. Gamma Knife surgery for patients with nonfunctioning pituitary macroadenomas: predictors of tumor control, neurological deficits, and hypopituitarism. J Neurosurg 2012;117:129–135.

Swearingen B, Biller BM, Barker FG 2nd, et al. Long-term mortality after transsphenoidal surgery for Cushing disease. Ann Intern Med 1999; 130:821–824.

37 Germinomas

Antonio Silvani, Andrea Salmaggi, and Paola Gaviani

INTRODUCTION

Central nervous system germ cell tumors (GCTs) are rare and account in the West for 0.3–3.4% of all tumors; in Asia, their frequency reaches 9–15%. GCTs are commonly diagnosed in the first and second decade of life, but they may be seen rarely also in adults. Typically they occur in the midline suprasellar or pineal region of the brain. Tumors of the pineal area comprise 50–60% of CNS GCTs; those of the suprasellar region, 30–40%. CNS GCTs may rarely occur in the basal ganglia, thalamus, and cerebral hemispheres.

Based on histological classification, CNS GCTs are divided into germinomas and nongerminomatous GCTs (Table 37.1). Germinoma is the most common subtype of CNS GCTs and accounts for two-thirds of them.

Another classification system proposed by Sawamura and de Tribolet splits histological variants into three therapeutic groups based on their prognosis (Table 37.2).

CLINICAL PRESENTATION

Clinical presentation is related to the location, volume of the tumor, and the patient's age. Endocrine abnormalities, headache, vomiting, and visual changes are among the most common symptoms. A typical presentation is Parinaud syndrome, due to compression on the tectum with paralysis of upward gaze, loss of light perception and accommodation, nystagmus, and failure of convergence. Many patients with unrecognized CNS GCTs may have had a long history of endocrinological symptoms such as diabetes insipidus. Diagnosis in such cases may be delayed for several years

DIAGNOSIS

MRI of the brain and spine with and without gadolinium is the gold standard imaging study, for the diagnosis of GCT. Usually, germinomas are homogeneous and show isointensity or slightly low signal intensity on T1-weighted images, and isointensity or high intensity both on T2-weighted and FLAIR images (Figures 37.1 and 37.2), with enhancement after contrast administration. Both NGGCTs and malignant teratomas are more heterogeneous with small hemorrhages and cysts.

Some central nervous system CGT produce tumor markers that can be detected in both serum and cerebrospinal fluid. These markers can be helpful for identification of

Table 37.1 WHO Classification for Central Nervous System Germ Cell Tumors

GGCTs	NGGCTs
Germinoma—pure and with syncytiotrophoblasts	Teratoma (mature and malignant)
	Embryonal carcinoma
Germinoma with syncytiotrophoblast areas	Yolk sac tumor/endodermal sinus tumor
	Choriocarcinoma

Table 37.2 Prognosis of Central Nervous System Germ Cell Tumors

Good Prognostic Group (5-year OS > 90%)	Intermediate Prognostic Group (5-year OS ≈ 70%)	Poor Prognostic Group (5-year OS < 50%)
Germinoma	Immature teratoma	Teratoma with malignant transformation
Mature teratoma	Mixed germ cell tumors consisting of germinoma with either mature or immature teratoma	Embryonal carcinoma
		Yolk sac tumor
		Choriocarcinoma
		Mixed germ cell tumors including a component of embryonal carcinoma, yolk sac tumor, choriocarcinoma, or other malignant neoplasms such as squamous cell carcinoma

OS = overall survival

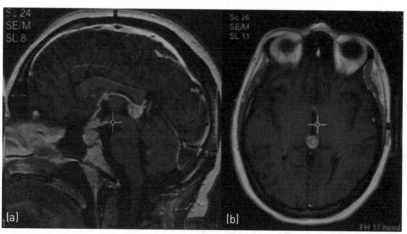

FIGURE 37.1
MRI T1-weighted gadolinium images: (a) synchronous pineal and suprasellar germinoma and (b) pineal germinoma.

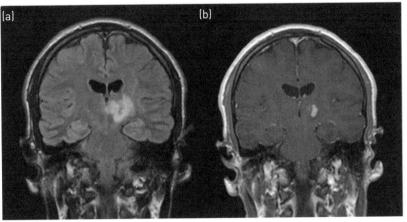

FIGURE 37.2
MRI FLAIR and T1-weighted gadolinium images of a rare thalamic germinoma.

histological subtypes. Choriocarcinoma produces the human chorionic gonadotropin (βHCG) and yolk sac tumor produces α-fetoprotein.

Germinoma with syncytiotrophoblastic areas produces βHCG, but the serum titer of this variant of germinoma is usually less than 100 IU/mL, while in choriocarcinoma patients is more than 500 IU/mL in most cases.

In the past, patients with imaging findings suggestive of CNS germinoma were treated empirically with radiotherapy, but now the recommendation for all patients with pineal and suprasellar tumors is to undergo endoscopic/stereotactic biopsy or open biopsy for histological confirmation.

The diagnostic work-up for CNS GCTs should include measurement of the tumor markers βhCG and AFP in both serum and CSF, CSF cytology and testicular ecography, and brain and spinal contrast-enhanced MRI.

TREATMENT

Surgery

Many patients with pineal tumors present with symptoms and signs of obstructive hydrocephalus, and this necessitates either a ventriculoperitoneal shunt or an endoscopic third ventriculostomy.

For germinoma, there is no clear benefit of partial or even gross total resection compared with biopsy alone. Conversely, NGGCTs frequently are resistant to conventional radio-chemotherapy, and then a total resection by second-look surgery could be effective in disease control. Sometimes, malignant teratomas are responsive to chemoradiotherapy; however, a residual disease often composed of mature teratoma component may grow (growing teratoma syndrome), in these cases a new radical surgery is the sole effective treatment.

Radiotherapy and Chemotherapy

Germ cell tumors are highly responsive to radiation therapy and historically, craniospinal irradiation (CSI) has been used to treat these tumors, but due to high rate of long-term neurotoxicities, reduced volume radiotherapy with or without chemotherapy are now used. The optimal radiation dose and the field of treatment are controversial. In a recent study, Haas-Kogan et al. reported the outcome of a group of germinoma patients treated by whole-ventricular irradiation (WVI) alone. The results of this study suggest that focal treatment with WVI does not result in a greater number of relapses than with CSI. Only patients with disseminated disease could receive 24 Gy to the craniospinal axis.

Several studies of RT versus neoadjuvant chemotherapy plus response-based RT are ongoing. In germinoma patients, the addition of chemotherapy to RT permits the use of a lower radiation dose, reducing the risk of long-term neurotoxicities with excellent survival rates; conversely chemotherapy alone without radiation therapy has proven less effective (overall response rate and OS) compared to chemotherapy and radiation combination or radiotherapy alone.

In patients with NGGCTs, the use of more aggressive treatment combining chemotherapy with radiation therapy is planned to improve the poor outcome of these patients.

The chemotherapeutic agents that have shown the best activity against CNS GCTs are platinum-derivate, VP16, vinblastine, ifosfamide, and bleomycin.

GGT and NGGCT patients with relapsed or progressive disease have a poor prognosis. Treatments for recurrent GCTs include surgery, focal or whole neuroaxis irradiation, and chemotherapy. Some authors reported efficacy of high-dose chemotherapy (usually thiotepa based) followed by autologous stem cell transplant.

SUGGESTED READING

Louis DN, Ohgaki H, Wiestler O, et al, editors. Third Edition. Albany, NY: WHO Publication Center; 2007. WHO Classification of Tumours of the Central Nervous System; p. 197–204.

Haas-Kogan DA, Missett BT, Wara WM et al. Radiation therapy for intracranial germ cell tumors. Int J Radiat Oncol Biol Phys 2003;56:511–518.

Matsutani M. Treatment for intracranial germinoma: final results of the Japanese Study Group. Neuro Oncol 2005; 7:519

Kamoshima Y, Sawamura Y. Update on current standard treatments in central nervous system germ cell tumors. Curr Opin Neurol. 2010;23:571–575

38 Primary Central Nervous System Lymphomas

Antonio Silvani, Paola Gaviani,
and Andrea Salmaggi

INTRODUCTION

Primary CNS lymphoma (PCNSL) is a highly aggressive variant of extranodal non-Hodgkin lymphoma accounting for 1–4% of all intracranial malignancies. Several authors have confirmed the increasing incidence of PCNSL also in immunocompetent patients. Neither an environmental causative factor nor any other predisposing factors than an immunocompromised status have been identified. The vast majority of PCNSL are diffuse large B-cell lymphomas with T-cell lymphomas being very rare. The most common location is in cerebral hemispheres, with a preference for the periventricular white matter, basal ganglia, and corpus callosum. Rarely the PCNSLs affect: cerebellum, brainstem. and spinal cord. The lesions are solitary in 60–70% of the cases; immunodeficient patients more frequently have multiple lesions at diagnosis.

Ocular involvement is seen in 20–25% of the patients at first diagnosis. Occult systemic disease has been reported in up to 8% of patients initially thought to have PCNSL.

CLINICAL PRESENTATION

Clinical symptoms of PCNSL consist more frequently of cognitive dysfunction, psychomotor slowing, personality changes, and disorientation; raised intracranial pressure, headache, and focal symptoms affect about half of cases; seizures due to particular localization of PCNSL are present only in a minority of patients.

DIAGNOSIS

Initial evaluation for the diagnosis of PCNSL routinely includes cranial magnetic resonance imaging (MRI), ophthalmologic examination including slit lamp, computed tomography (CT) scanning of chest, abdomen, and pelvis, bone marrow biopsy, human immunodeficiency virus (HIV) testing, and CSF studies when possible (Table 38.1).

In immunocompetent patients, PCNSL is normally a solitary and supratentorial lesion. In MRI images, PCNSL is typically iso-hypointense on T1-weighted imaging and it is iso-hypointense to grey matter on T2-weighted imaging. Contrast

Table 38.1 Diagnostic Procedures In Patients With Suspected CNS Lymphomas

	Clinical Evalutation	Imaging	Laboratory-Pathology
Mandatory	Neurological examination Complete physical examination Ophthalmological examination with slit lamp	MRI with gadolinium Contrast-enhanced CT (chest, abdomen and pelvis) Testis ultrasound	Biopsy Vitrectomy HIV serology CSF pathology Bone marrow aspirate
Optional		PET-FdG	PCR of rearranged immunoglobulin genes in CSF

enhancement tends to be homogeneous. Both ring-enhancing lesions and ependymal spread are more frequently seen in immunosuppressed patients. Diffusion-weighted imaging (DWI) and apparent diffusion coefficient (ADC) are influenced by the tumor cellularity; the ADC ratio in the brain relative to normal is lower in lymphoma than in high-grade gliomas. Spectroscopic imaging (MRS) may show a rising of choline peak and a reduction of N-acetylaspartate. However, MRS does not show a specific pattern in lymphoma, but preliminary data suggest that the baseline lipid and/or lactate level could have prognostic significance (Table 38.2).

Table 38.2 Imaging Findings

Location	90% supratentorial; frontal and parietal localization more common, frequently cross the corpus callosum and extended along ependymal surfaces. Deep gray nuclei commonly affected. Infrantentorial, pineal and sellar localizations are uncommon
Morphology	Solitary mass or multiple lesions (more frequent in HIV+) may be infiltrative or circumscribed
CT findings	Hyperdense more frequently, may be isodense, necrosis more frequent in immunocompromised patients. Enhancement moderate, uniform, Ring enhancement is rare (+ immunocompromised). Rarely, non enhancing lesions mimic white matter disease
MRI findings	T1WI: homogeneous, isointense-hypointense to cortex T2WI: homogeneous, isointense-hypointense to cortex FLAIR: homogeneous, isointense-hypointense to cortex, mild surrounding edema DWI: restricted diffusion MR perfusion: increased rCBV C.E.MRI: Strong homogeneous enhancement, non enhanced lesions are very rare. Peripheral enhancement with central necrosis more frequent in immunocompromised pts Lymphomatosus meningitis more frequent in CNS localizations from systemic disease MRS: NAA decreased, Cho elevated, lipid and lactate peaks reported

In PCNSL patients, a well-known finding is the impressive initial response to steroids, which occurs after often only 48 hours of treatment. Imaging demonstrates the dramatic reduction in both tumor size and peritumoral edema; however, almost all patients relapse. Some authors suggest that a disappearing tumor after steroids treatment is pathognomonic of PCNSL, but also multiple sclerosis and neurosarcoidosis respond to steroid and they can mimic the imaging and clinical evolution of PCNSL.

CSF cytology reveals tumor cells in less than 15% of patients when lumbar puncture is done, more frequently CSF analysis reveals only nonspecific abnormalities, such as increased protein concentration. The use of flow cytometry could provide an improved diagnostic sensitivity as compared to cytopathology alone. Rarely, demonstration of clonal immunoglobulin gene arrangement can increase the yield of CFS analysis. Otherwise, in immunodeficient patients, the detection of EBV DNA by PCR of the CSF is a specific diagnostic indicator.

In the suspicion of a PCNSL established by imaging, histological diagnosis of PCNSL remains mandatory. Stereotactic biopsy is the most common approach for these patients, surgery is not generally considered helpful therapeutically.

Since the tumor cells of PCNSL are highly sensitive to steroids and will undergo apoptosis, precluding diagnosis, steroids administration before biopsy should be avoided unless the patient is in imminent danger of cerebral herniation. If corticosteroid treatment is unavoidable and non diagnostic biopsy is obtained, steroids should be withdrawn and the re-biopsy of the tumor attempted. Close observation is required, because after suspension of steroid impressive tumor growth has been observed.

PROGNOSTIC FACTORS

The International Extranodal Lymphoma Study Group developed a prognostic scoring system, which categorizes patients into three risk groups. In this system, five independent patient- and lymphoma-related predictors were identified: age >60 years, ECOG performance status >1, increased serum LDH level, increased CSF protein concentration, and the involvement of deep regions of the brain. Patients with 0 to 1, 2 to 3, and 4 to 5 of these unfavorable variables had 2-year overall survival rates of 80%, 48%, or 15%, respectively.

TREATMENT

PCNSL is a highly radiosensitive tumor and whole brain radiotherapy achieves complete remission in 60% of patients, but recurrence takes place approximately 1 year after RT conclusion. Usually, radiotherapy is delivered to the whole brain, because of the widespread infiltration of the disease; variable doses (ranging from 20 to 55 Gy) and modalities (with or without a boost on the tumor bed) are used. Present recommendations suggest whole brain radiotherapy of 45 Gy without a boost. In case of ocular involvement the eyes receive 36 to 40 Gy of radiation.

Actually, the role of radiotherapy is increasingly questioned due to increased amount of long-term survivors and the evidence of severe long-term neurotoxicity. However, a decreased dose or suppression of radiotherapy, also after chemotherapy, seems to decrease progression-free survival (PFS) with a variable impact on overall survival (OS). At the moment combined modality therapy of chemotherapy and radiotherapy

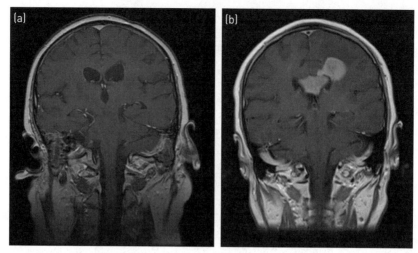

FIGURE 38.1

T1-weighted post gadolinium MRI: Complete response after 2 cycles of MTX (3500 mg/square meter).

has been shown to be the most effective treatment. Usually, chemotherapy is delivered before radiotherapy, with this schedule non responder patients to CHT can be early identified and radiotherapy rescue can be initiated. Moreover, chemotherapy administration before radiotherapy reduces the risk of neurotoxicity.

High-dose methothrexate (HDMTX) is now recognized as the drug of choice for initial treatment of PCNSL. The typical treatment is the intravenous injection of 3.5 to 8 g/m^2 every 10 to 21 days with leucovorin rescue. HDMTX achieved therapeutic level in CSF obviating the need for intrathecal administration. Response rates vary considerably from 30% to 80% (Figure 38.1), but a large amount of responder PCNSL patients will suffer progression or relapse, with a rate of 25% to 55% within a median follow-up of 13 to 83 months. HD-MTX treatment is associated with mild to moderate, and in most cases reversible, toxicity in fewer than 10% of cases. The most frequent adverse events related to HDMTX treatment are leukoencephalopathy, anemia, leukopenia, thrombocytopenia, and hepatic dysfunction.

In several studies. MTX has already been combined with one or more of the following chemotherapy drugs: cytosine arabinoside (AraC), vincristine, procarbazine, dexamethasone, carmustine, lomustine, etoposide, and methylprednisolone (Table 38.3).

The most studied and used combination is HDMTX plus HD-AraC. For this combination several authors reported an improvement both in overall response rate and PFS in comparison to HDMTX monotherapy. But, it should be emphasized as the HDMTX+HD-AraC combination increases significantly the frequency and severity of side effects. The most common and relevant side effects of this combination are: neutropenia, thrombocytopenia, and infectious complications.

In 2012 a Cochrane systematic review confirmed results in terms of ORR and PFS of this combination, but reported that there was no evidence that OS is statistically improved in patients receiving methotrexate plus cytarabine combination compared to those receiving methotrexate alone.

Table 38.3 Results of Prospective Trials of Combined Modality therapy as Upfront Treatment in Immunocompetent Patients With PCNSL

Chemotherapy	WBRT	Intrathecal Treatment	CR (%)	OS months
MTX (3.5 g/m^2) Glass J, 1994	30 Gy	No	56	33
MTX (1 g/m^2), Ara-C De Angelis LM 1992, Abrey LE 1998	40 Gy + 14 Gy boost	MTX	87	42
MTX (3 g/m^2), ADR, Ara-C, CFX, VCZ, MPS Blay Y 1995	20 Gy + 30 Gy boost	MTX, Ara-C	56	2 yrs 70%
MTX (3 g/m^2), VP26, BiCNU Poortmans PM 2003	30 Gy +10 Gy boost	MTX, Ara-C	69	46
MTX (3.5 g/m^2), PCB, VCZ, Ara-C Abrey L 2000	45 Gy in <60 y old	MTX	56	51
MTX (3.5 g/m^2) ± Ara-C Ferreri AJ 2009	Dose depended on age, response, participating center	No	MTX, 18 MTX + ara-C 46	3 y: MTX, 32%; MTX + ara-C, 46%
MTX (3.5 g/m^2), rituximab, PCB, VCZ, Ara-C Shah GD 2009	23.4 Gy if CR; 45 Gy if not CR	No	77	2 y OS 67%

ADR, adriamycin; CFX, cyclophosphamide; PCB, procarbazine; VCZ, vincristine; MPS, methylprednisolone.

At the moment, high-dose chemotherapy followed by hematopoietic stem cell transplantation remains an experimental procedure with insufficient data to guide clinicians.

In conclusion, combined modality therapy using high-dose MTX and whole brain radiotherapy has improved response rates compared to chemotherapy o radiotherapy alone, but the crucial limitation is significant risk of delayed neurotoxicity, presenting as dementia and ataxia. This risk is highest in patients over the age of 60 years and leads to considerable morbidity and mortality.

In PCNSL, response criteria have not been consistent between studies, for this reason, the IPCG proposed standard guidelines for monitoring response to therapy in the setting of clinical trials. Response criteria would take into account imaging, corticosteroid dose, CSF cytology, and ophthalmologic examination (Table 38.4).

At the end of treatment, the IPCG recommended assessment of the patient every 3 months for 2 years, then every 6 months for 3 years, and then every 12 months for 5 years.

Table 38.4 Standardized Baseline Evaluation and Response Criteria for Primary CNS Lymphoma

Response	Imaging	Steroids	OFT examination	CFS
CR	No contrast-enhancing disease	–	Negative	Negative
Unconfirmed CR	No contrast-enhancing diseaseMinimal enhancing disease	Any Any	Negative Minor RPE abnormality	Negative Negative
PR	50% decrease in enhancementNo contrast-enhancing disease	NA NA	Negative or minor RPE abnormality Decrease in vitreous cells or retinal infiltrate	Negative Positive Suspicious
PD	25% increase in enhancing disease Any new site of disease	NA	Recurrent or new disease	Positive
SD	All scenarios not covered by responses above			

RPE, retinal pigment epithelium.

SUGGESTED READING

Abrey LE, Batchelor TT, Ferreri AJ, et al. Report of an international workshop to standardize baseline evaluation and response criteria for primary CNS lymphoma. J Clin Oncol 2005;23:5034–5043.

Abrey LE, DeAngelis LM, Yahalom J. Long-term survival in primary CNS lymphoma. J Clin Oncol 1998;16(3):859–863.

Abrey LE, Yahalom J, DeAngelis LM. Treatment for primary CNS lymphoma: the next step. J Clin Oncol 2000;18(17):3144–3150.

Baraniskin A, Deckert M, Schulte-Altedorneburg G, et al. Current strategies in the diagnosis of diffuse large B-cell lymphoma of the central nervous system. Br J Haematol. 2012;156:421–432.7

Bergner N, Monsef I, Illerhaus G, et al. Role of chemotherapy additional to high-dose methotrexate for primary central nervous system lymphoma (PCNSL) Cochrane Database Syst Rev 2012 Nov 14;11.

Blay JY, Bouhour D, Carrie C, Bouffet E, Brunat-Mentigny M, Philip T, Biron P. The C5R protocol: a regimen of high-dose chemotherapy and radiotherapy in primary cerebral non-Hodgkin's lymphoma of patients with no known cause of immunosuppression. Blood 1995 Oct 15;86(8):2922–2929.

Brastianos PK, Batchelor TT. Primary central nervous system lymphoma: overview of current treatment strategies. Hematol Oncol Clin North Am 2012;26:897–916.

Ferreri AJM, Reni M, Foppoli M, et al. High-dose cytarabine plus high dose methotrexate versus high-dose methotrexate alone in patients with primary CNS lymphoma: a randomised phase 2 trial. Lancet 2009;374:1512–1524.

Glass J, Gruber ML, Cher L, Hochberg FH. Preirradiation methotrexate chemotherapy of primary central nervous system lymphoma: long-term outcome. J Neurosurg 1994 Aug;81(2):188–195.

Guha-Thakurta N, Damek D, Pollack C, Hochberg FH. Intravenous methotrexate as initial treatment for primary central nervous system lymphoma: response to therapy and quality of life of patients. Journal of Neuro-oncology 1999; 43(3):259–268.

Sutherland T, Yap K, Liew E, et al. Primary central nervous system lymphoma in immunocompetent patients: a retrospective review of MRI features. J Med Imaging Radiat Oncol ;56:295–301.

39 Brain Tumors in Childhood

Veronica Biassoni, Cecilia Casali, Elisabetta Schiavello, Francesco Di Meco, and Maura Massimino

INTRODUCTION

Tumors of the central nervous system (CNS) are the second most common neoplasm after hematopoietic cancers and the most common solid tumor in childhood. As such, they are the leading cause of death in the pediatric population.

Advances in surgery, radiation, and chemotherapy have led to better treatment outcomes over the past decades. Nonetheless, some types of brain tumors (BTs) still present many challenges.

EPIDEMIOLOGY

The US Central Brain Tumor Registry reports an average annual incidence of 4.3 cases/100000 person-year in the USA. Age at diagnosis is variable, with a peak between 4 and 8 years and a slight preponderance in males.[1]

Higher risks of developing a primary CNS tumor in childhood have been associated with: 1. a history of previous radiation doses to the CNS; 2. certain genetic syndromes (i.e. Neurofibromatosis 1 and 2, Li-Fraumeni syndrome, bilateral retinoblastoma, Tuberous Sclerosis, Von Hippel–Lindau disease, Gorlin syndrome, Cowden syndrome, Turcot syndrome, Pierpont syndrome[2] and ataxia-telangiectasia). Taken together, these conditions account for 5% of childhood BTs. In attending to these patients, physicians are advised to consider the abovementioned risk factors and to watch for any sign or symptom suggestive of a CNS tumor.

Unlike in adults, who are mainly affected by high-grade astrocytomas (WHO grade 3 and 4), the most frequent childhood histotypes are low-grade gliomas and embryonic tumors (i.e. PNET and medulloblastoma), which constitute respectively 50% and 20% of CNS tumors in children < 15 years of age (Figure 39.1).[3]

CLINICAL PRESENTATION

The clinical signs and symptoms of CNS tumors depend on location, rate of growth[4] and patient age (see Table 39.1). Progressive neurological deficits, signs and symptoms caused by increased intracranial pressure, visual disturbances, behavioral disorders, seizures, endocrine disruption, and failure to thrive may occur in various

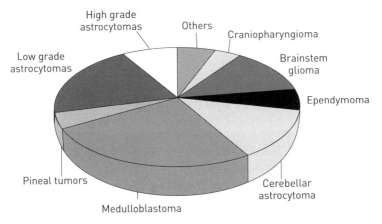

FIGURE 39.1
Childhood BT incidence according to histology.

Table 39.1 Relationship Between Tumor Site and Clinical Manifestations of Supratentorial Neoplasms

	Frontal	*Parietal*	*Temporal*	*Occipital*
SYMPTOMS	Late becoming symptomatic Raised ICP Psychomotor retardation Behavioral changes Urination disturbances Epileptic seizures Motor apraxia Language disturbances	Raised ICP Visual field alteration Space and time disorientation Apraxia— Agnosia Epileptic seizures	Speech disturbances Hearing disturbances Comprehension disturbances Uncinate seizures (unpleasant smell perceptions) Epileptic seizures with olfactory manifestations, déjà vu and déjà veçu	Partial epileptic seizures sometimes with visual hallucinations Frequent alterations of the visual field
MOTOR	Controlateral Hemiparesis	Weakness Muscle atrophy of the controlateral hemisoma Involuntary movements	Possibile motor disturbances	Late motor disturbances due to functional deterioration of adjacent areas

Adapted from "Medicina Oncologica" 8th edition, Bonadonna, Robustelli della Cuna, Valagussa, Ed. Elsevier Masson; modified.

combinations. The median duration of symptoms and signs before diagnosis is approximately 60 days—a reflection of the insidious nature of pediatric BTs.[5,6] Lesions in the posterior fossa are notoriously difficult to diagnose for primary care physicians due to the absence of focal neurological signs.

RAISED INTRACRANIAL PRESSURE (ICP)

Children with BTs may present an acute or chronic history of raised ICP, depending on the growth rate and location of the tumor. The classic presentation includes daily headaches worsening with Valsalva maneuver or lying flat. Vomiting is more common during the night or early morning. Hydrocephalus can also cause papilloedema, optic disk pallor, and vision loss. "Sunsetting eyes," or sixth nerve palsies, can be "false-localizing" signs indicating raised ICP rather than a cranial nerve involvement. The extreme presentation of a rapidly rising ICP is a decreased level of consciousness and the "Cushing's triad" (raised blood pressure, bradycardia, and altered pattern of respiration) that requires urgent treatment (medical, dexamethasone, mannitol and hyperventilation, and surgical as soon as possible). Neurosurgical CSF diversion techniques (third ventriculostomy, ventriculoperitoneal shunt or external ventricular drain) are often needed to stabilize the patient before or during surgery. Infants usually do not present the classical signs of raised ICP due to the plasticity of their skull bones before the closure of fontanels and suture lines; therefore, a close monitoring of head circumference and fontanel size may be precociously diagnostic. Making a diagnosis in older children is often difficult, because symptoms may resemble other diseases with physical and psychological causes.[4,7,8]

Headache

Headache related to BTs is mostly accompanied by signs/symptoms of obstructive hydrocephalus. Some slow growing tumors will cause headache by direct compression of the surrounding structures (skull, meninges). However, many BTs will present without headache, because the brain parenchyma largely lacks pain receptors.

Vomiting

Vomiting secondly to a BT is mostly related to some degree of obstructive hydrocephalus; isolated vomiting can otherwise be caused by a tumor irritating the "vomiting center" or the chemoreceptor trigger zone ("area postrema" on the floor of the IVth ventricle), both located in the medulla oblongata.[9]

Signs and Symptoms Related to Tumor Location

Children are able to balance neurological deficits. For example, a "head tilt" can be a way to correct diplopia from cranial nerve palsy, and many children with diplopia will be able to watch television or read without any problem. Special signs, such as an "uneven smile" or ptosis, may develop so gradually they go almost unnoticed.

Diencephalic syndrome is a combination of signs and symptoms related to hypothalamic dysfunction due to hypothalamic tumors, often pilocytic and pilomyxoid astrocytomas, in children usually aged <12 months. Clinical features include: weight loss leading to severe emaciation despite a normal calorie intake, hyperalertness, hyperkinesis, and euphoria.[10] Growth rates usually remain linear. Additional symptoms, such as nystagmus, hydrocephalus, and vomiting, have also been reported as possible manifestations of the syndrome.

Parinaud's syndrome is typical in patients with pineal or upper brainstem tumors.[11,12] These patients have supranuclear upgaze palsy, and pupils reactive to accommodation but not to direct light.

Primitive or secondary spinal cord tumors can present with back pain, scoliosis, neuropathic pain, numbness or limb weakness. Bowel or bladder signs usually occur late and may be a cause for concern. Acute spinal cord compression warrants an immediate neurosurgical consultation; steroids should be started while further treatment planning occurs. When surgical resection or debulking cannot be performed, radiation therapy or chemotherapy may be used to save the spinal cord function.[13]

Seizures

Tumors located in the cerebral cortex can present with seizures and very few other accompanying symptoms. Seizures can be difficult to control and multiple anticonvulsants may be required. If the epileptogenic zone is localized, surgical resection may be curative.

It is advisable to conduct an adequate presurgical evaluation, including electroencephalography and extensive neurophysiological monitoring, in order to plan an appropriate surgical strategy.[14]

Endocrine Disorders

Endocrinopathies could be the only presenting symptom of a childhood BT involving/compressing the hypothalamic–pituitary axis. Endocrine symptoms, such as polyuria or polydipsia (diabetes insipidus), precocious puberty (PP), diencephalic cachexia, and changes in weight, height and growth velocity, can occur long before the diagnosis of a hypothalamic-pituitary lesion. This might require a more careful history and clinical evaluation as well as a timely reevaluation as the occurrence of other neurologic, ophthalmic or endocrine signs and symptoms may suggest the presence of an underlying hypothalamic-pituitary lesion.[15]

DIAGNOSIS

Imaging

Computerized Tomography (CT) and Magnetic Resonance Imaging (MRI)

CT of a suspected BT should be reserved for emergency situations, such as to assess hydrocephalus and/or bleeding in unstable patients. Once a brain lesion is suspected by clinical examination and/or initial imaging, the diagnostic gold standard is MRI with and without gadolinium.[16,17] Compared to CT, this provides more details on the topography, size, and solid/cystic components of the tumor. MRI does not expose patients to radiations and avoids bone-related artifacts. T1 weighted sequences provide good anatomical details, but differences between normal and pathological tissue can be highlighted by T2 images. Fluid Attenuation Inversion Recovery (FLAIR) and

T2 sequences show areas of interruption of the blood–brain barrier (BBB), areas of neoplastic infiltration, and edema.

In the young pediatric population, achieving high quality MRI, given the long execution time and high sensitivity to motion artifacts, may necessitate sedation or general anesthesia.

Nowadays, neuroimages allow the preoperative localization of eloquent cortical areas and subcortical tracks/networks by functional MRI (fMRI) and tractography or Diffusion Tensor Imaging fiber tracking MRI (DTI MRI). DTI allows the study of pathways of anatomical connectivity in vivo. The use of the diffusion tensor makes it possible to calculate the degree of diffusion, the directionality of motion (anisotropy), and the principal orientation(s) of diffusion of each voxel.

Transfontanellar Ultrasound (Transfontanellar US)

As an initial test to detect the tumor in the first year of life (prior to the closure of the fontanels), Transfontanellar US may be safer than CT, especially in patients presenting with acute symptoms.

Positron Emission Tomography (PET)

PET is potentially useful to distinguish tumor recurrence from radionecrosis especially when the tumor has a high metabolic activity: malignant tumors tend to be hypermetabolic compared to surrounding tissues, while the necrotic tissue shows a reduced metabolism. This distinction poorly applies to childhood BTs. It can also be used to highlight unresectable brain areas that are functionally important in children. SPECT (Single Positron Emission Computed Tomography) is easier to access than PET, and can be equally useful.

TREATMENT

Multidisciplinary Team Approach

For pediatric solid tumors, treatment relies on a combination of surgery, radiation, and medical therapy. The primary treating team should include a neuro-oncologist, a neurosurgeon, and a radiation-oncologist.

Surgery

Surgery is an important component of the overall treatment of pediatric BTs. Surgical treatment, in particular, is aimed at obtaining a histopathological diagnosis (HP) and, when possible, maximal resection of tumor tissue with minimal consequences for the patient.

It has repeatedly been demonstrated that the extent of resection in some tumor subtypes directly correlates with patient survival, even when faced with a benign histological diagnosis, as in pilocytic astrocytoma.[18,19] Although a few studies[20] dispute this, citing a lack of any statistical difference between the survival of children who underwent total resection and those who underwent subtotal resection, the majority of the literature recommends removing as much tumor tissue as possible.[21]

The practice of repeated surgery for residual tumor, as well as the concept of second-look surgery for ependymoma, has gained considerable popularity in recent years.[22]

Over the past decades, various techniques have been attempted to achieve higher, or closer-to-radical, rates of tumor resection as well as lower rates of morbidity. Among them, the gold standard is the pre- and peri-operative evaluation of the functional structures involved. Studies have been conducted to improve the identification of the location of functional structures close to, or directly involved with, the tumor, both pre- and intra-operatively. Intra- and peri-operatively, the best practice is to perform electrocortical stimulation mapping (ESM) under awake or asleep conditions. However, the results obtained demonstrate a good but incomplete correspondence between fMRI or DTI MRI results and ESM.

Navigational Systems

Neuronavigation is currently the most commonly used tool in neurosurgery. Navigational systems, be they frame-based or frameless, can be combined with preoperative CT and/or MRI images to produce dynamic spatial information of the brain in a three dimensional frame.

Neuronavigation makes it possible to locate eloquent, or "noble," structures in advance and to plan and/or change the surgical approach accordingly. These systems facilitate the adoption of an optimal orientation during the initial stages of surgery, which allows for a more precise surgical cut with minimal craniotomy as well as for a reliable navigation on relaxed brain tissues. During the various stages of surgery, however, accuracy may be significantly compromised by brain or tumor shifts occurring secondary to the resection of the tumor, the drainage of the cerebrospinal fluid (CSF), or the mechanical forces acting on the brain matter during surgical manipulation. This can lead to the incomplete resection of the tumor and/or encroachment into normal brain tissues.

Intraoperative Imaging Techniques

New intraoperative imaging techniques, such as CT,[21] or dyes, such as 5-ALA, have recently been introduced.[22] These methods, however, may be limited by such factors as the low specificity of imaging, the poor vascularization of tumor tissue and the fact that their use is limited to only a few, often rare, histotypes in pediatric patients.

Ultrasound

Following improvements in the definition of ultrasound images, the use of intraoperative ultrasonography has become increasingly popular. With the exception of a few centers,[23] however, its use is not widespread in the field of neurosurgery. The major benefit of medical ultrasound scanning lies in the real-time fidelity of the image, the ease of use compared to CT scanners, and the low costs per image. To date, due to the lack of a routine diagnostic cerebral ultrasound, the ultrasound imaging of BTs is poorly defined. For this reason, the latest generation of US scanner are equipped with a navigation software. Combining the ultrasound scan with this form of anatomical mapping helps to improve the reading of the image, particularly in difficult cases.

Intraoperative MRI

Intraoperative MRI (ioMRI) is currently the gold standard in neurosurgical practice. This is a technical solution based on the use of an integrated MR placed inside the operating room and interfaced with a sophisticated neuronavigation system and a surgical microscope. The integration of these tools helps the neurosurgeon to reach brain lesions with high precision and to choose the best path for radical excision, thereby minimizing postoperative complications. When deemed appropriate, operators can interrupt surgery and perform an ioMRI to identify any near-real-time structural and functional changes in the brain, obtain a new 3D dataset for neuronavigation, and check the actual extent of tumor removal.[24,25]

There are a number of obstacles to the large-scale deployment of this method, and chief among them is the sheer cost of the equipment. Neurosurgeons often adopt a combination of the various neuronavigational systems available. This approach allows surgeons to enjoy the advantages of each approach and stretch the limits of any single system when used on its own.

Intraoperative Neurophysiological Monitoring (IONM)

IONM allows the identification and preservation during surgery of functional cortical and subcortical sites, which helps to maximize surgical resection and to decrease postoperative morbidity.[26]

The role of surgery is very limited for lesions in critical areas, such as the brainstem and the optic pathway, as well as for some histotypes, such as germinoma, which is highly radio- and chemo-sensitive. Such cases can only warrant a biopsy to obtain just enough tissue for a histopathological diagnosis and the planning of appropriate treatment strategies.

Neuroendoscopic biopsy is widely accepted as the first choice for tissue biopsy of pediatric intra- or periventricular tumors. It is also suitable when these are accompanied by ventriculomegaly, which can be easily resolved by additional endoscopic procedures such as endoscopic third ventriculostomy (ETV), septostomy, and the fenestration of cystic tumors. Neuroendoscopic biopsy allows for direct visualization of the biopsy site and achieves effective control of tumor bleeding.[27] Navigation-assisted neuroendoscopy has substantially increased the accuracy and safety of endoscopic procedures, even in the case of tumors without ventriculomegaly, which was previously considered a contraindication. This technique can also be employed for endoscopic tumor removal, but only in cases of soft tumors not exceeding 2 cm in diameter.[28,29]

When the tumor is not a proper candidate for neuroendoscopic surgery, stereotactic surgery or open craniotomy biopsy can be considered. Stereotactic surgery for tumor biopsy has a high tumor-sampling success rate with minimally invasive approaches, but it does not allow to control tumor bleeding and treat any associated hydrocephalus simultaneously. Conventional open surgery shows relative high mortality and morbidity and must be considered only as a last option to obtain a decompression of the lesion.

Treatment of Hydrocephalus

No consensus exists regarding the management of hydrocephalus in children with posterior fossa tumors before, during or after surgery.[30] In most cases the treatment of hydrocephalus is made simultaneously to the surgical treatment of the tumor lesion.

Only rarely is it carried out in the previous days to stabilize the patient and to allow further investigations in the event of acute deterioration.

Treatment options include either ETV (a small stoma made in the semiopaque membrane of the tuber cinereum between the infundibular recess and the paired mammillary bodies) or external ventricular drainage, which is removed after the stabilization of intracranial pressure. Sometimes, a ventriculoperitoneal shunt is placed to relieve persistent ventriculomegaly.

The factors that can predict persistent postoperative hydrocephalus are: short duration of the symptoms (less than 3 months); severity of the preoperative hydrocephalus (Evan's index and frontal and occipital horn ratio); location of the tumors in the midline (as opposed to laterally); medulloblastoma and ependymoma as tumor subtypes; and postsurgical meningitis and/or pseudomeningocele. It is imperative that the surgeon be aware of these factors during the surgical planning as well as the postoperative clinical and radiological monitoring.

Radiotherapy

It aims to prevent local recurrence and dissemination. Due to the known long-term side effects on a developing brain, it is recommended to delay radiotherapy after 3–5 years of age, whenever possible. Currently all patients with BT receive radiotherapy based on a treatment plan where MRI and CT scans are fused in a three-dimensional view. When using adjuvant chemotherapy before radiotherapy, one must consider that some drugs have a toxicity potentially enhanced by radiotherapy itself (i.e. neurotoxicity of methotrexate, ototoxicity of cisplatin). According to histology, the target volume may include the tumor bed (50–55 Gy), or the tumor with the neuraxis (30–35 Gy). Conventional fractioning consists of daily 1.6–1.8 Gy applications 5 days a week. Hyperfractioning (two applications per day, with each dose reduced to 1.1–1.3 Gy every 6–8 hours) aims to increase the radiobiological dose while reducing side effects. Proton-beam radiation is an emerging technique that aims at delivering the same doses to the tumor while sparing the normal surrounding tissue. Even so, it cannot be considered the standard of care for childhood BTs.[31,32] Irradiating a child requires more time than it does an adult because it calls for absolute immobility; this can be obtained by giving simple explanations to the child, a drug premedication, or a short general anesthesia.

Chemotherapy

Due to the presence of the BBB, the effectiveness of chemotherapy in BTs is lower than in other solid tumors.[33] Drugs easily cross the BBB either as small soluble ionized particles or carried by drug-binding plasma proteins. The BBB is not homogenously intact (areas of discontinuity can be found in the periventricular zone), nor is its permeability constant within the tumor itself: it is quite intact in small tumors and in the peripheral areas of large tumors, but almost permeable in the central areas of most lesions. The main drugs used in the treatment of pediatric BTs are: nitrosoureas, vincristine, procarbazine, derivatives of platinum, epipodophyllotoxins, high-dose methotrexate, and other antimetabolites. Chemotherapy and radiotherapy are delivered as soon as possible after surgery, on the assumption that the postoperative anatomical alterations can facilitate the passage of drugs through the BBB. The use of steroids appears to reduce the penetration of drugs, while high-dose radiation seems to increase their transcapillary transport. Low-grade gliomas benefit from lower-dose chemotherapy administered over extended periods: this schedule has been shown to slow or stop their growing rate.[34] High-dose chemotherapy followed by peripheral blood stem cells transplantation is being widely used in infants to prevent/delay radiotherapy.[35] Chemotherapy agents may also be used as radiosensitizers during radiotherapy to increase its effectiveness.

New drugs

The characterization of molecular pathways involved in tumor growth and differentiation has ushered in a new era in cancer therapeutics. The diagnosis and management of BTs will be progressively based on molecular stratification, allowing for patient- and tumor-tailored therapies.

Tumorigenesis involves multiple pathways with significant crosstalk between pathways. Therefore, targeting multiple pathways via broader-ranging agents or combinations of agents may prove necessary.

Most of these novel biologic agents have cytostatic activity, and may need to be combined with conventional cytotoxic chemotherapy and radiotherapy for maximal tumor response. These agents have potentially better CNS penetration and lower toxicity profiles compared with conventional chemotherapy.

Molecular pathways implicated in pediatric BTs, agents that target these pathways, and current clinical trials are summarized in Table 39.2.[36,37]

Table 39.2 Biologic Agents in Pediatric CNS Tumor Trials

Target	Drug
Epidermal growth factor receptor	Monoclonal antibodies: cauximab and nimotuzumab
Platelet-derived growth factor receptor	Small molecule inhibitors: erlotinib, gefitinib,
Ras/Raf/MEK/ERK pathway	and lapatinib
Farnesyltransferase inhibitors	Imatinib and sunitinib
Raf inhibitors MEK inhibitors	Tipifarnib and lonafarnib
Phosphatidylinositol 3-kinase/mTOR or AktmTOR pathway	Sorafenib and sunitinib (multikinase inhibitors)
	AZD6244
	MK-2206
Akt inhibitors	Sirolimus, temsirolimus, and everolimus
mTOR inhibitors	
Angiogenesis inhibitors	
VEGF pathway	Monocolonal antibody: bevacizumab Small
VEGF and basic fibroblast growth factor	molecule inhibitors: pazopanib.
Protein kinase C-β inhibitors	PTC299, and AZD2171
αvβ3 and αvβ5 integrin inhibitors	VEGF Trap
Histone deactylase inhibitors	Thalidomide and lenalidomaide Enzastaurin
Sonic Hedgehog pathway	Cilengitide
SMO inhibitor	Suberoylanilide hydroxamic acid,
Notch signaling pathway	depsipeptide, and valproic acid
Gamma-secretase inhibitor	GDC0449
	RO4929097

(continued)

Table 39.2 Continued

401

Brain Tumors in Childhood

Target	Drug

Abbreviations:

Akt = Protein kinase B

CNS = Central nervous system

ERK = Extracellular regulated mitogen-activated protein kinase

MEK = Mitogen-activated protein kinase-extracellular regulated mitogen-activated protein kinase

mTOR = Mammalian target of rapamycin

SMO = Smoothened

VEGF = Vascular endothelial growth factor

Nageswara Rao AA, Scafidi J, Wells EM, Packer RJ. Biologically targeted therapeutics in pediatric brain tumors. Pediatr Neurol 2012 Apr;46(4):203–211. Review

MAIN CATEGORIES OF CHILDHOOD CNS TUMORS

- Glial tumors
  - Astrocytoma and other gliomas
    - Low-grade
    - High-grade
  - Ependymoma
- Embryonal tumors
  - Medulloblastoma
  - CNS primitive neuroectodermal tumor
  - Atypical teratoid rhabdoid tumor
- Choroid plexus tumors
  - Papilloma
  - Carcinoma
- Germ cell tumors
  - Germinoma
  - Nongerminomatous germ cell tumor
- Craniopharyngiomas
- Meningiomas

LOW-GRADE GLIOMAS (LGGS)

WHO grade I and II astrocytomas:

- Pilocytic astrocytoma, WHO grade I
- Pilomyxoid astrocytoma WHO grade II
- Subependymal giant cell astrocytoma, WHO grade I
- Pleomorphicxanthoastrocytoma, WHO grade II
- Diffuse astrocytoma, WHO grade II 20% of BTs in children (most frequent BT in childhood)
- Potentially in any area of the brain/spine (in children, mostly in posterior fossa or optic pathway)

Surgery

- Maximally safe resection (generally achievable for hemispheric or cerebellar locations) has significant prognostic implications in these tumors; typically well-circumscribed, they quite frequently include a subtle component, which may be hard to differentiate from the normal surrounding brain tissue. Thus, real-time imaging, combined with navigational capabilities, may be helpful in these operations insofar as it maximizes resection control
- Deep midline, optic pathway/hypothalamic, and brainstem locations should undergo subtotal resection or biopsy only

Chemotherapy

- Not always necessary (surgical resection is the goal of treatment)
- Several clinical trials have demonstrated a role for chemotherapy in stabilizing or shrinking low-grade gliomas;[38,39] it is therefore used in progressive or unresectable tumors[40]
- Most widely used CT regimens: carboplatin and vincristine, cisplatin and etoposide, vinblastine[41,42]

Radiotherapy

- Not as a first choice (due to its long-term side effects in populations with excellent prognoses)
- Radio-induced tumors are of concern in patients with LGG associated to genetic syndromes, such as phacomatosis

Prognosis and Follow-Up

- Very good prognosis: 5-year OS > 90%[43]
- Complete and often curative surgical resection
- Follow-up with MRI (due to high frequency of local relapse/progression) with closer controls in the event of residual disease ± ophthalmologic assessment for optic pathway gliomas ± endocrinological assessment according to the site of interest

HIGH GRADE GLIOMA (HGG)

- WHO grade III (anaplastic astrocytoma) or IV (glioblastoma multiforme)
- 10–20% of childhood BTs
- Most often originates from the supratentorial area, rarely from the cerebellum
- Growing pattern: infiltrative, high growth rate, frequent recurrence after treatment

Surgery

- At present, the strongest indicator of prognosis is extent of resection;[44,45] nevertheless, radical surgery often not feasible due to the infiltrative pattern and the tumor location frequently involving thalamus and pons[46]

- In case of diffuse intrinsic pontine gliomas (DIPG) or gliomatosis cerebri, biopsy is recommended to ascertain their biological characteristics and to enhance the understanding and targeting of treatments, especially in clinical trials[47,48]

Radiotherapy

- High-dose focal radiation after maximal surgery is the best treatment strategy[49]
- Craniospinal radiation is unnecessary as these tumors do not tend to spread into the CSF

Chemotherapy

- No strategy can be considered a gold standard
- According to the largest randomized published trial, the addition of prednisone, vincristine, and CCNU gave better results than radiotherapy alone[50] (different schedules have been used: preradiation, concomitant, and post radiation for maintenance)
- Myeloablative CT is not standard but is used for either firstly diagnosed or relapsed tumors, with variable results[51,52]
- Temozolomide, the standard CT in adult HGG, has been investigated in the pediatric population[53,54] and is still widely used
- Target therapies (gefitinib, erlotinib, imatinib, nimotuzumab) in combination with conventional therapies are currently being evaluated[55,56]

Prognosis and Follow-Up

- Poor prognosis: 5–20% of 5-year OS with a median survival of 11–24 months[57]

EPENDYMOMA

- 6% of all childhood BTs; patients are mostly under 5 years at diagnosis except for spinal cord localization (10% of cases), which is predominant during adolescence
- Arises from the ependymal lining of the ventricles (mostly in the fourth ventricle)
- Myxopapillary (WHO grade I, spinal location), classical form (WHO grade II), anaplastic (WHO grade III)[58]
- Typically presents as unifocal disease, in 10% of cases[59] it can spread throughout the brain or spine, and very rarely outside of the CNS[60]

Surgery

- Gross-total safe resection has a primary prognostic role: 5-year survival is about 70% for almost complete resection and about 30% for subtotal resection; second-look surgery is justified when postoperative imaging suggests residual disease, or during treatment[61,62]
- Increased risk of persistent hydrocephalus

Radiotherapy

- Essential even after complete resection[63]
- No effective advantage of hyperfractionated RT compared to conventional RT (total dose tumor bed 59.4 Gy); consolidated role of boost to the residual disease

Chemotherapy

- Not really chemosensitive
- Adjuvant CT is recommended if residual disease or unfavorable histology (anaplastic ependymoma) are present, to obtain a reduction of the residue, or to shrink the residual tumor and allow total resection in a second-look surgery[64]

Prognosis and Follow-Up

- 5-year OS goes from 80% for children with complete surgery to less than 40% when total resection is not achieved
- Late recurrences can occur for which complete surgery is always the goal
- A long follow-up is needed[65]

MEDULLOBLASTOMA

- 10–20% of BTs and 40% of tumors of the posterior fossa
- Often arises from cerebellar vermis or the fourth ventricle
- Various subtypes (classic, nodular/desmoplastic, large cell/anaplastic) that relate to prognosis and have traditionally been used to guide treatment
- Other molecular subtypes and genetic patterns predictive of the outcome emerged from recent studies, i.e., *ERB-B2, TRKC, PDGFRA, MYCC, and MYCN* expression of β-catenin: these will be incorporated in the incoming clinical trials[66,67]
- Possible seeding into the subarachnoid space, the CSF, or in supratentorial sites, rarely into the bone marrow, bones, and liver

Surgery

- Maximal safe resection is the mainstay. Postoperative staging allows to classify patients into a standard risk group (residual disease ≤1.5 cm^2, no metastasis) and a high risk group (residual >1.5 cm^2 and/or metastasis)

Chemoradiotherapy

- CT/RT are both mandatory after surgery
- RT aims at controlling residual disease and avoiding subarachnoid dissemination
- Localized disease: standard treatment includes CSI (23.4 Gy) plus a boost on the tumor site (30.6 Gy) and CT according to various schedules (vincristine, high-dose methotrexate, cisplatin, etoposide, carboplatin, cyclophosphamide and nitrosourea)[68,69]
- Metastatic disease: the current strategy at our Institute includes preradiant intensive chemotherapy and hyperfractionated accelerated radiotherapy (HART) whether

followed by consolidation with myeloablative chemotherapy or not; the related EFS at 5 years rises from 50% to 70% with this treatment[70]

Prognosis and Follow-Up

- Most relapses in the 5 years after diagnosis
- Follow-up should also include evaluation of the CSI-related sequelae: neurocognitive development and endocrine profile

CHOROID PLEXUS TUMOR

- Rare, 2% of BTs
- Three subtypes: papilloma (grade I WHO), atypical choroid plexus papilloma (WHO II) and choroid plexus carcinoma (CPC, WHO grade III); frequently located in the lateral ventricles, rarely in the fourth ventricle with infiltration of the surrounding parenchyma
- Li-Fraumeni syndrome (p53 mutation) may be associated with CPC.[71] This calls for a more detailed family history

Treatment

- WHO grade I and II tumors receive gross total resection only
- Operative management is often hindered by excessive bleeding and significant CSF production; preoperative embolization should be considered a useful adjunct[72]
- The schedule of treatment of CPC is aggressive: surgery, radiotherapy and adjuvant CT; intensive CT is often used with the aim of delaying/avoiding radiation, so the CT-only approach is appealing in very young patients.[73,74] Unfortunately, GTR has only a modest effect on survival in this patient cohort[75]
- The rarity of choroid plexus tumors makes it difficult to establish exact relapsing rates; however prognosis of choroid plexus papillomas is excellent after surgery, while prognosis of CPC is still poor (only 40% with a 5-year OS)[76]

GERM CELL TUMORS (GCT)

- Predominantly in males; median age: 12 years
- 2 subtypes: pure germinomas (comprising two-thirds of all GCTs) and "nongerminomatous germ cell tumors" (a more heterogeneous group further subclassified into: embryonal yolk sac tumors, choriocarcinomas, endodermal sinus tumors, and malignant teratomas); the latter subtype can be associated to pathological αFP/βhCG serum/CSF findings[77]
- Generally grow in the suprasellar and pineal region as well as in the third ventricle
- Symptoms may last several months before diagnosis; midline lesions can present with visual disturbances, hydrocephalus, endocrinopathies, personality alterations, school performances decline, headaches, or seizures; Parinaud syndrome is very common at presentation
- GCTs can spread into CSF; spinal metastases can occur at diagnosis

Surgery

- Surgical removal not recommended because of their high chemoradiosensitivity
- Surgery is important in establishing the histological diagnosis as well as in the treatment of hydrocephalus
- Biopsy is mandatory for diagnosis if αFP/βhCG in serum/CSF are not pathological
- Debulking procedures may be advocated in NGGCT as they are often resistant to chemotherapy

Radiochemotherapy

- GCTs are very sensitive to RT, so radiation alone may even be curative
- In order to reduce/eliminate radiation exposure, chemotherapeutic regimens (platin-based) are used with good results;[78] current radiotherapy fields should include whole ventricular systems
- In case of metastatic disease, RT alone could be curative[79]

Prognosis and Follow-Up

- Germinomas have a long-term survival rates >90%
- Nongerminomatous GCTs have a worse prognosis: 5-year OS for 60–70%[80] and treatment must include both platinum-based regimens and radiation therapy
- Endocrinological sequelae should be carefully monitored during the follow-up together with markers detection when pathological at diagnosis

ATYPICAL TERATOID RHABDOID TUMOR (ATRT)

- Aggressive neoplasm with a dismal prognosis characteristic of infancy[81]
- 1–2% of CNS tumors in children of all ages, but 10–20% in patients less than 3 years old
- Usually located in the posterior fossa and the cerebral hemispheres
- It has been recently recognized as a separate entity[82] from PNET/medulloblastoma due to the presence of rhabdoid cells and components of mesenchymal and epithelial malignant cells; monosomy of 22q11 is the cytogenetic feature (*hSNF/INI1* gene involved)[83]
- A consistent fraction of cases carries de novo *SMARCB1* constitutional mutations in the setting of the "rhabdoid tumor predisposition syndrome" and the outcome is worst in infant syndromic ATRT patients

Surgery

- The role of the extent of surgery in different locations is also unclear; some authors have recommended aggressive surgical excision to achieve gross total resection, including second surgery where feasible. However, the prognosis without adjuvant therapy has not improved

Chemotherapy

- Multiple therapeutic approaches have been attempted over the last two decades to increase survival, without success
- Intrathecal chemotherapy may have a role[84] in patients not referred for radiation. There is no accepted standard chemotherapy; however, intensive alkylator-based chemotherapy regimens, high-dose methotrexate, and regimens that include HDCT with stem cells rescue may prove more effective[85,86]

Radiotherapy

- Focal radiation is a crucial treatment; nevertheless, the higher frequency of ATRT in patients less than 3 years of age makes it difficult to draw an optimal treatment strategy, also considering that they have shorter survival than older patients with the same tumor[87]

Prognosis and Follow-Up

- OS is less than 12 months and 1 year PFS less than 20%
- Infant age, metastasis at diagnosis and the status of carrier of rhabdoid tumor predisposition syndrome lead to lethal outcome[88].

PNET-PINEOBLASTOMA

- Embryonal tumor are often broadly referred to as PNET—"primitive neuro-ectodermal tumors" (as distinct from "peripheral neuro-ectodermal tumors," which refer to certain extracranial sarcomas)
- Although histologically indistinguishable from infratentorial medulloblastoma, they have a typical/different genetic pattern and often poorly respond to medulloblastoma-tailored therapies
- When located in the pineal region they are called "pineoblastoma," in other sites "central nervous system PNET"
- They constitute 2–3% of pediatric CNS tumors
- Mostly hemispheric location with a wide local extension; less than 10% originates from the midline structures and less than 5% in the spinal cord
- Frequently present with leptomeningeal dissemination

Surgery

- Maximal safe removal is associated with a more favorable prognosis but is often not feasible due to tumor location and diffuse infiltrative behavior; the survival rate of 40% for patients with residual less than 1.5 cm^3 falls to 13% for incomplete resections

Radiochemotherapy

- Adjuvant therapy consists of radiation to the tumor bed (40–60 Gy) and, in selected cases to the neuraxis (30–35 Gy), associated with chemotherapy (nitrosoureas, procarbazine, cyclophosphamide, vincristine, cisplatin, and carboplatin); it has recently intensified with the use of myeloablative schedules in order to reduce radiation doses/fields and improve prognosis

Prognosis and Follow-Up

- 1 year OS of children with PNET is 65%, while only 35% are alive at 5 years
- Pineal location is usually associated with better prognosis
- Better results were also achieved with radiotherapy in nonconventional fractionation (hyperfractionated accelerated) and myeloablative-chemotherapy
- The overall prognosis for these patients depends on several factors including the extent of resection, age at diagnosis, CSF dissemination, and site in the supratentorial space.

CRANIOPHARYNGIOMA

- It is classified as a WHO grade I tumor but can cause a number of long-term complications primarily due to its location in the suprasellar region which disrupts the hypothalamic–pituitary axis and can lead to a large spectrum of endocrinopathies (i.e., growth deficiencies, visual changes/loss, adrenal crisis, headaches or seizures)
- It usually does not disseminate throughout the CNS axis

Surgery

- The treatment of craniopharyngiomas includes surgery as well as radiotherapy. Surgical strategies may range from complete resection to biopsy, according to tumor location and extension. Constant evaluation of surgical complications must be made
- Diencephalic obesity is related to surgical manipulation of hypothalamic tissue
- Combined surgical approaches are sometimes required to provide a durable remission

Radiotherapy

- Radiation can prevent recurrence in unresectable cases[89]

Chemotherapy

- Has a minor role
- High-dose chemotherapy has not proven efficacy. Some studies have pointed to the benefit of injecting chemotherapy directly into the tumoral cysts[90]

Prognosis and Follow-Up

- A Craniopharyngioma often progresses into a chronic condition with significant morbidity
- Severe problems with sleep, learning, vision and weight gain are not uncommon; these patients definitely benefit from a multidisciplinary team approach[91].

MENINGIOMAS

- They occur mainly in adults, rarely in children
- The most frequent molecular alteration is the loss of chromosome 22 with deletion of the *NF2*-gene; in patients with NF2, with a germinal mutation, meningiomas have an elevated incidence, often with multiple locations
- Surgical excision remains the treatment of choice in symptomatic patients
- Adjuvant radiotherapy is used only in selected cases

SPINAL CORD TUMORS

- They account for 5–6% of CNS tumors
- Patients are frequently over 8 years of age; equal incidence in males and females
- Astrocytomas or ependymomas are usually histologically identical to their intracranial counterpart; mixopapillary ependymoma is typicalliy located in the spine
- Very rare tumors with rather high degree of malignancy
- The most frequent localization is dorsal, followed by the cervical and lumbar spine
- Growth is usually slow with involvement of multiple vertebral segments and compression of normal tissue; multiple tumor localizations are suggestive of NF2
- They are slow-growing, often causing weakness, pain, paresthesia, abnormal gait and sphincter functions; weakness is variable up to tetraparesis; the pattern of pain may occasionally suggest involvement of the spinal, plexus, or nerve roots

Surgery

- The surgical goal is to perform as gross total a resection as possible following multilevel laminotomy. Intraoperative electrophysiology, including somatosensory-evoked potential monitoring is mandatory to preserve the spinal functions.

Chemoterapy/Radioterapy

- The impact of adjuvant treatment on progression and survival is still unclear; presently, the decision to initiate non-surgical treatment depends primarily on the WHO grade of the tumor and the extent of resection
- For incomplete resection, postoperative local radiotherapy may be recommended

Prognosis and Follow-Up

- OS for low-grade astrocytomas is 70% at 5 years and 55% at 10 years. Following complete excision, the prognosis appears to be 100% at 5 years. The worst prognosis is that of high-grade/anaplastic tumors, whose survival is in the order of few months.

BRAIN STEM TUMORS

- These tumors are mostly astrocytomas and account for 10–15% of intracranial tumors and 20% of posterior fossa tumors.
- They have different degrees of malignancy and extensively infiltrate the brain stem.
- The onset of symptoms is often insidious, with headache, cervical pain, gait disturbances, dysphagia and cranial nerve palsies. Usually symptoms are rapidly progressive.
- We can distinguish three patterns of brainstem lesions:
  - diffuse, infiltrating pontine glioma (DIPG)
  - localized with a nodule or cyst
  - exophytic into the lumen of the fourth ventricle or ponto-cerebellar angle (often low-grade gliomas curable with surgery alone)

TREATMENT

Due to the high rate of morbidity/mortality related to surgery with no changes in prognosis, only a cycle of 5 to 7 weeks of radiotherapy (54 Gy) is recommended. This improves symptoms in around 70% of cases and results in an objective radiological response.

Neither standard adjuvant CT nor high-dose CT were able to modify the prognosis. A high EGFR expression on DIPG has recently been highlighted. Presently, therapeutic trials with anti-EGFR antibodies are on-going; it is expected that these will lead to extended EFS and OS as well as improved quality of life.

PROGNOSIS AND FOLLOW-UP

The results of standard therapies remain discouraging, with a 5-year survival under 5%.

SUGGESTED READING

1. Dolecek TA, Propp JM, Stroup NE, Kruchko C. CBTRUS. Statistical report: primary brain and central nervous system tumors diagnosed in the United States. In 2005-2009 Central Brain Tumor Registry of the United States, 2005. NeuroOncol 2012 Nov;14Suppl 5:v1–49.
2. Vadivelu S, Edelman M, Schneider SJ. Choroid plexus papilloma and Pierpont syndrome Case report. J Neurosurg Pediatrics 11:115–118, 2013.
3. Fleming AJ, Chi SN. Brain tumors in children. Curr Probl Pediatr Adolesc Health Care 2012 Apr;42(4):80–103.

4. Reulecke BC, Erker CG, Fiedler BJ. Brain tumors in children: Initial symptoms and their influence on the time span between symptom onset and diagnosis. J Child Neurol 2008;23:178–183.

5. Mehta V, Chapman A, McNeely PD. Latency between symptom onset and diagnosis of pediatric brain tumors: an Eastern Canadian geographic study. Neurosurgery 2002;51:365–372, discussion 372–373.

6. Monteith SJ, Heppner PA, Woodfield MJ. Paediatric central nervous system tumours in a New Zealand population: A 10-year experience of epidemiology, management strategies and outcomes Journal of Clinical Neuroscience 2006;13:722–729.

7. Wilne S, Koller K, Collier J. The diagnosis of brain tumours in children: A guideline to assist healthcare professionals in the assessment of children who may have a brain tumour. Arch Dis Child 2010;95: 534–539.

8. Wilne SH, Ferris RC, Nathwani A, Kennedy CR. The presenting features of brain tumours: A review of 200 cases. Arch Dis Child 2006;91:502–506.

9. Baker PC, Bernat JL. The neuroanatomy of vomiting in man: Association of projectile vomiting with a solitary metastasis in the lateral tegmentum of the pons and the middle cerebellar peduncle. J Neurol Neurosurg, Psychiatry 1985;48: 1165–1168.

10. Sardi I, Bresci C, Schiavello E. Successful treatment with a low-dose cisplatin—etoposide regimen for patients with diencephalic syndrome. J Neurooncol 2012 Sep;109(2):375–383.

11. Gropman AL, Packer RJ, Nicholson HS. Treatment of diencephalic syndrome with chemotherapy: Growth, tumor response, and long term control. Cancer 1998;83:166–172.

12. Cho BK, Wang KC, Nam DH, Kim DG, Jung HW, Kim HJ, et al. Pineal tumors: Experience with 48 cases over 10 years. Childs Nerv Syst 1998;14:53–58.

13. Bertsch H, Rudoler S, Needle MN. Emergent/urgent therapeutic Irradiation in pediatric oncology: Patterns of presentation, treatment, and outcome. Med Pediatr Oncol 1998;30:101–105.

14. Sandberg DI, Ragheb J, Dunoyer C. Surgical outcomes and seizure control rates after resection of dysembryoplastic neuroepithelial tumors. Neurosurg Focus 2005;18:E5.

15. Taylor M, Couto-Silva AC, Adan L. Hypothalamic-pituitary lesions in pediatric patients: endocrine symptoms often precede neuro-ophthalmic presenting symptoms. J Pediatr. 2012 Nov;161(5):855–863.

16. Panigrahy A, Blüml S. Neuroimaging of pediatric brain tumors: From basic to advanced magnetic resonance imaging(MRI). J Child Neurol 2009;24:1343–1365.

17. Luh GY, Bird CR. Imaging of brain tumors in the pediatric population. Neuroimaging Clin N Am 1999;9:691–716.

18. Albright AL, Wisoff JH, Zeltzer PM. Effects of medulloblastoma resections on outcome in children: a report from the Children's Cancer Group. Neurosurgery 1996; 38:265–271.

19. Massimino M, Solero CL, Garrè ML. Second-look surgery for ependymoma: the Italian experience. J Neurosurg Pediatr 2011; 8(3):246–250.

20. Modha A, Vassilyadi M, George A. Medulloblastoma in children—the Ottawa experience. Childs Nerv Syst 2000;16:341–350.

21. Gwinn R, Cleary K, Medlock M. Use of a portable CT scanner during resection of subcortical supratentorial astrocytomas of childhood. Pediatr Neurosurg 2000; 32:37–43.

22. Stummer W, Novotny A, Stepp H. Fluorescence-guided resection of glioblastoma multiforme by using 5-aminolevulinic acid-induced porphyrins: a prospective study in 52 consecutive patients. J Neurosurg 2000; 93:1003–1013.

23. Nimsky C, Ganslandt O, Hastreiter P, Fahlbusch R. Intraoperative compensation for brain shift. SurgNeurol 2001; 56:357–365.

24. Hall WA, Truwit CL. Intraoperative MR imaging. Magn Reson Imaging Clin N Am 2005;13:533–543.

25. Rutka JT, Kuo JS, Carter M. Advances in the treatment of pediatric brain tumors. Exp Rev Neuro ther 2004;4:879–893.

26. Jahangiri FR, Minhas M, Jane J Jr. Preventing lower cranial nerve injuries during fourth ventricle tumor resection by utilizing intraoperative neurophysiological monitoring. Neurodiagn J 2012 Dec;52(4):320–332.

27. Reinacher PC, van Velthoven V Intraoperative ultrasound imaging: practical applicability as a real-time navigation system. ActaNeurochirSuppl 2003; 85:89–93.

28. Gaab MR, Schroeder HW (1998) Neuroendoscopic approach to intraventricular lesions. J Neurosurg 88:496–505.

29. Souweidane MM, Luther N. Endoscopic resection of solid intraventricular brain tumors. J Neurosurg 2006;105:271–278.

30. Gopalakrishnan CV, Dhakoji A, Menon G. Factors Predicting the Need for Cerebrospinal Fluid Diversion following Posterior Fossa Tumor Surgery in Children. Pediatr Neurosurg 2012;48:93–101.

31. DeLaney TF. Clinical proton radiation therapy research at the Francis H. Burr Proton Therapy Center. Technol Cancer Res Treat 2007;6:61–66.

32. Merchant TE, Hua CH, Shukla H. Proton versus photon radiotherapy for common pediatric brain tumors: Comparison of models of dose characteristics and their relationship to cognitive function. Pediatr Blood Cancer 2008;51:110–117.

33. Palmer SL, Reddick WE, Gajjar A. Understanding the cognitive impact on children who are treated for medulloblastoma. J Pediatr Psychol 2007;32:1040–1049.

34. Massimino M, Spreafico F, Cefalo G. High response rate to cisplatin/etoposide regimen in childhood low-grade glioma. J ClinOncol 2002;20:4209–4216.

35. Geyer JR, Sposto R, Jennings M. Multiagent chemotherapy and deferred radiotherapy in infants with malignant brain tumors: A report from the Children's Cancer Group. J Clin Oncol 2005;23: 7621–7631.

36. Qaddoumi I, Sultan I, Broniscer A. Pediatric low-grade gliomas and the need for new options for therapy: Why and how? Cancer Biol Ther 2009;8:4–10.

37. Gottardo NG, Gajjar A. Chemotherapy for malignant brain tumors of childhood. J Child Neurol 2008;23:1149–1159.

38. Packer RJ, Ater J, Allen J. Carboplatin and vincristine chemotherapy for children with newly diagnosed progressive low-grade gliomas. J Neurosurg 1997;86:747–754.

39. Gururangan S, Fisher MJ, Allen JC. Temozolomide in children with progressive low-grade glioma. NeuroOncol 2007;9:161–168.

40. Heath JA, Turner CD, Poussaint TY, Scott RM. Chemotherapy for progressive low-grade gliomas in children older than ten years: The Dana-Farber experience. Pediatr Hematol Oncol 2003;20:497–504.

41. Fouladi M, Hunt DL, Pollack IF. Outcome of children with centrally reviewed low-grade gliomas treated with chemotherapy with or without radiotherapy on Children's Cancer Group high-grade glioma study CCG-945. Cancer 2003 Sep 15;98(6):1243–1252.

42. Listernick R, Darling C, Greenwald M. Optic pathway tumors in children: the effect of neurofibromatosis type 1 on clinical manifestations and natural history. J Pediatr 1995;127:718–722.

43. Sievert AJ, Fisher MJ. Pediatric low-grade gliomas.J Child Neurol 2009;24:1397–1408.

44. Pollack IF. The role of surgery in pediatric gliomas. J NeuroOncol 1999;42:271–288.

45. Wisoff JH, Boyett JM, Berger MS. Current neurosurgical management and the impact of the extent of resection in the treatment of malignant gliomas of childhood: A report of the children's Cancer Group trial no. CCG-945. J Neurosurg 1998;89:52–59.

46. MacDonald TJ, Aguilera D, Kramm CM. Treatment of high-grade glioma in children and adolescents. NeuroOncol 2011 Oct;13(10):1049–1058.

47. Broniscer A, Baker JN, Baker SJ, Chi SN. Prospective collection of tissue samples at autopsyin children with diffuse intrinsic pontine glioma. Cancer 2010;116:4632–4637.

48. Walker DA, Liu J, Kieran M. A multi-disciplinary consensus statement concerning surgical approaches to low-grade, high-grade astrocytomas and diffuse intrinsic pontine gliomas in childhood (CPN Paris 2011) using the Delphi method. NeuroOncol 2013 Apr;15(4):462–468.

49. Cohen KJ, Broniscer A, Glod J. Pediatric glial tumors. Curr Treat Options Oncol 2001;2:529–536.

50. Sposto R, Ertel, IJ, Jenkin, RD. The effectiveness of chemotherapy for treatment of high grade astrocytoma in children: Results of a randomized trial. A report from the Children's Cancer Study Group. J Neurooncol 1989; 7: 165–177.

51. Heideman, R.L., Douglass, E.C., Krance, R.A. High-dose chemotherapy and autologous bone marrow rescue followed by interstitial and external beam radiotherapy in newly diagnosed pediatric malignant gliomas. J. Clin. Oncol 1993;11, 1458–1465.

52. Massimino M, Biassoni V. Use of high-dose chemotherapy in front-line therapy of childhood malignant glioma. Expert Rev Anticancer Ther 2006 6:709–717.

53. Qaddoumi I, Sultan I, Gajjar A. Outcome and prognostic features in pediatric gliomas: a review of 6212 cases from the Surveillance, Epidemiology, and End Results database. Cancer 2009;115:5761–5770.

54. Chinot OL, de La Motte Rouge T. AVAglio: Phase 3 trial of bevacizumab plus temozolomide and radiotherapy in newly diagnosed glioblastomamultiforme. Adv Ther 2011 Apr;28(4):334–340.

55. Lee DW, Barrett DM, Mackall C. The future is now: chimeric antigen receptors as new targeted therapies for childhood cancer. Clin Cancer Res 2012 May 15;18(10):2780–2790.

56. Bouffet E, Tabori U, Huang A, Bartels U. Possibilities of new therapeutic strategies in brain tumors. Cancer Treat Rev 2010 Jun;36(4):335–341.

57. Cage TA, Mueller S, Haas-Kogan D, Gupta N. High-grade gliomas in children. Neurosurg Clin N Am 2012 Jul;23(3):515–523.

58. Louis DN, Ohgaki H, Wiestler OD. The 2007 WHO classification of tumours of the central nervous system. Acta Neuropathol 2007;114: 97–109.

59. Robertson PL, Zeltzer PM, Boyett JM. Survival and prognostic factors following radiation therapy and chemotherapy for ependymomas in children: A report of the Children's Cancer Group. J Neurosurg 1998;88:695–703.

60. Fangusaro J, Van Den Berghe C, Tomita T. Evaluating the incidence and utility of microscopic metastatic dissemination as diagnosed by lumbar cerebro-spinal fluid (CSF) samples in children with newly diagnosed intracranial ependymoma. J Neuro Oncol 2010;103:693–698.

61. Ridley L, Rahman R, Brundler MA. Multifactorial analysis of predictors of outcome in pediatric intracranial ependymoma. Neuro Oncol 2008;10:675–689.

62. Hukin J, Epstein F, Lefton D, Allen J. Treatment of intracranial ependymoma by surgery alone. Pediatr Neurosurg 1998;29:40–45.

63. Merchant TE, Li C, Xiong X, Kun LE. Conformal radiotherapy after surgery for pediatric ependymoma: A prospective study. Lancet Oncol 2009;10: 258–266.

64. Needle MN, Goldwein JW, Grass J. Adjuvant chemotherapy for the treatment of intracranial ependymoma of childhood. Cancer 1997;80: 341–347.

65. Zacharoulis S, Ashley S, Moreno L. Treatment and outcome of children with relapsed ependymoma: A multi-institutional retrospective analysis. Childs Nerv Syst 2010;26:905–911.

66. Northcott PA, Korshunov A, Witt H. Medulloblastoma comprises four distinct molecular variants. J Clin Oncol 2010;29:1408–1414.

67. Gibson P, Tong Y, Robinson G. Subtypes of medulloblastoma have distinct developmental origins. Nature 2010;468:1095–1099.

68. Lannering B, Rutkowski S, Doz F. Hyperfractionated versus conventional radiotherapy followed by chemotherapy in standard-risk medulloblastoma: results from the randomized multicenter HIT-SIOP PNET 4 trial. J Clin Oncol 2012 Sep 10;30(26):3187–3193.

69. Gottardo NG, Gajjar A. Chemotherapy for malignant brain tumors of childhood. J Child Neurol 2008 Oct;23(10):1149–1159.

70. Gandola L, Massimino M, Cefalo G. Hyperfractionated accelerated radiotherapy in the Milan strategy for metastatic medulloblastoma. J ClinOncol 2009 Feb 1;27(4):566–571.

71. Krutilkova V, Trkova M, Fleitz J. Identification of five new families strengthens the Link between childhood choroid plexus carcinoma and germline TP53 mutations. Eur J Cancer 2005;41:1597–1603.

72. Haliasos N,Brew S,Robertson F. Preoperative embolization of choroid plexus tumours in children: part I-does the reduction of perioperative blood loss affect the safety of subsequent surgery? Childs Nerv Syst.2013 Jan;29(1):65–70.

73. Wrede B, Liu P, Wolff JE. Chemotherapy improves the survival of patients with choroid plexus carcinoma: A metaanalysis of individual cases with choroid plexus tumors. J NeuroOncol 2007; 85:345–351.

74. Lafay-Cousin L, Mabbott DJ, Halliday W. Use of ifosfamide, carboplatin, and etoposide chemotherapy in choroid plexus carcinoma. J Neurosurg Pediatr 2010;5:615–621.

75. Bettegowda C,Adogwa O,Mehta V Treatment of choroid plexus tumors: a 20-year single institutional experience. J Neurosurg Pediatr 2012 Nov;10(5):398–405.

76. Chow E, Reardon DA, Shah AB, Jenkins JJ, Langston J, Heideman RL, et al. Pediatric choroid plexus neoplasms. Int J Radiat Oncol Biol Phys 1999;44:249–254.

77. Kamoshima Y, Sawamura Y. Update on current standard treatment in central nervous system germ cell tumors. Curr Opin Neurol 2010;23:571–575.

78. Echevarría ME, Fangusaro J, Goldman S. Pediatric central nervous system germ cell tumors: A review. Oncologist 2008;13:690–699.

79. Janmohamed S, Grossman AB, Metcalfe K. Suprasellar germ cell tumours: Specific problems and the evolution of optimal management with a combined chemoradiotherapy regimen. ClinEndocrinol (Oxf) 2002;57:487–500.

80. Jubran RF, Finlay J. Central nervous system germ cell tumors: Controversies in diagnosis and treatment. Oncol Williston Park 2005;19:705–711.

81. Hilden JM, Meerbaum S, Burger P. Central nervous system atypical teratoid/rhabdoid tumor: results of therapy in children enrolled in a registry. J Clin Oncol 2004:22, 2877–2884.

82. Radner H, Blumcke I., Reifenberger G., Wiestler O.D. The new WHO classification of tumors of the nervous system2000.Pathologyandgenetics. Pathologe 2002: 23, 260–283.

83. Dunham C. Pediatric brain tumors: A histologic and genetic update on commonly encountered entities. Semin Diagn Pathol 2010;27:147–159.

84. Chi SN, Zimmerman MA, Yao X. Intensive multimodality treatment for children with newly diagnosed CNS atypical teratoid rhabdoid tumor. J Clin Oncol 2009;27, 385–389.

85. Pai Panandiker AS, Merchant TE, Beltran C. Sequencing of local therapy affects the pattern of treatment failure and survival in children with atypical teratoid rhabdoid tumors of the central nervous system. Int J Radiat Oncol Biol Phys 2011;82, 1756–1763.

86. Park ES, Sung KW, Baek HJ. Tandem high-dose chemotherapy and autologous stem cell transplantation in young children with atypical teratoid/rhabdoid tumor of the central nervous system. J Korean Med Sci 2012;27, 135–140.

87. Chen YW, Wong TT, Ho DM. Impact of radiotherapy for pediatric CNS atypical tera-toid/rhabdoid tumor (single institute experience). Int J Radiat Oncol Biol Phys 2006;64, 1038–1043.

88. Ginn KF, Gajjar A. Atypical teratoid rhabdoid tumor: current therapy and future direc-tions. Front Oncol 2012;2:114.

89. Habrand JL, Bolle S, Datchary J. Proton beam therapy in pediatric radiotherapy. Cancer Radiother 2009;13:550–555.

90. Hukin J, Steinbok P, Lafay-Cousin L. Intracystic bleomycin therapy for craniopharyn-gioma in children: The Canadian experience. Cancer 2007;109:2124–2131.

91. Waber DP, Pomeroy SL, Chiverton AM. Everyday cognitive function after craniopha-ryngioma in childhood. Pediatr Neurol 2006;34:13–19.

40 Metastatic Brain Disease

Anna Fiumani and Andrea Salmaggi

INTRODUCTION

Brain metastases are the most common intracranial tumor in adults, and the incidence of brain metastasis is believed to be increasing due to improved imaging techniques with an increased ability to detect smaller tumors and improvement in the treatment of many tumors leading to prolonged survival.[1] Incidence is estimated to range from 100,000 to 300,000 patients per year in the United States. In adults, lung cancer is the main cause of brain metastasis (50–60%), followed by breast cancer (15–20%) and melanoma (5–10%).

The resection of a single brain metastasis is considered to be a standard option in patients with accessible lesions, good functional status, and absent/controlled extracranial disease.[2] According to evidence-based medicine data, Level I evidence supports the use of surgical resection plus postoperative WBRT (whole brain radiation therapy) compared with WBRT alone or with surgery alone in patients with good performance status (functionally independent and spending less than 50% of time in bed) and limited extracranial disease.[3]

The standard management of patients with brain metastases has been optimized over time, due to technical improvements in surgery and radiation therapy and a better definition of prognostic factors that has led to a more accurate patient selection.

However, the outcome for patients with brain metastases is generally poor, with median survivals following WBRT alone in the range of 3–6 months. Given this poor prognosis, considerable efforts have been made to explore additional or alternative treatment modalities that have the potential to improve survival, quality of life, and local tumor control.

The medical management for patients with brain metastases includes corticosteroids and/or anticonvulsants to alleviate symptoms. New areas of research include definition of the role of conventional and novel chemotherapy and targeted agents, radiation sensitizers, stem cell–associated therapies and methods, and agents to decrease cognitive morbidity. The large avaiability of these new treatment approaches has raised the need to tailor therapy to appropriate subgroups, based on expected survival. In 1997, Gaspar et al.[4] published a seminal report on a prognostic index for patients with brain metastases, the Radiation Therapy Oncology Group's (RTOG) Recursive Partitioning Analysis.

The Graded Prognostic Assessment (GPA) is a newer prognostic index for patients with brain metastases.[5]

Compared with the recursive partitioning analysis data that had identified three risk classes with 2, 4, and 7 months as median survival times according only to age, performance status, and presence of extra-CNS metastatic disease, the GPA has included other potentially relevant factors in prognosis (i.e., histotype of primitive tumor and number of brain metastases).

The overall MST for all patients was 7.16 months, but the MST varied from 2.79 to 25.30 months depending on diagnosis and GPA. The overall median survival time (MST) by histology for the various GPA classes were: non–small-cell lung cancer (NSCLC), 7.00 months (range, 3.02–14.78 months); small-cell lung cancer (SCLC), 4.90 months (range, 2.79–17.05 months); melanoma, 6.74 months (range, 3.38–13.32 months); renal cell carcinoma, 9.63 months (range, 3.27–14.77 months); breast cancer, 13.80 months (range, 3.35–25.30 months); and GI cancers, 5.36 months (range, 3.13–13.54 months).

Of note, in patients with different primary, different prognostic factors were detected: for instance, only performance status and number of brain metastases influenced survival in melanoma patients, whereas both age and Karnofsky performance scores (KPS) and number of brain metastases and presence of extracerebral metastatic disease were prognostic factors in lung cancer. Only performance status affected survival in patients with brain metastases from gastrointestinal tumors, whereas age, performance status, and histological subtype influenced survival in breast cancer patients (with luminal B subtype having the worst prognosis).

The MSTs for all patients with GPA scores of 0–1.0, 1.5–2.0, 2.5–3.0, and 3.5–4.0 were 3.10, 5.40, 9.63, and 16.73 months, respectively.

Diagnosis

Diagnosis of brain metastasis is often a presumptive one in the context of an established diagnosis of extra-CNS malignancy.

However, especially for (but not only for) patients presenting with a single lesion and having a history of controlled systemic cancer or of long-established remission of systemic disease (although some histotypes do develop late CNS metastases, among these breast and kidney cancers), histology of the brain lesion should be carefully taken into consideration in order to exclude other conditions deserving different treatments.

In patients without a known history of cancer and displaying 1 to 3 brain lesions suggestive for metastatic lesions, the NCCN 2012 guidelines recommend to perform chest/abdominale/pelvic CT and/or body FDG-PET in order to detect sublicinal disease sites amenable to less risky histological assessment.

Contrast-enhanced MRI is more sensitive than computed tomography in the detection of brain metastases, especially for small lesions and for those located in the posterior fossa.

THE ROLE OF MEDICAL TREATMENT FOR SYMPTOM MANAGEMENT IN NEWLY DIAGNOSED BRAIN METASTASES

For adults with brain metastases who have not experienced a seizure due to their metastatic brain disease, routine prophylactic use of anticonvulsants is not recommended.[6]

Only a single underpowered randomized controlled trial (RCT), which did not detect a difference in seizure occurrence, provides evidence for decision-making purposes.[7] This study, by Forsyth et al., is a RCT of anticonvulsants versus no anticonvulsants in 100 patients with newly diagnosed brain tumors (diagnosis <1 month from study entry). Patients were stratified for primary (n = 40) or metastatic (n = 60) pathology. Of patients with brain metastasis, 26 were treated with anticonvulsants, usually phenytoin (n = 25) or phenobarbital (n = 1) using oral loading and conventional maintenance dosing; 34 patients received no anticonvulsants. The primary outcome reported was seizure occurrence at 3 months postrandomization. The trial was terminated early because the seizure rate in the no anticonvulsant arm was only 10%, which put the anticipated seizure rate of 20% outside the 95% confidence interval. The only outcome reported specifically for the subgroup of patients with brain metastases was seizure incidence, and there was no significant difference between those who received anticonvulsant prophylaxis and those who did not (log rank test; $P = 0.90$).

There is a dichotomy between this Level 3 recommendation not to use routine prophylactic anticonvulsants and the ubiquity of anticonvulsant use for prophylaxis of seizures associated with metastatic brain disease. Future studies should be planned to allow better control, recording and analysis of anticonvulsant dosing and response to allow a more robust analysis of the risk to benefit ratio of various agents.

Glucocorticoids have typically been used to assist in controlling cerebral edema in the early supportive care of the patient with newly diagnosed metastatic brain disease.[8]

Dexamethasone is generally considered the steroid of choice because of its minimal mineralocorticoid effect and long half-life, although any other corticosteroid can be effective if given in equipotent doses. Steroids have been used alone for palliation of symptoms and in combination with radiotherapy as an initial course of therapy. Data in literature indicate that the majority of these patients have been managed with starting doses of 4–8 mg/day and it has been stated that up to 75% of patients with brain metastases show marked neurological improvement within 24–72 hours after beginning dexamethasone.

Despite the widespread use of steroids in the management of brain metastases, only two publications meet the criteria to establish recommendations. The first[9] of the two studies described a randomized study of 4, 8, and 16 mg/day dosing of dexamethasone and found no advantage to higher dosing in patients who were not felt to be in impending danger of cerebral herniation. Vecht et al. published their findings from two consecutively executed double-blind randomized trials in patients with brain metastases and KPS of 80 or less which were designed to evaluate the minimum effective dose of oral dexamethasone.

Initially a dexamethasone dosage of 8 mg/day (Group 1) was compared with 16 mg/day (Group 2), followed by a comparison of 4 mg/day (Group 3) versus 16 mg/day (Group 4). The outcomes of interest were alteration in KPS and the frequency of side effects at days 0, 7, 28, and 56. The authors conclude that for the majority of patients, the lower doses of 4 and 8 mg dexamethasone per day have an equivalent effect on improving neurological performance when compared with a dose of 16 mg/day at 1 and 4 weeks of treatment, in moderately symptomatic patients without signs of impending herniation.

Wolfson et al.[10] prospectively studied 12 patients with histologically confirmed malignancies and radiographically documented brain metastases and attempted to evaluate the indications for glucocorticoids. Patients were scored for general performance status and neurological function Class. All subjects received 24 mg/ day of intravenous dexamethasone for 48 hours and after an assessment, were randomized to receive either 4 mg of oral dexamethasone every 6 hours (Group 1) or no steroids (Group 2) during radiotherapy (30 Gy in 10 fractions). Due to the small size and lack of any statistical analysis, it is impossible to reach any conclusion based on this study; therefore, no recommendations will be made based on this small trial.

In 2006, the results of a series of systematic reviews with the stated purpose "to establish evidence-based guidelines and identify controversies regarding the management of patients with brain metastases" were published by Soffietti et al.[11] This was conducted by a multidisciplinary task force of the European Federation of Neurological Societies and includes a review of data obtained from the Cochrane Library, bibliographic databases, overview papers, and previous guidelines from scientific societies and organizations. Under the section on supportive care and steroids only the publication by Vecht is cited, reviewed and used to support the recommendation that, in most cases, initial dexamethasone doses should not exceed 4–8 mg/day. However, in patients with more severe symptoms related to increased intracranial pressure, doses of 16 mg/day or higher should be considered (Level of Evidence B).

Dexamethasone is indicated as the corticosteroid of choice and twice daily dosing was thought to be sufficient (Good Practice Point). Tapering of steroid dosing within 1 week of starting therapy and discontinuation within 2 weeks if possible was encouraged (Good Practice Point). Finally, patients who do not have signs or symptoms of increased intracranial pressure do not have to be treated with steroids (Good Practice Point).

THE ROLE OF SURGICAL RESECTION IN THE MANAGEMENT OF NEWLY DIAGNOSED BRAIN METASTASES

For patients with a single accessible brain metastasis, surgical resection followed by postoperative WBRT has been compared with WBRT alone in three randomized controlled trials (RCTs)[12–14] (refer to next paragraph).

One RCT[15] evaluated surgical resection alone compared with surgery plus postoperative WBRT for the initial management of a single brain metastasis.

Fewer patients who received postoperative WBRT experienced a recurrence in the brain compared with those who had surgical resection alone.

Recurrence in the surgery + WBRT group was less frequent both at the original site of the brain metastasis and at distant sites in the brain compared with patients who did not receive postoperative WBRT.

The time to any recurrence in the brain was significantly longer in the group that had postoperative WBRT compared with the group that did not.

Fewer patients in the surgery + WBRT group died as a result of neurological causes than did patients in the surgery-alone group.

However, overall survival did not differ significantly between the two groups. Median survival in the surgery + WBRT group was 48 weeks compared with 43 weeks in the group that received no further treatment following surgical resection.

In conclusion, Class I evidence is available to support a Level 1 recommendation for patients with a single brain metastasis amenable to surgical resection. The Class I evidence supports the use of WBRT following surgical resection.

Recurrences in the brain, at the original site or at distant brain sites, were all significantly lower in the group that received adjuvant postoperative WBRT than the group undergoing surgical resection alone. However, both overall survival and time spent in an independent status (KPS > 70) did not differ significantly between the groups. Of note, cognitive aspects were not specifically analyzed in this trial.

There is insufficient evidence to make a recommendation for patients with poor performance scores, advanced systemic disease, or multiple brain metastases.

The advent of stereotactic radiosurgery (SRS) has provided a new and less invasive local treatment modality that, like surgical resection, has the ability to treat brain metastases while sparing healthy brain tissue.

A small multicenter RCT conducted in Germany by Muacevic et al.[16] specifically compared resection plus postoperative WBRT to SRS alone for the initial treatment of a newly diagnosed brain metastasis. A total of 64 adult patients with single, small (≤3 cm) operable brain metastases and a KPS ≥70 were randomized to receive SRS alone (n = 31) or surgical resection followed by WBRT (n = 33).

The primary outcome was overall survival and did not differ significantly between the two groups. However, the Muacevic RCT closed early and only enrolled approximately one-quarter of the proposed participants and was thus underpowered to detect a survival difference, if in fact one exists. Median survival in the surgery + WBRT group was 9.5 months, compared with 10.3 months in the group that received SRS. In terms of secondary outcomes, duration of freedom from local recurrence did not significantly differ between the two groups. The 1-year local control rate was 82% in the surgery + WBRT group and 96.8% in the SRS group. Freedom from recurrence at distant brain sites was significantly longer in the group that had surgical resection plus WBRT compared with the group that received SRS. Finally, the overall number of neurological deaths was not significantly different between the groups.

Data from retrospective cohort studies[17,18] that compared surgical resection plus WBRT to SRS plus WBRT yield conflicting results in terms of overall survival and duration of freedom from local recurrence, anyway most of them demonstrated that overall survival did not differ significantly between the resection plus WBRT group compared with the group that received SRS plus WBRT. So, Class II evidence does suggest that larger lesions (>3 cm in maximum diameter) or those causing significant mass effect (>1 cm midline shift) may have better outcomes with surgical resection. Radiosurgery is recommended for single surgically inaccessible lesions measuring <3 cm in maximum diameter.

The value of postsurgical WBRT compared with observation has been assessed in the EORTC 22952-26001 study in patients with one to three brain metastases. This trial also included patients treated with stereotactic radiosurgery; overall, the results showed that there were no significant differences in survival in patients treated with WBRT at disease progression in the brain compared with those treated immediately after surgery/radiosurgery. However, immediate postsurgical WBRT did reduce intracranial relapses, despite not improving survival or time spent in functionally independent status. The results of this trial show that careful follow-up in patients operated on for one to three brain metastases (excluding patients with SCLC) may allow delaying WBRT at tumor relapse/progression in the brain without affecting overall survival.[19]

No studies were concluded for comparison between surgical resection ± WBRT versus surgical resection + SRS and as such, no evidence-based recommendations can be made regarding one approach compared with the other.

Conclusion

Surgical resection continues to play a crucial role in the multidisciplinary management of single brain metastases.[20] It allows the rapid debulking of a large, immediately life-threatening tumor, making it beneficial to patients with neurological signs and symptoms related to metastatic disease. Surgery relieves mass effect and symptomatic intracranial hypertension, restores CSF flow, and lowers steroid dependence through a reduction in peritumoral edema. Surgery can provide seizure relief. Additionally, patients with improved functional status after surgery may get better outcomes with adjunct treatments. Surgery has the advantage of providing or confirming a pathological diagnosis. Class I evidence suggests that surgical resection followed by WBRT represents a superior treatment modality, in terms of improving tumor control at the original site of the metastasis and in the brain overall, when compared with surgical resection alone. As reviewed by Gaspar et al.,[21] Class I evidence also supports the use of surgical resection plus postoperative WBRT in patients with good performance status and limited extracranial disease compared with WBRT alone. Class II evidence suggests that larger lesions (>3 cm) or those causing significant mass effect (>1 cm midline shift) may have better outcomes with surgical resection, whereas radiosurgery may offer slightly better local control rates for radioresistant lesions (i.e., melanoma, renal cell, etc.). However, because of underpowered Class I evidence in the resection + WBRT versus SRS alone comparison, the authors could only make a Level 3 recommendation suggesting that SRS alone may provide equivalent functional and survival outcomes compared with resection + WBRT for patients with single brain metastases.

While surgical resection of more than one brain metastasis has been performed in cases of significant mass effect from more than one lesion, and in cases where two or more lesions are accessible through the same craniotomy approach, no robust comparative data exists to evaluate the role of surgical resection for multiple brain metastases. Future studies incorporating the role of resection for more than one brain metastasis, with or without additional adjuvant therapy, will also help clarify whether the benefits of resection discussed above apply to multiple lesions.

In patients with a single brain metastasis (except from SCLC) and PS WHO of 0 to 2, careful monitoring after surgery alone may allow deferring WBRT at disease recurrence in the brain.

THE ROLE OF WHOLE BRAIN RADIATION THERAPY IN THE MANAGEMENT OF NEWLY DIAGNOSED BRAIN METASTASES

WBRT has long been a standard treatment for patients with brain metastases.[15] The outcome for patients with brain metastases is generally poor, with a median survival following WBRT alone of only 3–4 months regardless of primary tumor histology (SCLC excepted).[22]

Indeed, after WBRT, 50% of patients still succumb to their brain tumor. For patients with a single accessible brain metastasis, surgical resection followed by postoperative

WBRT has been compared with WBRT alone in three RCTs.[12-14] Two of three are in agreement to demonstrate that there was a statistically significant increase in survival in the surgical group. In addition, the time to recurrence of brain metastases, freedom from death due to neurological causes, and duration of functional independence were significantly longer in the surgical resection group. Regarding the question if there is an optimal dosing/fractionation schedule of WBRT when used, Gaspar et al.[21] reviewed 23 studies that met the eligibility criteria for this question. The radiation dosages have been expressed in terms of the tumor response biologically effective dose (BED) in order to quantitatively capture the observed biological effect between treatment arms.

There is Class I evidence that altered dose/fractionation schedules of WBRT do not result in significant differences in median survival, local control or neurocognitive function when compared with "standard" WBRT dose/fractionation (i.e., 30 Gy in 10 daily fractions or a BED of 39 Gy).[10]

Conclusion

Whole brain radiotherapy remains the primary management approach for brain metastasis in eloquent areas, for lesions too large for SRS and not amenable to resection, and for multiple (i.e, more than three) metastases in which SRS or surgical resection have not demonstrated a survival advantage. Also, for certain tumors that have a high propensity for microscopic dissemination (e.g., SCLC), WBRT remains the standard practice. Based on the available Class I and Class II evidence, surgical resection followed by early or delayed WBRT is an effective treatment for patients with single, surgically accessible, brain metastases who have controlled extra-cranial disease and are in good general condition. Good general condition in the relevant studies was defined as functional independence and spending less than 50% of time in bed. Patients with disease progression in the 3 months preceding the diagnosis of the brain metastases have a relatively poor survival and poor functional status but still had a significant improvement in survival as a result of surgical resection. Due to the risk of fourth ventricle compression and the subsequent increase in intracranial pressure, surgery should be particularly considered prior to WBRT if there is a brain metastasis situated within the posterior fossa.

Despite the widespread use of WBRT after diagnosis of multiple (more than three) brain metastases and after surgery/SRS for one to three brain metastases, in the last years concern over the medium- and long-term neurotoxicity has been growing; in a randomized controlled trial, Chang et al.[23] have shown that patients undergoing WBRT after SRS for one to three brain metastases suffered from marked impairment in learning and memory functions at 4 months compared with patients treated with SRS alone.

THE ROLE OF STEREOTACTIC RADIOSURGERY IN THE MANAGEMENT OF NEWLY DIAGNOSED BRAIN METASTASES

Approximately 37–50% of solid tumor patients present with single brain metastases while roughly 50–63% have multiple tumors at initial presentation.[23] Lesions amenable to SRS are typically defined as measuring less than 3 cm in maximum diameter and producing minimal (less than 1 cm of midline shift) mass effect.[24] Given that SRS can treat more than one tumor per session, and that most tumors are detected while small in size, the percentage of patients who are potential candidates for SRS is quite large. The number of tumors that can be effectively treated with SRS in a given patient is an area still under study.

For patients with single accessible brain metastases, surgical resection followed by postoperative WBRT has been compared with WBRT alone in three RCTs.[12-14] Outcomes for patients with single solid metastatic brain tumors amenable to either surgical resection or SRS have been shown to be roughly equivalent for both local control and overall patient survival. Open surgery has the potential for better overall outcomes for lesions >3 cm in diameter in locations amenable to resection with acceptable risk, and better and/or faster outcomes for smaller lesions causing symptomatic edema or mass effect. On the other hand, SRS may result in superior local control rates for radioresistant lesions (e.g., renal cell, melanoma, etc.), and may allow WBRT to be deferred for subsequent salvage treatment without adverse sequelae. SRS has the ability to treat lesions that may not be safely resectable.

Patients are generally considered candidates for SRS if the tumor(s) in question is less than 10 cc in volume (<3 cm average diameter).

Two prospective RCTs (Class I evidence) (26–27) evaluated WBRT alone versus WBRT + SRS for the initial management of patients with solid metastatic brain tumors. The first study was stopped at the 60% accrual point due to an overwhelmingly positive tumor control difference at interim analysis. The latter demonstrated significantly better survival for patients with single metastatic tumors ($P = 0.01$), superior local control for patients with one to three metastatic brain tumors ($P = 0.01$), and improved KPS for patients with one to three metastatic brain tumors in the WBRT +SRS arm. There was no significant difference between groups in median survival for patients with two or three brain tumors, MMSE at 6 months, incidence of neurological cause of death, or adverse therapeutic events.

One prospective RCT (Class I evidence) (28) evaluated SRS alone versus WBRT + SRS for the initial management of patients with solid metastatic brain tumors. Results revealed no significant difference between study groups for median survival (8.0 versus 7.5 months), 1 year local control rate (72.5 versus 88.7%), neurological cause of death, 1 year KPS score, MMSE score, or acute or late neurotoxicity.

No RCTs were conducted to compare SRS alone versus WBRT alone. Several prospective and retrospective cohort studies (Class II evidence) evaluated SRS alone versus WBRT alone for the initial management of patients with solid metastatic brain tumors, with different results in term of median survival.

In the prospective RCT EORTC 22952-26001 trial, adjuvant whole brain radiotherapy (WBRT) was compared with observation after either surgery or radiosurgery in patients with one to three cerebral metastases; this trial has shown that adjuvant WBRT following either surgery or radiosurgery does reduce intracranial relapses and neurological deaths, but does not prolong duration of functional independence or overall survival.[19]

One prospective RCT (Class I evidence)[16] evaluated SRS alone versus resection + WBRT for the initial management of patients with solid metastatic brain tumors. There was no significant difference in outcome between the two groups in terms of functional performance outcome, rate of neurological death, or median survival (9.5 months surgery + WBRT versus 10.3 months SRS). However, the study was stopped early at only 25% accrual and was therefore underpowered to detect <15% differences in outcome between groups. The SRS patients did experience an increased number of distant tumor recurrences (25.8% versus 3%), but these occurrences did not impact overall outcome when subsequent salvage SRS was taken into account. The resection + WBRT group did experience a significantly larger number of grade 1 or 2 early and late complications compared with the SRS group.

No RCTs or prospective studies were conducted to compare resection plus WBRT versus resection plus SRS.

Conclusion

There is Class I evidence from two RCTs with similar inclusion criteria that single-dose SRS + WBRT provides significantly superior local tumor control compared with WBRT alone for patients with one to three brain metastases.[25,26] One of the RCTs also showed improved KPS score results for the single dose SRS + WBRT regimen. These results were achieved without an increased incidence of adverse therapeutic events.[26] There is Class I evidence from one RCT[25] that single-dose.

SRS + WBRT provides a significantly superior survival benefit compared with WBRT alone for patients with single brain metastases. Whether or not a survival advantage might also exist for patients with >2 brain metastases remains controversial.

In one RCT,[28] and prospective as well as retrospective cohort studies support equivalent survival results for single-dose SRS alone versus WBRT + single-dose SRS. Regarding local recurrence risk, the RCT demonstrated that a single-dose SRS alone strategy led to a higher risk of local recurrence at the treated site compared with WBRT + single-dose SRS.

Three Class I studies have demonstrated that WBRT lowers the risk of distant recurrence compared with local tumor therapies (SRS or surgical resection) used in isolation.[15,21,28]

There is, however, disagreement among Class I and II studies regarding the risk of distant recurrence outside the treatment volume if single-dose SRS is used in isolation as opposed to WBRT + single-dose SRS. The RCT demonstrated a significantly increased risk of either distant brain or overall brain recurrence when single dose SRS is utilized in isolation and no advantage to SRS alone when assessing neurocognitive sequelae from radiation. Given these results, prudence warrants regular careful surveillance at 2–3 month intervals with neuroimaging if single-dose SRS is used in isolation.

Comparison of SRS alone versus WBRT alone has been the issue of Class II evidence studies: some have demonstrated a statistically significant survival advantage for single-dose SRS alone compared with WBRT alone for patients with either single or multiple brain tumors. While different studies evaluated patients with differing numbers of brain metastases, all studies included patients with up to three metastatic brain tumors. Given the relative paucity and weakness of the data, and despite relatively consistent results, only a Level 3 recommendation is warranted.

Almost all retrospective cohort studies (Class II evidence) that evaluated SRS + WBRT versus resection + WBRT for the initial management of patients with solid metastatic brain tumors demonstrated no significant survival differences between the two strategies.

One Class I evidence study evaluated the comparison between SRS alone versus resection plus WBRT, revealing no significant difference in functional performance outcome, neurological death outcome or median survival for patients with single brain metastases, even if with method limitations exposed above.

THE ROLE OF CHEMOTHERAPY IN THE MANAGEMENT OF NEWLY DIAGNOSED BRAIN METASTASES

The primary therapeutic approach for disseminated systemic disease remains chemotherapy, so it could be expected that is the logical choice for brain metastases as well. However, there are limitations for the application of chemotherapy in this context. One issue concerns the ability of chemotherapeutic agents to cross the blood–brain barrier (BBB). Many chemotherapeutic agents are relatively excluded from the brain, and the ones that do penetrate, may reach insufficient concentrations. There is also the longstanding observation that intracranial response rates to chemotherapy are typically lower than in the extracranial compartment, and a common hypothesis for this finding is that patients are preexposed to cytotoxic therapies, and it is the chemoresistant clones that metastasize to the brain.[29]

However, data in newly diagnosed, previously untreated patients with SCLC suggest that intracranial response rates remain significantly lower than extracranial response rates, thereby suggesting that chemoresistant clones alone do not necessarily explain this dichotomy.[30] Some types of metastatic brain tumors may respond to chemotherapy to some degree, including breast cancer, germ cell cancer, and ovarian cancer in addition to SCLC. The role of chemotherapy in the management of brain metastases has been explored in a very limited number of controlled comparative trials, and therefore the Class of evidence and hence the Level of recommendations have limited applicability.

In 2004,[31] a multi-institutional, RCT of palliative radiation with concomitant carboplatin for patients with brain metastases from NSCLC, with overall survival as the primary endpoint showed no statistically differences in median survival (4.4 versus 3.7 months). Prior chemotherapy or brain radiotherapy were exclusion criteria, patients were not susceptible or refused surgery. The trial was terminated early due to low patient accrual, thus limiting the ability to draw statistically significant conclusions.

In 2002, Antonadou et al.[32] reported a phase II RCT in which patients with brain metastases were randomized to WBRT alone or WBRT plus temozolomide. This RCT of 48 patients did not show a survival improvement with the addition of temozolomide chemotherapy, but showed a statistically significant improvement in response rates and an improvement in neurological function with the addition of temozolomide to WBRT, which constitutes Class I evidence.

In 2003, Mornex et al.[33] published results of a prospective randomized phase III trial of fotemustine plus WBRT (n = 37) versus fotemustine alone (n = 39) in patients with cerebral metastases from malignant melanoma and stated that there was no difference in cerebral response or control or in overall survival between the two groups. There was a statistically significant difference in time to cerebral progression favoring the WBRT + fotemustine group ($P = 0.028$) with that group having a median time to objective cerebral progression of 56 days compared with 49 days in the chemotherapy alone group. This constitutes Class I evidence.

In 2000 Postmus et al.[34] reported on a phase III randomized study comparing teniposide versus teniposide with WBRT in patients with brain metastases from SCLC. Results did not demonstrate a prolongation of overall survival. However the response rate in the combined modality group was significantly higher than in the teniposide alone group: time to progression in the brain significantly longer in the combined modality group. This RCT constitutes Class I evidence.

In 2001 Robinet et al.[35] published a randomized trial evaluating the use of systemic chemotherapy for the treatment of inoperable brain metastases from NSCLC with early WBRT versus WBRT delayed until progression.

In the first group patients were treated with cisplatin and vinorelbine used concurrently with WBRT and the second group was treated with the same chemotherapy, but with WBRT delayed for at least two cycles. There was no significant difference between the groups with regard to overall survival. This study provides Class I evidence for the similarity in outcome in the treatment of brain metastases from NSCLC with chemotherapy with concurrent versus delayed WBRT.

In 2008 Lee et al.[36] published a randomized trial testing the use of systemic chemotherapy first followed by WBRT versus WBRT first followed by systemic chemotherapy for the treatment of advanced NSCLC with synchronous brain metastases. There was no difference in overall response rates between the two arms. With a median follow up of 40 months, there was no difference in progression free survival (PFS) or overall survival. This study provides a Class I evidence for the similarity in outcome in the treatment of brain metastases from NSCLC with either chemotherapy with delayed WBRT or WBRT followed by chemotherapy.

Conclusion

The role of chemotherapy in the management of brain metastases has been explored in a very limited number of controlled comparative trials, and therefore the Class of evidence and hence the Level of recommendations have limited applicability.[37] These recommendations do not apply to the exquisitely chemosensitive tumors, such as germinomas metastatic to the brain. Additionally, these studies have been conducted mostly in patients with NSCLC and extrapolating to other histological types would be considered inadequately supported by the data.

These data can be summarized as follows:

The lack of clear and robust survival benefit with the addition of chemotherapy to WBRT.

enhanced response rates, specifically in NSCLC with the addition of chemotherapy to WBRT.

A single trial provides evidence that outcome is similar whether WBRT is delivered upfront with chemotherapy or delayed by up to 2 cycles, but the data remains too limited to support definitive recommendations for the delay of radiation therapy, especially given the lack of any known survival advantage with chemotherapy.

The inherent question (does it matter if chemotherapy precedes WBRT or vice versa?) has been inadequately addressed and the data are too sparse to make definitive conclusions.

THE ROLE OF TARGETED THERAPY IN THE MANAGEMENT OF NEWLY DIAGNOSED BRAIN METASTASES

The huge amount of information on new molecular compounds and the advances in understanding the molecular pathways that mediate brain colonization have led to an increase of interest in preclinical and clinical investigations in the field of brain metastases.[38] Targeted therapies have been initially employed in primary cancers, based on the identification of molecular targets critical for tumor growth. In the past, patients with brain metastases have been largely excluded from clinical trials with antiangiogenic agents based on concerns regarding the risk of central nervous system (CNS) hemorrhage. However, recent reviews of large clinical trial datasets, retrospective and prospective studies have shown that patients with and without CNS metastases are at a similar risk of bleeding into the brain (0.8–3.3%), independent of antiangiogenic therapy.[39]

Over time, clinical trials have increasingly investigated new agents that target specific molecular pathways in specific tumor types.

Brain metastases from NSCLC have been shown to respond to oral EGFR (epidermal growth factor receptor) and TKIs (tyrosine kinase inhibitor) gefinitib and erlotinib. Response rates (complete and partial) after gefinitib range from 10% to 38% with a median duration of response of 9–13.5 months, and the latency between the start of treatment and appearance of response is short (about 1 month).[40] Similar findings have been documented with erlotinib.[41] As for extracranial disease, response to EGFR inhibitors is highly dependent on the presence of activating EGFR mutations. EGFR inhibitors can be safely administered concurrently with WBRT.

The risk of developing brain metastases among patients with breast cancer is higher for tumors that are *HER2* positive or triple negative (i.e., lacking expression of *HER2*, estrogen and progesterone receptors). *HER2*-positive patients (up to 25% of the overall population) have the greatest risk (especially if estrogen/progesterone receptor negative). The frequency of brain metastases among *HER2*-positive patients treated with trastuzumab (a monoclonal antibody targeting *HER2*) in the metastatic setting is between 25% and 40%[42]; similarly, when analyzing large phase III trials in the adjuvant setting, CNS metastases are significantly increased in the trastuzumab-containing treatment arms compared with the non–trastuzumab-containing arms.[43] A combination of factors likely explains the increased incidence of CNS disease in these patients, including a high propensity of *HER2* cells for brain colonization, and improved control of systemic disease with trastuzumab, which has poor BBB penetration, and therefore is not able to target micrometastases that are protected by an intact BBB.

Up to 60% of melanomas carry an activating mutation in the gene encoding BRAF, a serine-threonineprotein kinase. More than 85% of BRAF mutations are of the V600E type, which leads to constitutive kinase activity of BRAF and downstream activation of mitogen-activated protein kinase (MAPK) pathway, thereby enhancing the proliferative and metastatic capacity of the tumor. Vemurafenib, a specific inhibitor of BRAF V600E mutated protein, has yielded response rates of up to 70% with improved PFS and OS in BRAF V600E mutated metastatic melanoma patients.[44]

Another novel approach to treat advanced melanoma is the blockade of cytotoxic T-lymphocyte antigen-4 (CTLA-4), a molecule that downregulates the pathways of T-cell activation. Ipilimumab is a fully human monoclonal antibody that blocks cytotoxic T-lymphocyte antigen-4 and potentiates antitumor immune responses. In two phase III trials, ipilimumab has shown a statistically significant improvement in OS as monotherapy in previously treated patients[45] and in combination with dacarbazine in treatment-naïve patients.[46]

Conclusion

At present, definite data on the clinical activity of targeted agents in brain metastases are lacking, as virtually no well designed clinical trials have been performed. There is a need to understand novel targets and secondary resistance mechanisms. Overall, responses of established brain metastases to targeted agents have not been achieved in the majority of patients, and the reasons are multifactorial.[47] Targeted agents may have still a limited capacity to cross the BBB. Drug efflux pumps markedly contribute to the lack of brain permeability of compounds such as gefinitib, erlotinib, lapatinib, sunitinib and sorafenib. Many molecular therapeutics are cytostatic and not cytotoxic, and thus not enough tumor cells in a lesion are killed to achieve a clinical response. Moreover, the increased interstitial fluid pressure from edema limits drug distribution.

SUGGESTED READING

1. Shaffrey ME, Mut M, Asher AL, et al. Brain metastases. Curr Probl Surg 2004;41:665–741.
2. Modha A, Shepard SR, Gutin PH. Surgery of brain metastases—is there still a place for it? J Neurooncol 2005;75:21–29.
3. Kalkanis SN, Kondziolka D, Gaspar LE, et al. The role of surgical resection in the management of newly diagnosed brain metastases: a systematic review and evidence-based clinical practice guideline. J Neurooncol 2010; 96: 33–43.
4. Gaspar LE, Scott C, Rotman M, et al. Recursive partitioning analysis (RPA) of prognostic factors in three Radiation Therapy Oncology Group (RTOG) brain metastases trials. Int J Radiat Oncol Biol Phys 1997;37:745–751.
5. Sperduto PW, Kased N, Roberge D, et al. Summary Report on the Graded Prognostic Assessment: An Accurate and Facile Diagnosis-Specific Tool to Estimate Survival for Patients With Brain Metastases. J Clin Oncol 2012;30(4):419–425.
6. Mikkelsen T, Paleologos NA, Robinson PD, et al. The role of prophylactic anticonvulsants in the management of brain metastases: a systematic review and evidence-based clinical practice guideline J Neurooncol 2010;96:97–102.
7. Forsyth PA, Weaver S, Fulton D, et al. Prophylactic anticonvulsants in patients with brain tumour. Can J Neurol Sci 2003;30:106–112.
8. Ryken TC, McDermott M, Robinson PD, et al. The role of steroids in the management of brain metastases: a systematic review and evidence-based clinical practice guideline J Neurooncol 2010;96:103–114.
9. Vecht CJ, Hovestadt A, Verbiest HB, et al. Dose-effect relationship of dexamethasone on Karnofsky performance in metastatic brain tumors: a randomized study of doses of 4, 8, and 16 mg per day. Neurology 1994;44(4): 675–680.

10. Wolfson AH, Snodgrass SM, Schwade JG, et al. The role of steroids in the management of metastatic carcinoma to the brain. A pilot prospective trial. Am J Clin Oncol 1994;17(3):234–238.
11. Soffietti R, Cornu P, Delattre JY, et al. EFNS guidelines on diagnosis and treatment of brain metastases: report of an EFNS task force. Eur J Neurol 2006;13(7): 674–681.
12. Patchell RA, Tibbs PA, Walsh JW, et al. A randomized trial of surgery in the treatment of single metastases to the brain. N Engl J Med 1996;322(8):494–500.
13. Mintz AH, Kestle J, Rathbone MP, et al. A randomized trial to assess the efficacy of surgery in addition to radiotherapy in patients with a single cerebral metastasis. Cancer 1996;78(7):1470–1476.
14. Vecht CJ, Haaxma-Reiche H, Noordijk EM, et al. Treatment of single brain metastasis: radiotherapy alone or combined with neurosurgery? Ann Neurol 1993;33(6):583–590.
15. Patchell RA, Tibbs PA, Regine WF, et al. Postoperative radiotherapy in the treatment of single metastases to the brain: a randomized trial. JAMA 1998;280(17):1485–1489.
16. Muacevic A, Wowra B, Siefert A, et al. Microsurgery plus whole brain irradiation versus Gamma Knife surgery alone for treatment of single metastases to the brain: a randomized controlled multicentre phase III trial. J Neurooncol 2008;87(3):299–307.
17. Schoggl A, Kitz K, Reddy M, et al. Defining the role of stereotactic radiosurgery versus microsurgery in the treatment of single brain metastases. Acta Neurochir 2000;142(6):621–626.
18. O'Neill BP, Iturria NJ, Link MJ, et al. A comparison of surgical resection and stereotactic radiosurgery in the treatment of solitary brain metastases. Int J Radiat Oncol Biol Phys 2003;5(5):1169–1176.
19. Kocher M, Soffietti R, Abacioglu U, et al. Adjuvant whole-brain radiotherapy versus observation after radiosurgery or surgical resection of one to three cerebral metastases: results of the EORTC 22952–26001 Study. J Clin Oncol 2011;29:134–141.
20. Mut M. Surgical treatment of brain metastasis: A review. Clinical Neurology and Neurosurgery 2012;114: 1–8.
21. Gaspar LE, Mehta MP, Patchell RA, et al. The role of whole brain radiation therapy in the management of newly diagnosed brain metastases: A systematic review and evidence-based clinical practice guideline. J Neurooncol 2009;96:17–32.
22. Deutsch M, Parsons JA, Mercado R. Radiation therapy for intracranial metastases. Cancer 1974;34:1607–1611.
23. Chang EI, Wefel JS, Hess KR, et al. Neurocognition in patients with brain metastases treated with radiosurgery or radiosurgery plus whole-brain irradiation: a randomized controlled trial. Lancet Oncol 2009;10:1037–1044.
24. Gavrilovic IT, Posner JB. Brain metastases: epidemiology and pathophysiology. J Neurooncol 2005;75(1):5–14.
25. Linskey ME, Andrews DW, Asher AL, et al. The role of stereotactic radiosurgery in the management of newly diagnosed brain metastases: a systematic review and evidence-based clinical practice guideline. J Neurooncol 2010;96:45–68.
26. Kondziolka D, Patel A, Lunsford LD, et al. Stereotactic radiosurgery plus whole brain radiotherapy versus radiotherapy alone for patients with multiple brain metastases. Int J Radiat Oncol Biol Phys 1999;45(2):427–434.
27. Andrews DW, Scott CB, Sperduto PW, et al. Whole brain radiation therapy with or without stereotactic radiosurgery boost for patients with one to three brain metastases: phase III results of the RTOG 9508 randomised trial. Lancet 2004;363(9422):1665–1672.
28. Aoyama H, Shirato H, Tago M, et al. Stereotactic radiosurgery plus whole-brain radiation therapy vs stereotactic radiosurgery alone for treatment of brain metastases: a randomized controlled trial. JAMA 2006;295(21):2483–2491.

29. Mehta MP, Paleologos NA, Mikkelsen T, et al. The role of chemotherapy in the management of newly diagnosed brain metastases: a systematic review and evidence-based clinical practice guideline J Neurooncol 2010;96:71–83.

30. Seute T, Leffers P, Wilmink JT, et al. Response of asymptomatic brain metastases from smallcell lung cancer to systemic first-line chemotherapy. J Clin Oncol 2006;24(13):2079–2083.

31. Guerrieri M, Wong K, Ryan G, et al. A randomised phase III study of palliative radiation with concomitant carboplatin for brain metastases from non-small cell carcinoma of the lung. Lung Cancer 2004;46(1):107–111.

32. Antonadou D, Paraskevaidis M, Sarris G, et al. Phase II randomized trial of temozolomide and concurrent radiotherapy in patients with brain metastases. J Clin Oncol 2002;20(17):3644–3650.

33. Mornex F, Thomas L, Mohr P, et al. A prospective randomized multicentre phase III trial of fotemustine plus whole brain irradiation versus fotemustine alone in cerebral metastases of malignant melanoma. Melanoma Res 2003;13(1):97–103.

34. Postmus PE, Haaxma-Reiche H, Smit EF, et al. Treatment of brain metastases of small-cell lung cancer: comparing teniposide and teniposide with whole-brain radiotherapy—a phase III study of the European Organization for the Research and Treatment of Cancer Lung Cancer Cooperative Group. J Clin Oncol 2000;18(19):3400–3408.

35. Robinet G, Thomas P, Breton JL, et al. Results of a phase III study of early versus delayed whole brain radiotherapy with concurrent cisplatin and vinorelbine combination in inoperable brain metastasis of non-small-cell lung cancer: Groupe Francais de Pneumo-Cancerologie (GFPC) Protocol 95-1. Ann Oncol 2001;12(1):59–67.

36. Lee DH, Han JY, Kim HT, et al. Primary chemotherapy for newly diagnosed nonsmall cell lung cancer patients with synchronous brain metastases compared with whole-brain radiotherapy administered first: result of a randomized pilot study. Cancer 2008;113(1):143–149.

37. Mehta M, Paleologos NA, Mikkelsen T, et al. The role of chemotherapy in the management of newly diagnosed brain metastases: a systematic review and evidence-based clinical practice guideline J Neurooncol 2010;96:71–83 DOI 10.1007/s11060-009-0062-7.

38. Soffietti R, Trevisan E, Rudà R. Targeted therapy in brain metastasis Curr Opin Oncol 2012, 24:679–686.

39. Besse B, Lasserre SF, Compton P, et al. Bevacizumab safety in patients with central nervous system metastases. Clin Cancer Res 2010;16:269–278.

40. Namba Y, Kijima T, Yokota S, et al. Gefitinib in patients with brain metastases from nonsmall-cell lung cancer: review of 15 clinical cases. Clin Lung Cancer 2004; 6:123–128.

41. Porta R, Sanchez-Torres JM, Paz-Ares L, et al. Brain metastases from lung cancer responding to erlotinib: the importance of EGFR mutation. Eur Respir J 2011; 37:624–631.

42. Brufsky AM, Mayer M, Rugo HS, et al. Central nervous system metastases in patients with HER2-positive metastatic breast cancer: incidence, treatment, and survival in patients from registHER. Clin Cancer Res 2011; 17:4834–4843.

43. Yin W, Jiang Y, Shen Z, et al. Trastuzumab in the adjuvant treatment of HER2-positive early breast cancer patients: a meta-analysis of published randomized controlled trials. PLoS One 2011; 6:e21030.

44. Chapman PB, Hauschild A, Robert C, et al. Improved survival with vemurafenib in melanoma with BRAF V600E mutation. N Engl J Med 2011; 364:2507–2516.

45. Hodi FS, O'Day SJ, McDermott DF, et al. Improved survival with ipilimumab in patients with metastatic melanoma. N Engl J Med 2010; 363:711–723.
46. Robert C, Thomas L, Bondarenko I, et al. Ipilimumab plus dacarbazine for previously untreated metastatic melanoma. N Engl J Med 2011; 364:2517–2526.
47. Steeg PS, Camphausen KA, Smith QR. Brain metastases as preventive and therapeutic targets. Nat Rev Cancer 2011; 11:352–363.

Index